DISASTER PSYCHIATRY

Readiness, Evaluation, and Treatment

Committee on Disasters and Terrorism
Group for the Advancement of Psychiatry

Disaster Psychiatry Outreach
Board of Directors

DISASTER PSYCHIATRY

Readiness, Evaluation, and Treatment

Edited by

Frederick J. Stoddard Jr., M.D.
Anand Pandya, M.D.
Craig L. Katz, M.D.

Committee on Disasters and Terrorism
Group for the Advancement of Psychiatry

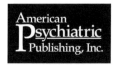

American Psychiatric Publishing, Inc.

Washington, DC
London, England

Note: The authors have worked to ensure that all information in this book is accurate at the time of publication and consistent with general psychiatric and medical standards, and that information concerning drug dosages, schedules, and routes of administration is accurate at the time of publication and consistent with standards set by the U.S. Food and Drug Administration and the general medical community. As medical research and practice continue to advance, however, therapeutic standards may change. Moreover, specific situations may require a specific therapeutic response not included in this book. For these reasons and because human and mechanical errors sometimes occur, we recommend that readers follow the advice of physicians directly involved in their care or the care of a member of their family.

The findings, opinions, and conclusions of this report do not necessarily represent the views of the officers, trustees, or all members of the American Psychiatric Association. The views expressed are those of the authors of the individual chapters.

Copyright © 2011 American Psychiatric Association
ALL RIGHTS RESERVED

Manufactured in the United States of America on acid-free paper
15 14 13 12 11   5 4 3 2 1
First Edition

Typeset in Adobe Galliard and ITC Officina Sans.

American Psychiatric Publishing, Inc.
1000 Wilson Boulevard
Arlington, VA 22209-3901
www.appi.org

Library of Congress Cataloging-in-Publication Data
Disaster psychiatry : readiness, evaluation, and treatment / edited by Frederick J. Stoddard Jr., Anand Pandya, Craig L. Katz. — 1st ed.
     p. ; cm.
   Includes bibliographical references and index.
   ISBN 978-0-87318-217-1 (pbk. : alk. paper)   1. Psychic trauma—Treatment. 2. Disasters—Psychological aspects. 3. Crisis intervention (Mental health services) I. Stoddard, Frederick J. II. Pandya, Anand A. III. Katz, Craig L.
   [DNLM: 1. Stress Disorders, Post-Traumatic—therapy. 2. Crisis Intervention. 3. Disasters. 4. Emergency Services, Psychiatric. 5. Survivors—psychology.   WM 172]
   RC552.P67D529 2011
   616.85′21—dc22

                                                            2011004790

British Library Cataloguing in Publication Data
A CIP record is available from the British Library.

Contents

Frederick J. Stoddard Jr., M.D.
Anand Pandya, M.D.
Craig L. Katz, M.D.

Part I
Readiness
Anand Pandya, M.D., Section Editor

Edward M. Kantor, M.D.
David R. Beckert, M.D.

Frederick J. Stoddard Jr., M.D.

Joseph P. Merlino, M.D., M.P.A.

Craig L. Katz, M.D.

Part II
Evaluation
Craig L. Katz, M.D., Section Editor

Part III
Intervention

Frederick J. Stoddard Jr., M.D., Section Editor

Part IV
Emerging and Other Topics
*Frederick J. Stoddard Jr., M.D., Anand Pandya, M.D.,
and Craig L. Katz, M.D., Section Editors*

Appendixes

Contributors

Volume Editors

Frederick J. Stoddard Jr., M.D.
Associate Clinical Professor of Psychiatry, Harvard Medical School, Massachusetts General Hospital, and Shriners Hospitals for Children, Boston, Massachusetts; Chair, Committee on Disasters and Terrorism of the Group for the Advancement of Psychiatry

Anand Pandya, M.D.
Vice Chair, Psychiatry and Behavioral Neurosciences, Cedars-Sinai Medical Center, Los Angeles, California; Associate Clinical Professor of Psychiatry, David Geffen School of Medicine at UCLA, Los Angeles, California; Vice President, Disaster Psychiatry Outreach

Craig L. Katz, M.D.
Clinical Associate Professor of Psychiatry and Medical Education, Mount Sinai School of Medicine, New York, New York; President, Disaster Psychiatry Outreach

Other Contributing Authors

David R. Beckert, M.D.
Assistant Professor, Department of Psychiatry and Behavioral Sciences, and Assistant Director, Psychiatry Residency Training Program, Medical University of South Carolina, Charleston, South Carolina

Grant H. Brenner, M.D.
Clinical Assistant Professor, Albert Einstein College of Medicine; Director, Trauma Service, William Alanson White Institute of Psychiatry, Psychoanalysis and Psychology, New York, New York

Frank G. Dowling, M.D.
Clinical Associate Professor of Psychiatry, SUNY at Stony Brook School of Medicine, Stony Brook, New York

Kristina Jones, M.D.
Instructor in Psychiatry, New York University School of Medicine, New York, New York; Assistant Professor of Psychiatry, Weill Cornell Medical College, New York, New York

Edward M. Kantor, M.D.
Associate Professor, Department of Psychiatry and Behavioral Sciences, and Director, Psychiatry Residency Training Program, Medical University of South Carolina, Charleston, South Carolina

Chad M. Lemaire, M.D., R.N., B.S.N.
Staff Psychiatrist, Legacy Community Health Services, Houston, Texas; Clinical Instructor, The Menninger Department of Psychiatry and Behavioral Sciences, Baylor College of Medicine, Houston, Texas; Fellow, Group for the Advancement of Psychiatry

Joseph P. Merlino, M.D., M.P.A.
Deputy Executive Director and Director of Psychiatry, Kings County Hospital Center; Professor of Clinical Psychiatry, State University of New York Downstate Medical College, Brooklyn, New York

David J. Mysels, M.D., M.B.A.
Staff Psychiatrist, Outpatient Addictions Service, Cambridge Health Alliance; Instructor in Psychiatry, Harvard Medical School, Boston, Massachusetts; Clinical Research Fellow, Division on Substance Abuse, Columbia University/New York State Psychiatric Institute, New York, New York

Anthony T. Ng, M.D.
Medical Director, Acadia Hospital Psychiatric Emergency Services, Bangor, Maine; Assistant Professor of Psychiatry, Uniformed Services University of the Health Sciences, Bethesda, Maryland

Srinivasan S. Pillay, M.D.
Assistant Clinical Professor, McLean Hospital/Harvard Medical School, Belmont, Massachusetts

Kenneth Sakauye, M.D.
Professor and Co-Chair of Psychiatry, University of Tennessee Health Science Center, Memphis, Tennessee

Heather L. Shibley, M.D.
Fellow in Child and Adolescent Psychiatry, Brown University School of Medicine, Providence, Rhode Island

Maria A. Sullivan, M.D., Ph.D.
Associate Professor of Clinical Psychiatry, Division on Substance Abuse, Columbia University/New York State Psychiatric Institute, New York, New York

DISCLOSURE OF INTERESTS

The following contributors to this book have indicated a financial interest in or other affiliation with a commercial supporter, a manufacturer of a commercial product, a provider of a commercial service, a nongovernmental organization, and/or a government agency, as listed below:

Anand Pandya, M.D.   *Honoraria:*   Ortho-McNeil-Janssen.

Srinivasan S. Pillay, M.D.   *Consultant:* Novartis (executive coach on non–medication-related issues).

Frederick J. Stoddard Jr., M.D.   *Honoraria:* Massachusetts General Hospital Psychiatry Academy, activities of which are supported through Independent Medical Education grants from AstraZeneca, Eli Lilly, and Janssen.

The following contributors stated that they had no competing interests during the year preceding manuscript submission:

David R. Beckert, M.D.; Grant H. Brenner, M.D.; Frank G. Dowling, M.D.; Kristina Jones, M.D.; Edward M. Kantor, M.D.; Craig L. Katz, M.D.; Chad M. Lemaire, M.D., R.N., B.S.N.; Joseph P. Merlino, M.D., M.P.A.; David J. Mysels, M.D., M.B.A.; Anthony T. Ng, M.D.; Kenneth Sakauye, M.D.; Heather L. Shibley, M.D.; Maria A. Sullivan, M.D., Ph.D.

Preface and Acknowledgments

This publication is the fruition of the aims of two organizations to produce a clinical manual of disaster psychiatry for those interested in responding to the broad need for disaster mental health services. They joined together to write it with the generous organizational support and feedback from the Group for the Advancement of Psychiatry (GAP) and its publications board, chaired by David Adler, M.D. Since its beginning in the post–World War II era of modern psychiatric care, GAP has served as a think tank operating through its committee structure of national experts to present reports and position statements that are disseminated nationally and internationally. Frederick J. Stoddard Jr., M.D., and C. Knight Aldrich, M.D., initiated the Committee on Disasters and Terrorism at GAP after 9/11 to offer GAP a committee addressing this critical area and to write a GAP publication on the topic for psychiatrists. Some of the contributors to this current text also authored chapters of the GAP committee's handbook for primary care clinicians, which was titled *Hidden Impact: What You Need to Know for the Next Disaster: A Practical Mental Health Guide for Clinicians* (Stoddard, Katz, and Merlino 2010).

The two organizations that joined to write this book are GAP and Disaster Psychiatry Outreach (DPO), a New York City–based charitable organization dedicated to training for and provision of disaster mental health services. Recognizing the need for disaster psychiatry training and services, Craig L. Katz, M.D., Anand Pandya, M.D., Lisa Chertkof, M.D., and Edward Kenney, M.D., founded DPO in 1989. Since then, DPO has been committed to utilizing the goodwill and expertise of psychiatrists to alleviate suffering in the aftermath of disasters. Its members have responded to disasters spanning from the 1998 airline crash of Swissair Flight 111, to 9/11 in 2001, to the earthquake in Haiti in 2010. DPO's training syllabus and other materials are important background sources for this manual. These include *Disaster Psychiatry: Intervening When Nightmares Come True* (Pandya and Katz 2004) and the *Psychiatric Clinics of North America* special issue "Disaster Psychiatry: A Closer Look" (Katz and Pandya 2004). Several DPO members, including Drs. Pandya and Katz, are also members of the GAP Committee on Disasters and Terrorism. Robert Ursano, M.D., although not a member of GAP, has generously served as a consultant to the GAP committee since its founding and chairs the American Psychiatric Association's Committee on Psychiatric Dimensions of Disaster.

Special recognition goes to the DPO Curriculum Committee, which developed the original DPO training curriculum in disaster psychiatry— "The Essentials of Disaster Psychiatry: A Training Course for Mental Health Professionals" (Disaster Psychiatry Outreach 2008)—that was an important starting point for this book. Chaired by Dr. John Sahs, the committee's members included Drs. Matthew Biel, Henry Kandler, Roger Nathaniel, Ilisse Perlmutter, Mark Schor, and Asher Simon. Special consultants to that committee included Drs. Linda Chokroverty, Anand Pandya, Craig L. Katz, and Carol North, as well as Mss. Lovdy Hamm and Anastasia Holmes. The DPO Response Guide (an unpublished document) also helped to shape this book and received major contributions from Drs. Anthony Ng, Grant Brenner, and Eric Cohen.

Disaster Psychiatry: Readiness, Evaluation, and Treatment updates and addresses many areas not covered in the American Psychiatric Association's online *Disaster Psychiatry Handbook* (Hall et al. 2004). Three contributors to this manual also worked on that earlier handbook: Drs. Anthony T. Ng, Anand Pandya, and Frederick J. Stoddard Jr.

The editors are grateful to the Disaster Task Force of the Massachusetts Psychiatric Society, which, encouraged by the work of the Disaster Committee of the American Psychiatric Association, has since the late 1990s contributed significantly to understanding, planning for, and participating in disaster response in New England and beyond. Among the task force participants were many psychiatrists from academic settings, the Massachusetts Department of Mental Health, and the uniformed services, who contributed to hospital and state disaster mental health planning, learning from an air disaster drill in May 1998, identifying areas of need, and responding to subsequent disasters. Many of these psychiatrists are regionally and nationally known for their work in disaster response or posttraumatic stress disorder (PTSD). Participants and contributors included Frederick J. Stoddard Jr., M.D., Chair; Ruth A. Barron, M.D., Pamela J. Beasley, M.D., Nancy Cinco, M.D., Ralph Cohen, M.D., James A. Chu, M.D., Donna M. Digioia, M.D., George Dominiak, M.D., Mary Ellen Foti, M.D., Dawn Gable, M.D., David Henderson, M.D., Judith L. Herman, M.D., Todd Holzman, M.D., Douglas H. Hughes, M.D., John J. Iwuc, M.D, Kathleen Lentz, M.D., Carlos Lopez, M.D., Lisa McCurry, M.D., Joseph Jankowski, M.D., Laurie Raymond, M.D., Victoria Russell, M.D., Kathy Sanders, M.D., Maria C. Sauzier, M.D., Susan Skea, M.D., Ramon Solhkhah, M.D., Bessel A. Van der Kolk, M.D., Charles Wasserman, M.D., and Janet Weisenberger, M.D.

Presubmission production assistance for this manuscript was provided by Shriners Hospitals for Children–Boston.

The editors are grateful for the careful guidance and support through the publication process of American Psychiatric Publishing, Inc., and Editor-in-Chief Robert E. Hales, M.D., Chief Executive Officer Ron McMillen, and Editorial Director John McDuffie.

References

Disaster Psychiatry Outreach: The Essentials of Disaster Psychiatry: A Training Course for Mental Health Professionals. New York, Disaster Psychiatry Outreach, 2008. Available as DPOCourseSyllabus_052108.pdf at: https://sites.google.com/a/disasterpsych.org/blog/File-Cabinet. Accessed December 21, 2009.

Hall RCW, Ng AT, Norwood AE; American Psychiatric Association Committee on Psychiatric Dimensions of Disaster (eds): Disaster Psychiatry Handbook. November 2004. Available at: http://www.psych.org/Resources/DisasterPsychiatry.aspx. Accessed October 12, 2010.

Katz CL, Pandya A (eds): Disaster psychiatry: a closer look. Psychiatr Clin North Am 27(special issue):391–610, 2004

Pandya AA, Katz CL (eds): Disaster Psychiatry: Intervening When Nightmares Come True. Hillsdale, NJ, Analytic Press, 2004

Stoddard FJ, Katz CL, Merlino JP (eds): Hidden Impact: What You Need to Know for the Next Disaster. A Practical Mental Health Guide for Clinicians. Sudbury, MA, Jones & Bartlett, 2010

Introduction

Frederick J. Stoddard Jr., M.D.
Anand Pandya, M.D.
Craig L. Katz, M.D.

Psychiatrists are increasingly active in disaster response. More than 700 psychiatrists responded to the 9/11 attacks alone (Disaster Psychiatry Outreach, personal communication, July 2010). With more recent disasters such as the Indian Ocean earthquake and tsunami in 2004, Hurricane Katrina in 2005, and the 2010 earthquake in Haiti, the numbers of psychiatrists involved in disaster work have increased. This book is what we believe to be the first clinical guide directed toward psychiatrists and other mental health professionals working in disaster psychiatry. It is more clinically oriented and practical than a textbook but explicit and practical in its discussion of the evidence base for recommendations for psychiatric evaluation and interventions.

There are varying definitions of *disaster*. The definition offered by the World Health Organization (1992) is brief and clear: a "severe disruption, ecological and psychosocial, which greatly exceeds the coping capacity of the affected community" (p. 2). Disasters may be caused by natural occurrences, or so-called acts of God (e.g., earthquakes, hurricanes, floods); human-made accidental or technological events (e.g., airline crash or power plant explosion); or willful human acts (e.g., mass shootings or terrorism).

Although depictions of the psychological and emotional impact of severe trauma on humans appear in ancient literature such as religious texts and Homer's *Iliad* and *Odyssey* (Shay 1994, 2002), approaches to clinical evaluation and treatment are relatively recent. *Soldier's heart*, a term dating from the Civil War era and a predecessor of what was later called *posttraumatic stress disorder*, was elegantly depicted in a film by that name shown on American public television in 2005. Although soldiers were initially the focus of clinical care, civilians eventually followed. After the 1942 Cocoanut Grove fire in Boston, which killed 492 people and left many relatives grieving the deaths of their young, papers on neuropsychiatric observations and complications and the symptomatology and management of acute grief by Erich Lindemann (1944), Stanley Cobb (Cobb and Lindemann 1943), and Alexandra Adler (1944) signaled the beginning of modern disaster psychiatry. However, even earlier classic work directly relevant to disaster psychiatry was done with both children and adults after the terror of the 1940 London Blitz (Freud and Burlingham 1943; Jones et al. 2006).

Today, the field of disaster psychiatry embraces a wide spectrum of clinical interests, ranging from public health preparations, to early psychological interventions, to psychiatric consultation to surgical units, to psychotherapeutic interventions to alleviate stress on children and families after school shootings, hurricanes, or civil conflict. Disaster psychiatry has an important role in emergency prevention, response, and recovery. Although disaster mental health is still a young field, research with adults and children is aiming to improve interventions. Research is slowly progressing in applying methods to accurately identify valid relationships, not merely associations, among preexisting risk factors, postdisaster mental health problems, and effective interventions (Norris et al. 2006; Pfefferbaum 1998; Pfefferbaum and North 2008).

Over the past two decades, the American Psychiatric Association (APA) has taken a leadership role in disaster preparedness and, at times, response, especially Robert L. Ursano, M.D., founder of the APA's Committee on Psychiatric Dimensions of Disaster, together with many other leaders in disaster response in the APA and internationally. Dr. Ursano, Ann E. Norwood, M.D., Carol S. Fullerton, M.D., and their colleagues at the Uniformed Services University of the Health Sciences played groundbreaking roles in educating mental health professionals about disasters, the need for disaster mental health training, and the need for their expertise. District branches of the APA in Massachusetts, New York, California, Louisiana, and several other states have actively contributed to training and responses to disasters near and far.

The APA has provided both basic and advanced training courses on disaster psychiatry. In times of disasters, the APA is a lead organization that works to coordinate and disseminate valuable and timely disaster psychiatry materials to those in the field and to facilitate the flow of information into and out of the organization.

In *Disaster Psychiatry: Readiness, Evaluation, and Treatment,* we synthesize information gathered from a variety of sources, including the peer-reviewed scientific literature; the clinical wisdom imparted by frontline psychiatrists, psychologists, and social workers; and the experiences of those who have organized disaster mental health services. The authors of the 21 chapters explain, utilizing a biopsychosocial model, what a disaster is, how it relates to mental health, and how psychiatrists and other mental health professionals can effectively intervene to reduce suffering in such circumstances. Many chapter authors provide brief case scenarios from past disasters, including mass trauma events, followed by discussion. Because one important goal of this volume is to inform mental health professionals about the evidence base for different best practices, chapters are extensively referenced and clearly present the level of scientifically validated research supporting each recommended intervention.

The book is divided into four parts for ease of use by psychiatric clinicians preparing for or responding to disasters: Readiness, Evaluation, Intervention, and Emerging and Other Topics. Each chapter ends with a list of Teaching Points followed by Review Questions to help reinforce the cardinal issues covered in the chapter. We close the book with an Appendix of Key Readings and Resources for readers seeking further information and in-depth knowledge.

As noted, many psychiatrists and other mental health professionals have become acquainted with disaster psychiatry, and many may be experiencing some "disaster fatigue" now, following the numerous massive disasters in only the past decade. From 9/11 in 2001 to the 2010 earthquake in Haiti, there has been little letup. The economic turmoil of the world markets and the vast oil disaster in the Gulf of Mexico add dimensions of uncertainty, not rare among disasters that may cause vast suffering over many years, but with such slow impact that the need for clinical disaster services, which tend to be acute and postacute, may not even be recognized. We hope that this clinical manual provides needed encouragement and support, based on accumulating evidence from treating disaster survivors, to those mental health professionals who may have experienced disaster fatigue as well as to those who have not.

References

Adler A: Neuropsychiatric complications in victims of Boston's Cocoanut Grove disaster. JAMA 123:1098–1101, 1943

Cobb S, Lindemann E: Neuropsychiatric observations after the Cocoanut Grove fire. Annals of Surgery 117:814–824, 1943

Freud A, Burlingham DT: War and Children. New York, Medical War Books, 1943

"The Soldier's Heart" (Frontline [WGBH Boston]; original airdate: March 1, 2005). Written, produced, and directed by Raney Aronson. Available at: http://www. pbs.org/wgbh/pages/frontline/shows/heart/. Accessed January 14, 2011.

Jones E, Woolven R, Durodie B, et al: Public panic and morale: Second World War civilian responses re-examined in light of the current anti-terrorist campaign. J Risk Res 9:57–73, 2006

Lindemann E: Symptomatology and management of acute grief. Am J Psychiatry 101:141–148, 1944

Norris FH, Galea S, Friedman MJ, et al: Methods for Disaster Mental Health Research. New York, Guilford, 2006

Pfefferbaum B: Caring for children affected by disaster. Child Adolesc Psychiatr Clin North Am 7:579–597, 1998

Pfefferbaum B, North CS: Research with children exposed to disasters. Int J Methods Psychiatr Res 17(suppl):S49–S56, 2008

Shay J: Achilles in Vietnam: Combat Trauma and the Undoing of Character. New York, Simon & Schuster, 1994

Shay J: Odysseus in America: Combat Trauma and the Trials of Homecoming. New York, Scribner, 2002

World Health Organization: Psychosocial Consequences of Disaster: Prevention and Management. Geneva, Switzerland, World Health Organization, 1992. Available at: http://whqlibdoc.who.int/hq/1991/WHO_MNH_PSF_91.3_REV.1.pdf. Accessed January 14, 2011.

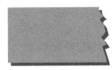

PART I

READINESS

Anand Pandya, M.D., Section Editor

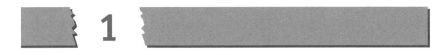

1

Preparation and Systems Issues

Integrating Into a Disaster Response

Edward M. Kantor, M.D.
David R. Beckert, M.D.

Dr. Greene, a community psychiatrist from Allentown, Pennsylvania, was moved by the devastation and the likely mental health needs of the population remaining in New Orleans following Hurricane Katrina in 2005. Having never volunteered in disaster work before, he was confused by the multiple groups, professional organizations, and federal agencies requesting volunteers. He had also heard about a nurse colleague who was organizing an ad hoc group of local medical volunteers. They were planning to rent a bus and set up a clinic somewhere outside the city. Additionally, he came across a public service announcement about something called the Medical Reserve Corps, looking for medical volunteers. He had no idea what the differences were between the groups and became frustrated trying to learn what might be right for him. By the time he figured out a plan of action, the group he contacted was only accepting volunteers with prior disaster experience. Weeks later he learned that the ad hoc group's bus was stopped by National Guard troops outside New Orleans and prevented from entering the disaster area. Initially frustrated, Dr. Greene found out that evacuees from Louisiana were being transported to a special resource center within easy driving distance from his home. Because Dr. Greene was a state employee, he was easily credentialed to participate in the state-run effort and provided on-site mental health support services until the evacuees found more permanent housing and were linked to new providers.

How does a person prepare for the unexpected? Even when aware of risk, is a person more likely to embrace the possibility and prepare, or to suppress the fear and carry on as usual? People tend to look at disasters and hope never to face one. Psychiatrists and mental health practitioners, however, are acutely aware of the importance of denial and avoidance in keeping painful material at arm's length. In fact, those strategies may be part of how people protect themselves during severe trauma. Beyond the superficial, individuals are aware that bad things happen and that preparing for the worst can influence the outcome in a positive way. For example, most people wear seat belts, many have quit smoking, and some are trying to avoid trans fats—all in the name of preparation and protection. More and more practitioners are washing their hands between patient visits or avoiding handshakes altogether. Most likely this change in behavior is not just due to hospital regulations and is at least partly due to concern and fear over the latest infectious threat. Still, it is rare for most of the population to be well prepared for disaster. Even with the wider availability of public safety information at Web sites such as www.ready.gov and an increase in local health campaigns, a significant portion of the population remains suspicious and questions the utility of immunizations and public health planning. An example of this was seen during the 2009 influenza immunization campaign, championed by the Centers for Disease Control and Prevention (CDC); despite the profound media blitz and the threat of a pandemic, only around 40% of all adults ages 18–65 years received a flu vaccine, compared with the projected goal of 60% (Centers for Disease Control and Prevention 2010).

Contemplating the Response

Sometimes, disaster responders are volunteers hoping to give back when something tragic happens in another community. At other times, they are victims of opportunity, thrust into these situations because of proximity. In any case, disaster responders are not immune from trauma. Psychiatrist responders need to be familiar with the four key considerations listed in Table 1–1. The first deals with *affiliation* with a recognized response group. Unaffiliated volunteers often become part of the problem and get frustrated in disaster events, not to mention having increased individual safety concerns and liability risks. Above all, it is important not to add to the confusion and become another mouth to feed or body to shelter. Affiliation with a group also helps prevent misunderstanding by establishing one's role and credentials, increasing the likelihood that one can actually function as a health care provider.

The second consideration involves fully up-to-date *knowledge,* including appropriate interventions and an awareness of important issues that impact those affected by disaster. What seems intuitive and simple on the surface may not be. For example, unsecured disaster areas are inherently

TABLE 1–1. Four major considerations for responders to disasters

Affiliation: Join a recognized organization with permission and resources to support the mission.

Knowledge: Keep up to date with appropriate interventions and be aware of major issues impacting those affected by disasters.

Purpose: Participate for the right reasons and understand one's own motivation for responding.

Function: Be in good health to operate in a variety of austere circumstances and not add to the local response burden by becoming a victim.

Source. Adapted from Kantor 2009.

dangerous, not only because of the event itself, but due to a loss of infrastructure, emerging disease, violence, and looting. As described in the case vignette at the beginning of this chapter, Dr. Greene's nurse colleague organized a mission of support, without an awareness of the postdisaster logistics and authority. The team was not affiliated and lacked sufficient knowledge of the response parameters, which frustrated the team and prevented participation.

The third issue addresses *purpose* and brings to light the issues of understanding one's own motivations for wanting to respond and the fact that a self-inventory can be useful prior to the actual response. Even for a highly trained psychiatrist responding to a disaster, there may be times when medical and psychiatric skills are not a priority and the most useful activities may be handing out water or sitting with a displaced child. Emphasizing the needs of the victims rather than a personal desire for recognition or to perform a specific job may help to minimize conflict in the chaotic aftermath of a major event.

The final point addressed in Table 1–1 is that one should be healthy enough to *function* in difficult conditions, including extremes of temperature, humidity, poor air quality, limited access to sanitation, and so forth. If a responder has a medical condition that may increase his or her own risk, staying back and helping the relief effort from a distance through fundraising, training others, or coordinating volunteers may be most appropriate.

Role Differentiation

Despite the usual goodwill of disaster responders, professional competition and conflict can arise among individual responders and disciplines. Many individuals who need and might benefit from mental health support are in fact experiencing what are truly "normal" reactions to extraordinary circumstances. As such, disaster psychiatry is not the same as trauma psychiatry or psychology, particularly in the immediate aftermath of an event. Although disasters can lead to individual psychopathology, the skills required early on in the response are different from those used in traditional trauma treatment, where specific pathology has been identified or illness is defined. At the outset, disaster psychiatry is not "office-based practice," and those impacted are not defined as "patients." Often, disaster survivors do not reach the threshold of diagnostic definition yet still require a supportive and connective approach for engagement, assessment, and psychosocial interventions. Consequently, the roles that a psychiatrist volunteer may be asked to fulfill are numerous and highly unpredictable. It is not uncommon for clinicians to step into other roles that include administrative, consultative, educational, and general medical duties. For example, handing out water and other resources can be useful activities, with the potential to facilitate contact with mental health personnel in a less threatening manner than direct referral. This can allow for early intervention, assessment, and triage for those most affected and in need of more formal mental health services.

The Response System

To be effective, disaster psychiatrists need to be aware of the roles of different organizations active in disaster response. In this section, we review some of the most important organizations and help psychiatrists understand their role within the context of a larger response.

Understanding the hierarchy in disaster response can be very helpful to psychiatrists and other practitioners who either are exposed to a disaster or choose to volunteer in a clinical capacity. Some aspects of this hierarchy are intuitive and can be navigated easily. Others unfortunately depend on at least a basic familiarity with the language, some common acronyms, and the basic rules of engagement. Knowing how the system typically works before an event will help to prevent confusion, minimize frustration, and improve one's ability to get things done. This holds true whether the goal is to protect oneself and one's family, to provide support and care for the patients in one's own practice, or to get involved as a volunteer provider in the disaster response itself.

Local Response

Barring certain military, federal, and aviation emergencies, the initial response to any emergency, including disaster, is the responsibility of local government. Additional resources from other organizations are requested only when necessary or clearly anticipated. Most local and all state government plans include emergency management officials, responsible for establishing an emergency operations center (EOC) and coordinating the community-wide response in disaster situations. Emergency management officials are the primary decision makers in a disaster response and determine the organization, function, and interrelation of the various activities. Examples of the major duties are outlined in Table 1–2.

During the acute phase of a disaster, emergency management officials and first responders focus on rescue operations, such as extinguishing fires, locating injured persons, extricating them, and providing on-site medical treatment, as well as managing hazardous materials and protecting responders. Other immediate operations include ensuring public safety by saving or restoring major infrastructure elements, such as transportation and telecommunications, public utilities, and the structural integrity of buildings. An additional responsibility is organizing care for victims and displaced persons with resources such as shelters, food, and potable water. Often, the need to provide emotional support for psychological trauma is not the primary focus for emergency managers and can be lost or forgotten in this chaotic environment (Disaster Psychiatry Outreach 2008).

National Response

The National Incident Management System (NIMS) is the federal infrastructure set up to navigate interagency and interjurisdictional cooperation during a disaster event. It is designed to be flexible and responsive regardless of the type of disaster and therefore is often referred to as "all-hazards" disaster planning and response. In the wake of lessons learned from recent disasters, an effort to further minimize the coordination problems between agencies and levels of government has grown into a new modified response structure called the National Response Framework (NRF). Implemented under the George W. Bush administration, NRF retains the core components of NIMS yet tries to emphasize partnerships and preplanning, in addition to procedures for communication and control at the time of an event. Under both plans, the scale of an event determines whether or not assistance is requested from other regional or even national resources and assets.

Incident Command System

The Incident Command System (ICS) (Federal Emergency Management Agency 2010a) is the most basic administrative and operational structure in all emergency responses. It exists to set forth clear lines of operation and facilitate cooperation between the various responding agencies, jurisdictions, and individuals. Since 2001, the concept of *incident command* has

TABLE 1–2.   Emergency management: major duties and responsibilities in disaster

1. Interagency coordination
2. Information sharing and education
3. Resource management and finances
4. Site safety hazardous materials
5. Search and rescue
6. Triage, tracking, transport, and evacuation
7. Management of volunteers
8. Disruption of utilities
9. Medical and mental health support
10. Food and shelter for victims and personnel

Source.   Disaster Psychiatry Outreach 2008; Federal Emergency Management Agency 2010b; Kantor 2010.

extended beyond emergency and disaster service organizations to include other local governmental and quasi-public agencies such as health departments, public schools, universities, and hospitals. In one of the newest groups to join the ICS structure, the hospital incident command system (HICS), command training is geared toward the needs of hospital staff and health care practitioners. Federal disaster support moneys require that localities and institutions orient staff to the ICS and NIMS and that they participate in local response planning and training efforts.

Under the ICS, each incident has an incident commander who is responsible for the entire event. Typically, the incident commander comes from the agency that first responded or that has primary responsibility for the type of event. For example, during a fire, the incident commander is typically a fire chief. If the fire is the result of a crime or terrorist event, the command may pass to the police or even a federal law enforcement agency. Larger or more complex disaster events, including those involving multiple agencies or jurisdictions, will establish a temporary command site, an EOC, near yet safely away from the event. Many EOCs are event specific and include the necessary expertise from participating agencies. As indicated in Figure 1–1, an ICS provides for expanding levels of control, depending on how big or complex an event becomes.

When an emergency is likely to tax the regular response system or requires resources beyond the capabilities of the jurisdiction where it occurred, government officials can "declare a disaster" and request state and/or federal assistance. Such assistance includes extra manpower, spe-

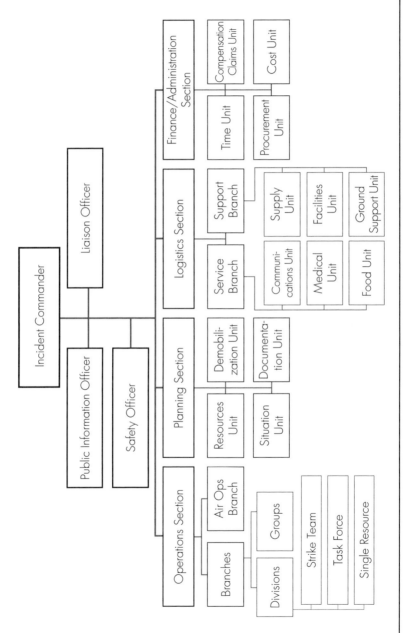

FIGURE 1–1. Incident command system organization.

Source. Federal Emergency Management Agency 2010c.

cialized expertise, and potential funding sources to support the communities and finance recovery operations. When resources are needed across state lines, they are available through an agreement known as an Emergency Management Assistance Compact (EMAC). Resources assigned this way often retain both legal authority to function and limited liability protection, depending on the activity and the states involved. Hurricane Katrina in 2005 is an excellent example of a disaster that overwhelmed the local infrastructure and required recovery operations that depended on personnel support and resources from other jurisdictions. In the case described at the beginning of the chapter, if Dr. Greene had already been affiliated with a response group, or at least had an understanding of what his role might have been ahead of time, he would have known whom to contact, what agency he would be part of, and how to engage the medical response structure in a more effective way.

Major Agencies and Response Groups

Since 2002, increased efforts have been made to include mental health needs in disaster planning at the federal level. Most states have taken some steps to include mental health issues as well. These actions have attempted to integrate sound mental health strategies into the overall response plans and to promote mental wellness and recovery as core components of the social and medical support efforts. Still, certain agencies and organizations tend to provide the majority of specific mental health care following a disaster. When it appears that a disaster could overwhelm local resources, assistance is requested by the incident commander through the local EOC. The Federal Emergency Management Agency (FEMA), now part of the Department of Homeland Security, is the lead federal agency for disaster planning, mitigation, coordination, and recovery, although many others offer various types of technical assistance and support.

In 2006, the National Disaster Medical System (NDMS), including Disaster Medical Assistance Teams (DMATs) and other medical resources, was administratively placed back under the U.S. Department of Health and Human Services. Much like mobile military hospital units, these fully functional mobile medical teams have specialized equipment that can be taken to a disaster site. A DMAT can be deployed across the country. Several teams specialize in mental health, and others support veterinary, mortuary, and pharmacy activities.

The American Red Cross, a nongovernmental organization, is charged with providing shelters, family assistance centers, social support, health screening, and basic mental health care during disasters. The Red Cross is organized by regions and divided into local chapters, each responsible for a particular geographic area yet coordinated through the national office, enabling it to respond to smaller events, such as house fires, or to larger events, such as hurricanes, providing mutual aid across jurisdictions (American Red Cross 2010).

Through the federal Citizen Corps program, several locally based volunteer programs were initiated in 2002. The two programs with relevance to disaster are the Community Emergency Response Teams (CERTs) and the Medical Reserve Corps (MRC), recently clarified by the U.S. Surgeon General's office as the *Civilian Volunteer* Medical Reserve Corps, to distinguish it from both the military reserve programs and the U.S. Public Health Service Commissioned Corps, which has revived its reserve program as well. Even so, the term *MRC* is still commonly used to describe the Civilian Volunteer Medical Reserve Corps. Both CERT and MRC programs have provided some grant funding and program guidance to support the start-up of sponsored volunteer corps to augment the disaster response capabilities of local communities. Future federal funding for the MRC program is unclear, as the initial demonstration grants have ended (Kantor 2010).

Although both are affiliated with the Citizen Corps, the national CERT program falls under FEMA within the U.S. Department of Homeland Security, whereas MRC operates out of the Office of the Surgeon General of the U.S. Public Health Service. The local units are registered with and connected to the federal government but are administered locally. CERT programs are typically multipurpose and can support a local disaster recovery with basic first aid, staff support, communication, and other nonspecialized activities. Originally, the main purpose of the MRC was to register and pre-credential volunteer health professionals to help fill the anticipated need for health care providers during public health emergencies and disasters in which additional health care support would likely be needed (pandemics, mass casualties, etc.). Although each unit is different, many MRC units have a mental health support component. As of May 2010, more than 820 recognized MRC units with over 206,000 individual volunteers were housed in a variety of agencies, including health departments, universities, and municipalities (Office of the Civilian Volunteer Medical Reserve Corps 2010).

There is an ongoing attempt to create a national advance registration program and single database for volunteer health professionals, although the initial effort stalled in 2007. States are still mandated through acceptance of federal disaster dollars to establish common registration systems that will ultimately work with the federal system. Although improvement has been seen in some areas of the country, in many other areas, registration practices and credentialing are not standardized across local groups, state organizations, the federal government, and nongovernmental organizations such as the Red Cross. Credentialing standards have been targeted as a compliance goal for the Department of Homeland Security as part of its NIMS compliance program (Kantor 2010; Federal Emergency Management Agency 2010b).

Each mental health care provider should become familiar with the specific response structure and protocols in his or her own community, because each locale is somewhat different, even though all basically adhere to the NRF in the United States. The disaster medical resources and the expected response can vary greatly by community, and each is heavily influenced by local tradition and the presence of specialized resources such as hospitals, National Guard units, and even medical schools (Kantor 2010).

Potential Roles for Mental Health Providers

The two major categories of volunteers in disaster response are termed *affiliated* and *unaffiliated*. These can be further modified to specify whether the responder is expected, oriented, and working with the system, or arrives on the scene with no plan and no credentials, disaster training, or security clearance. People who appear at disaster scenes on their own are known as *spontaneous volunteers* (also called spontaneous undocumented [or unaffiliated] volunteers, or SUVs for short). Regardless of status as affiliated or unaffiliated, mental health providers desiring to become future disaster volunteers should plan ahead, taking into consideration their personal interests, experience, licensure, and current work and family obligations. There are many anecdotes of frustrated clinicians who responded to calls for volunteers but were unable to function in their professional capacity because their credentials or individual skills could not be verified. For basic support functions, such as cleanup, feeding, and other unskilled activities, nonprofessional SUVs are fairly easy to credential on-site, assuming that a security clearance is unnecessary. For professionals who require licensing, credentialing, or a security clearance (e.g., for terrorist and disaster events), the process is much more complicated, and a clinician may have nothing to do or may feel underutilized. This situation can be a major source of frustration for both the volunteer and the system as a whole. Most experts and emergency preparedness agencies encourage advance registration and affiliation for health care volunteers.

Affiliated volunteers participate as members of recognized response groups. The organization is responsible for credentialing, screening, and even training the individual ahead of time or through organized, on-scene education known as *just-in-time training*. Because of the diversity of disaster events, even volunteers who have had prior training may still need just-in-time training related to the specific event. The federal government, along with the states and other national groups, is working at preregistration systems for medical volunteers. Even in the current age of high-speed electronic communication, if the infrastructure is damaged and communication is down, there may not be a way to verify credentials in the moment, and therefore precredentialing is critical. In the opening case vignette, Dr. Greene and his colleagues represent two types of spontaneous volunteers. His colleagues on the bus, both unaffiliated and spontaneous, were not allowed into the disaster area, preventing delivery of much-needed medical services. Dr. Greene, who was trying to affiliate before responding, was initially thwarted by the chaos and complexities of the multiagency and multijurisdictional disaster already in progress. Although unable to fulfill his initial goal at the disaster site, he was able to affiliate, serving in a much-needed medical role of caring for displaced survivors who were relocated to his home jurisdiction. If Dr. Greene had registered with a response agency ahead of time, precredentialing would have increased the likelihood that he could be part of the on-scene health and medical support efforts.

There are many other ways for psychiatrists and mental health care providers to affiliate as volunteers in disaster work. Finding the organization that fits one's interests, personality, and skill set is very important. Duties and expectations vary greatly across response groups, as does the likelihood of actually being called to respond to an event. A volunteer should be careful not to overcommit by affiliating with more than one response group. If a clinician might be critical to a local response group, he or she may not want to connect with a national group that is expected to respond out of the local area.

Even with the blossoming of online resources, word of mouth may be the best way to connect with local volunteer opportunities. Some local and state medical and specialty societies have disaster committees and offer training opportunities. They recommend that instead of responding independently, members connect with their local response organizations to ensure that the overall response structure is respected. In major disasters, however, the groups might call for additional volunteers, as happened after Hurricane Katrina. In that case, multiple health-related professional groups garnered volunteers from their membership lists and passed on willing names to the federal agencies.

National organizations, such as the American Red Cross and the MRC, often provide clear links to their local affiliates. Most have Web sites that provide sign-up instructions and outline the expectations for volunteers. Although the Red Cross is the most well-known agency for national response, traditionally its medical services have been limited in scope. During Hurricane Katrina, the Red Cross and the national MRC leadership developed a quick mechanism for utilizing MRC volunteers to fill Red Cross medical and mental health job functions. This was a first for both groups. Although MRC units are considered local assets, individual volunteers were allowed, with unit permission, to deploy if they had interest.

Training

Standardized disaster mental health training is an evolving issue. No agreed-upon standard training exists across federal agencies, nongovernmental organizations, states, or even individual disciplines. Many state and federal entities have considered the concept and implementation of guidelines and curricula, but confusion unfortunately remains regarding which course to take to function within a given organization's response framework. An individual volunteer, therefore, should first decide with which group to affiliate and then follow that group's training recommendations. At a bare minimum, most response organizations require a basic "introduction to disaster" and "incident command" orientation. Within the field of disaster behavioral health, there is movement toward the adoption of core concepts and competencies in training. The evidence-informed approach known as *Psychological First Aid* has gained acceptance among the disaster response community; the concept underlying this approach serves as a guiding principle for training and early response to the emotional and psychological needs of individuals affected by disasters and terrorism (see Chapter 12, "Psychological First Aid").

Conclusion

Choosing the right path to disaster response work is a very personal decision. Finding the right group or achieving the ideal role may require some personal research or practical exploration. Discussions with colleagues and local response groups can help an individual to find the right opportunity based on his or her personality, individual interests, and availability. It certainly makes sense to have basic disaster knowledge, whether a person is inadvertently affected at home or is choosing to help out in another community. Many of my colleagues have had fulfilling, even life-changing experiences through their work in disaster psychiatry. Understanding what to expect, working with a compatible group, and acquiring the requisite knowledge and skills are all likely to improve a person's perception of the experience.

■ Teaching Points

- Mental health professionals must examine their personal motivations for responding in a disaster.
- Familiarity with the basic hierarchy of the disaster response system in the United States is helpful when volunteering.
- Affiliating with an established group or agency before a disaster can facilitate involvement when a disaster occurs.
- An awareness of the different roles of organizations active in disaster response will help mental health practitioners understand where and how they can best contribute.
- Opportunities are available for training in disaster mental health support.

Review Questions

1.1 Disaster psychiatry is different from traditional office-based practice in which of the following ways?

   A. Individuals often are not suffering from a defined mental disorder.
   B. Interactions take place in a chaotic, unpredictable environment.
   C. Basic human needs such as hydration and food may take priority over mental health interventions.
   D. A and B only.
   E. All of the above.

1.2 True or False: Modern communication systems allow easy credentialing for psychiatrists with out-of-state licenses who arrive spontaneously at a disaster scene.

1.3 True or False: The Incident Command System varies greatly from state to state and has not yet evolved into a national response standard.

1.4 Organizations with specific roles for medical personnel include all of the following *except*

   A. American Red Cross.
   B. Medical Reserve Corps (MRC).
   C. Community Emergency Response Teams (CERTs).
   D. Disaster Medical Assistance Teams (DMATs).
   E. None of the above.

1.5   In larger or more complex disaster events, including those involving multiple agencies or jurisdictions, a temporary command site is typically established nearby—but at a safe distance from—the event. This site is known as

  A. A crisis planning and action center (CPAC).
  B. An emergency operations center (EOC).
  C. An emergency management assistance compact (EMAC).
  D. An emergency supervisory command (ESC).
  E. A strategic command center (SCC).

References

American Red Cross: Volunteer Portal. Washington, DC, American Red Cross, 2010. Available at: http://www.redcross.org/en/volunteer. Accessed January 3, 2011.

Centers for Disease Control and Prevention: Interim results: state-specific seasonal influenza vaccination coverage, United States, August 2009–January 2010. MMWR Morb Mortal Wkly Rep 59:477–484, 2010. Available at: http://www.cdc.gov/mmwr/preview/mmwrhtml/mm5916a1.htm. Accessed May 10, 2010.

Disaster Psychiatry Outreach: The Essentials of Disaster Psychiatry: A Training Course for Mental Health Professionals (Course Syllabus). New York, Disaster Psychiatry Outreach, 2008. Available as DPOCourseSyllabus_052108.pdf at: https://sites.google.com/a/disasterpsych.org/blog/File-Cabinet. Accessed May 7, 2010.

Federal Emergency Management Agency: Incident Command System (ICS) Resource Center. Washington, DC, Federal Emergency Management Agency, 2010a. Available at: http://training.fema.gov/EMIWeb/IS/ICSResource/index.htm. Accessed July 13, 2010.

Federal Emergency Management Agency: National Incident Management System Resources. Washington, DC, Federal Emergency Management Agency, 2010b. Available at: http://www.fema.gov/emergency/nims/index.shtm. Accessed July 13, 2010.

Federal Emergency Management Agency: Incident Command System Organization. Washington, DC, Federal Emergency Management Agency, 2010c. Available at: http://training.fema.gov/EMIWeb/IS/ICSResource/assets/ICSOrganization.pdf. Accessed January 3, 2011.

Kantor EM: Guidance for potential disaster health and mental health volunteers, in Haiti Updates. New York, Disaster Psychiatry Outreach, 2009. Available at: http://www.disasterpsych.org/updates/guidanceforpotentialdisasterhealth-andmentalhealthvolunteers/GuidanceforPotentialDisasterMedicalandMental-HealthVolunteers.pdf. Accessed July 13, 2010.

Kantor EM: The disaster response system in the United States, in Hidden Impact: What You Need to Know for the Next Disaster. A Practical Mental Health Guide for Clinicians. Edited by Stoddard FJ, Katz CL, Merlino JP. Sudbury, MA, Jones & Bartlett, 2010, pp 11–18

Office of the Civilian Volunteer Medical Reserve Corps: Home Page. Rockville, MD, Office of the Civilian Volunteer Medical Reserve Corps, 2010. Available at: http://www.medicalreservecorps.gov. Accessed July 13, 2010.

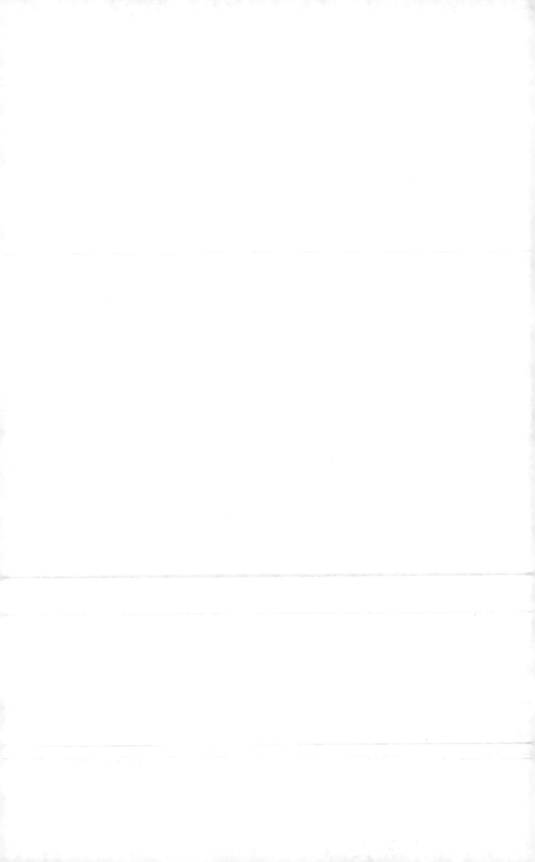

2

Communicating Risk Before, During, and After a Disaster

Frederick J. Stoddard Jr., M.D.

This chapter introduces a topic that mental health professionals have spent years studying and training for: communication, particularly verbal communication, but here, communicating about risk. Modes of communication, including visual, are expanding by the instant with the Internet, texting, YouTube, Twitter, Facebook, Skype, etc. Yet at present there is little education about how to improve our professional communication with our patients, the public, or our leaders in the disaster context. Together with case examples, this chapter introduces guiding principles for communicating about risk and offers relevant background material. The key topics include general principles of risk communication, relations with the media, and risk communication in preparation for, during, and after disasters. Contained within "during disasters" are the important issues of resilience and vulnerability and how communication about risk may lessen the vulnerability and improve the resilience of communities impacted by disaster.

General Principles for Communication About Risk

The term *risk communication* is used in disaster response planning to describe effective communication before, during, or after a crisis (Center for

Mental Health Services 2002). It encompasses exchange of information with individuals (e.g., patients), groups (e.g., schools), businesses (e.g., those impacted or threatened), public agencies (first responders such as police and fire departments), and the news media (via the Internet, radio, or TV). Psychiatrists and mental health teams may be consulted or hold leadership positions from which they may facilitate effective communication about risk (Norwood et al. 2005).

In 2002, the Center for Mental Health Services at the Substance Abuse and Mental Health Services Administration (SAMHSA) issued *Communicating in a Crisis: Risk Communication Guidelines for Public Officials* (Center for Mental Health Services 2002). In this document, *risk communication* is defined as "an interactive process of exchange of information and opinion among individuals, groups, and institutions; often involves multiple messages about the nature of risk or expressing concerns, opinions, or reactions to risk messages or to legal and institutional arrangements for risk management" (p. 14). In the same document, a *risk message* is defined as "a written, verbal, or visual statement containing information about risk; may or may not include advice about risk reduction behavior; a formal risk message is a structured written, audio, or visual packaged [*sic*] developed with the express purpose of presenting information about risk" (p. 20). Risk communication recommendations from the guidelines are summarized in Table 2–1.

A carefully constructed risk message is demonstrated by contrasting two different ways to communicate to the public a brief and effective message (point 5 in Table 2–1) about the risk for posttraumatic stress disorder (PTSD) following a disaster. The message to increase awareness of PTSD would get lost if all of the diagnostic criteria were recited. A better approach is to advise disaster victims to consider the possibility that they may have developed PTSD if they feel like their initial "fight-or-flight" reaction just will not go away.

TABLE 2–1.   Risk communication recommendations

---

1. Ease public concern.

2. Give guidance on how to respond.

3. Stay on message.

4. Deliver accurate and timely information.

5. Develop goals and messages that are simple, straightforward, and realistic. Deliver information with brevity, clarity, and effectiveness.

Source.   Adapted from Center for Mental Health Services 2002.

In disasters, public communication about mental health is essential, with helpful information provided by reliable sources, including psychiatrists and other health professionals. The lack of accurate, reliable public communication increases risk; leads to rumors and, in rare circumstances, panic; and may magnify the psychological trauma that survivors experience. Because of the current dependence on electronic communications, lack of public communication can occur when the power infrastructure is affected, as it was for a time after the 2004 Asian tsunami[1] and the 2010 Haitian earthquake.[2] Conversely, when the media conveys accurate news of a disaster and advice about what can be done, this may mitigate adverse effects and enable those who are exposed to the disaster to take protective actions. Finally, other news, such as repetitive showing of traumatic images on TV, may add to traumatization in the viewers, especially children. Most studies, such as that by Schlenger et al. (2002), found an association between the number of hours of watching terrorism-related TV programming and viewers' PTSD symptom levels.

The Media

Psychiatrists and other health professionals communicate about disaster risks to their patients, to their communities, and through the media. Their

---

[1]The Asian tsunami in 2004 was caused by an enormous earthquake, triggering a series of devastating tsunamis (massive waves) along the coasts of most land masses bordering the Indian Ocean, inundating coastal communities with waves up to 30 meters (100 feet) high. It was one of the deadliest natural disasters in recorded history. Indonesia was hardest hit with between 170,000 and 220,000 deaths, followed by Sri Lanka, India, and Thailand. According to the U.S. Geological Survey, approximately 228,000 people died, with other estimates much higher. Measured in lives lost, this is one of the 10 worst earthquakes in history. One-third of the dead appeared to be children, due to the high proportion of children in the populations affected and because they were the least able to resist the surging waters. Oxfam reported that up to 4 times more women than men were killed in some regions. It was estimated by the United Nations at the outset that the relief operation would cost over $7 billion, making this the costliest disaster in human history, and that reconstruction would probably take 5–10 years. Fear of a doubling of the death toll led to the massive humanitarian response. (This summary is adapted from sources quoted in "2004 Indian Ocean Earthquake and Tsunami" [2010].)

[2]The 2010 Haiti earthquake was a catastrophic 7.0 M_w earthquake with an epicenter 16 miles from Haiti's capital. The Haitian government estimated that 3 million people were affected by the quake, with 230,000 people dead, 300,000 injured, and 1 million made homeless. Additionally, 250,000 residences and 30,000 commercial buildings were severely damaged. An outpouring of medical, economic, and public safety assistance came from many governments and nongovernmental organizations ("2010 Haiti Earthquake" 2010).

first responsibility is to their patients, and communicating care to patients makes patients trust their doctors more. Therefore, it is first and foremost important for clinicians to hear, respect, and respond to their patients' worry, anxiety, and confusion. As community leaders, psychiatrists and other health professionals are often asked for advice and may provide advance information that helps to prepare their communities for disasters of various types (Beard and Kantor 2004; Bennett et al. 1999). They also may be consulted by journalists for health information to clarify risks (e.g., about PTSD) to their audiences, or for advice for parents or schools on what to tell and how to protect their children (Fassler 2003; Rauch 2009; Stoddard and Menninger 2004; Teichroeb 2006), or for advice to caretakers for protection and care of fragile elderly individuals.

Some psychiatrists and other health professionals might avoid speaking to a journalist because of concerns about being misquoted or about public exposure. Although a desire to avoid interviews is understandable, especially if previous interviewers misquoted the clinicians or lost their meaning, such avoidance may mean losing a valuable opportunity to convey needed information to many disaster survivors. Failure to skillfully exchange information with potentially targeted groups or the media may "greatly compromise a country's ability to address the devastating medical and psychosocial outcomes" that could result from a natural or human-caused disaster such as a biological attack (Tinker and Vaughn 2004, p. 308). Organizations such as the American Psychiatric Association, other professional societies, and hospitals periodically offer media training with expert faculty who teach skills about writing and delivering a constructive message, and such training may reduce concerns about media relations. Sample messages and recommendations are provided on the Web sites of the American Psychiatric Association (2010), the American Academy of Child and Adolescent Psychiatry (1999, 2002, 2008), and the National Child Traumatic Stress Network (2011).

Communication About Risk in Preparation for Disasters

Psychiatrists require preparation to adapt existing skills and build new ones to effectively respond to a disaster (Young et al. 2006). Toward this end, disaster training modules are increasingly being incorporated into medical schools, residency programs, and postgraduate courses. In particular, psychiatrists can promote the activities and interventions listed in Table 2–2.

Mental health professionals can prepare for possible leadership roles for crisis communication with community, state, and federal government offi-

---

TABLE 2–2.   Actions to promote in postdisaster messaging

1. Public health interventions and monitoring

2. Appropriate treatment for clinical populations

3. Public/risk communication, prevention, liaison, and ways to realistically lessen fear that may follow a terrorist act

4. Tabletop exercises, disaster drills, practice using protective equipment, and mass casualty exercises

5. Interventions to reduce stress in health care workers and other responders

6. Research

Source.   DiGiovanni 2001; Norris et al. 2006.

cials and the media (Institute of Medicine 2003). Preparation is needed for accurate and effective communication about specific aspects of disasters (e.g., the neuropsychological effects of biohazards such as anthrax or nerve gases, or of nuclear events). Experience from the 2002–2003 severe acute respiratory syndrome (SARS) epidemic indicated the need to communicate about and prepare for ethical dilemmas to relieve the stress of staff and patients (Nickell et al. 2004; Singer et al. 2003), and the H1N1 pandemic in 2009 presented potential challenges in the response to quarantine directives. One challenge is how staff can grapple with the conflict between professional duty and personal concerns for the safety and health of one's self and family during an epidemic. A related challenge of the emerging threats of toxic chemicals, biological agents, and radioactive materials is how to communicate in response to requests for "concrete, accurate and consistent information about actions needed for protection of self and family" (Wray et al. 2008, p. 2214).

Preparing to communicate with media and leaders is of critical importance. Mental health professionals should provide information about the human factors associated with the event, their time course, and ways to obtain help (Myers and Zunin 2000); educate about the stages of grief (disbelief and shock, symptoms of grieving, and acceptance of loss); and describe bereavement after unnatural death, marked by somatic, posttraumatic, depressive, and substance craving symptoms, as well as discuss the fact that it may be prolonged. Preparatory communications should also teach about the stresses of first responders and of those engaged in body recovery, and indicate how leaders and media representatives may best monitor and manage their own stress, educate others, and seek help when needed. Most important, public education is not beneficial if it creates a self-fulfilling prophecy of distress and dysfunction. It is important to refine messages that emphasize the fact that most survivors are resilient.

Communication About Risk During Disasters

> One of the major roles I played in running Bellevue's mental health clinics during 9/11 was keeping staff from burning out. Too many of our clinical staff were all too willing to work countless shifts in addition to always volunteering to take on more. They didn't like being told they couldn't go to "the pile" or to a firehouse or a family center. At times all I could do was to protect them from themselves. (Joseph P. Merlino, personal communication, April 15, 2010)

As is evident from the quotation above, part of communication about risk in the wake of disasters occurs among psychiatrists themselves to help them function effectively (see also Chapter 3, "Rescuing Ourselves"). Other risk communications need to address areas of vulnerability and strength among special populations within the community.

Anxiety, confusion, and scapegoating immediately postdisaster can be reduced through the dissemination of information that is as clear, consistent, and reassuring as possible (MacGregor and Fleming 1996; Newman et al. 2006). Table 2–3 offers guidelines that may help psychiatrists and other health professionals in communicating individually with patients and with others (Stoddard et al. 2010).

Because media organizations are often seeking images and descriptions that capture the traumatic nature of a disaster, individuals in the media are often highly exposed to experiences and images that can take a psychological toll. Therefore, when talking with journalists and other media representatives, mental health professionals may be able to help often-overlooked professionals who are expected to provide public service and who may value knowing how to readily access psychiatric evaluation and interventions to aid in coping with the stresses of their work and with their lives outside.

TABLE 2–3.   Guidelines for communicating with patients and other disaster survivors

---

1. Listen to, respect, and respond to the fears, anxieties, and uncertainties of patients; they want to know that the doctor cares before they care what the doctor knows.

2. Recognize that people are risk averse and, when upset, will often fixate on negatives; be extremely careful in offering up these five "N" words—*no, not, never, nothing, none*—and words with negative connotations that can add to rather than lessen fear.

3. Offer authentic statements of caring, empathy, and compassion while also taking time to listen, and back up your statements with actions.

4. Be honest, ethical, frank, and open, recognizing that there are limits on what needs to be disclosed.

5. Avoid mixed or inconsistent verbal and nonverbal messages.

Humans experience a range of vulnerability following disasters. The transient, even intense, psychological reactions of many victims include fear, anger, and distress. In addition, they are likely to experience physical, cognitive, behavioral, or spiritual changes. Trauma workers often refer to these phenomena as "normal responses to an abnormal situation." After disasters, a significant minority of survivors, many of whom have no history of prior psychiatric illness, develop PTSD or major depression (North et al. 1999). Survivors also report significant distress, isolation, and disruption of work or schoolwork. (See also Chapter 5, "Psychiatric Evaluation.")

Protective Factors

If the population's resilience could be reinforced by public education, both providing hope and enhancing resiliency, the primary prevention of adverse psychological consequences could conceivably render disasters less damaging to populations (Charney 2004; Shalev 2004; Stoddard 2009; Watson et al. 2006). The following case vignette illustrates successful dissemination of public education designed to reduce parental fears.

> Following 9/11, several news journalists, seeking help in writing their newspaper articles, called a child psychiatrist for guidance on what to tell parents to expect of children's responses and how to help them. The clinician described the range of reactions that might occur in children of different ages, depending on the children's proximity to the event, to adults impacted by the attack or to televised images of the attack and devastation. He explained that parents might observe their children for signs of distress, such as worrying, preoccupation with televised images, insomnia related to the attacks, or school difficulties. He suggested that parents help their children by encouraging them to express their feelings and concerns in words or drawings and by reassuring them honestly about their fears. If a child's symptoms were severe or persistent, or if a child had questions with which parents would like help, they were advised to consult a mental health professional or a pediatrician.

In the absence of fear, posttraumatic stress is much diminished. The immediate aftermath of disasters not only disrupts the lives of individuals but also has significant impact on families, communities, and societies. Clinicians who might publicly communicate about appropriate psychiatric care need to recognize that the consequences of disasters will depend to some extent on the social context of those affected. The levels of fear in the context of disasters seem to have reached new heights, especially in some urban areas that are especially vulnerable to natural disasters or terrorist events. To counter this fear, psychiatrists should consider the question, "What are the sources of hope upon which people draw to resist fear?" Hope can reside in many places. Most people will speak of finding hope in family, community, religion, culture, companionship, and nation. Accordingly, it is important to refine public communications to address the particular strengths, vulnerabilities, and needs of each population.

Vulnerable Populations

In public communications, mental health professionals should address the needs of vulnerable populations. Children (Fremont 2004), elderly persons, people with chronic mental illness and physical disabilities, and first responders are vulnerable populations that present specific developmental, psychiatric, medical, and professional challenges. For more details, see the chapters on special populations (Chapter 6), people with serious and persistent mental illness (Chapter 7), children and adolescents (Chapter 17), and geriatric persons (Chapter 18). In addition, people who are members of communities associated with the ethnicity or religion of perpetrators of mass violence (whether through stereotyping, racism, or actual affiliation) may have to face both the immediate stresses and increased stigmatization, and may benefit from interventions specifically adapted to ameliorating these stresses (Norris and Alegria 2006).

Outreach to underserved and vulnerable communities can be achieved by identifying and communicating with trusted figures in that community, such as religious leaders, supervisors, primary care physicians, and community leaders (Reissman et al. 2005). Public communication through psychoeducation can be a two-way street, with the psychiatrist assisting and advising these leaders while simultaneously learning about the distinct vulnerabilities and strengths of that community. Psychoeducation will also need to account for those factors that will especially affect those figures: the leaders' own disaster exposure, secondary traumatization, the burden of leadership in a time of crisis, and concerns about their own abilities to protect and provide community leadership.

Communication About Risk After Disasters

Although it is tempting to assume that psychological risk after disasters is proximal to the event, in this age of distance travel and electronic communications, the "proximal" areas to consider in providing public communication about the event may extend for long distances, even across the world. The commissioner of the Departments of Health and Mental Hygiene in New York, who served from 1998 to 2002, wrote that "one important lesson learned from [9/11] is that terrorism creates health impacts that reach far beyond the immediate boundaries of a disastrous event, because people will, whenever possible, seek to leave the immediate area and return to their homes" (Covello 2001). These victims may seek help in communities far from the event, and other people are affected by televised images or the Internet.

The following case vignette illustrates helpful communication after a disaster.

A shooting by an enraged employee occurred at a small technology company, and some people were killed, others wounded, and all emotionally traumatized. The company was closed temporarily due to the police investigation. Dr. Benson, a hospital psychiatrist with American Psychiatric Association disaster training and both clinical and research experience with PTSD, was asked by the hospital public relations department to speak to a TV journalist the next day. He was interviewed for about 10 minutes for airing on the evening news. Prior to the interview, Dr. Benson asked what to expect and was prepared by the public relations department to anticipate general questions about PTSD, the impact of such mass shooting events, and ways to help those who are impacted. He prepared for the interview by learning more about the shootings and asking the interviewer for her questions in advance.

As planned, the TV interviewer asked general questions about the attacker, the impact of such a terrible event on the victims and their families, and PTSD. Dr. Benson listened carefully to the journalist, appreciating her concern, and answered her specific questions with little elaboration. He acknowledged that he did not know directly about the event and that this appeared to be an emotionally devastating and very sad act of violence. In response to the first question, Dr. Benson said that he did not know the mental state of the shooter, that the individual may or may not have had a mental illness, that this would likely be evaluated because the shooter was in custody, and that it would be unprofessional and unethical for him to publicly speculate about the shooter's mental state because he had not personally examined him. In response to the second question, Dr. Benson explained that the company appeared to be using mental health consultants to help its staff cope as well as possible with the trauma and grief and the damage to its business. Finally, in response to further questions, Dr. Benson explained in some detail about symptoms of PTSD and bereavement, and that psychotherapeutic support would be helpful, if desired by workers at the company. He explained that the trauma to the families was likely to be great and that expert support to ease their suffering would also be helpful. The interviewer thanked Dr. Benson and concluded the interview.

In a postdisaster interview, a mental health professional should attempt to decrease public fears and confusion by providing clear and accurate information. Education about the actual risks, such as PTSD and depression (Bills et al. 2008), and instruction in how to decrease risk enhances feelings of control and familiarity with disasters. Instruction in active coping techniques is helpful. This is especially important with the threat of biological, chemical, and radiological agents, but also with all types of disasters. Collaboration between mental health professionals and primary health care providers is an important model for prevention and provision of services to large numbers of people. Learning to identify vulnerable locations and populations can assist in public communications that may be effective in countering the potential impact of disasters or terrorist events.

Journalists and media representatives do not always interact well with psychiatrists, and vice versa. Following 9/11, some psychiatrists volunteering for Disaster Psychiatry Outreach in New York City had problems that led the organization to write guidelines in its curriculum that are especially helpful to psychiatrists who do not have media training or experience (Disaster Psychiatry Outreach 2008). The advice presented in that curriculum does not conflict with the content of this chapter but qualifies it greatly, especially for inexperienced, apprehensive psychiatrists with no media training, who should do absolutely no media work until they become trained. Types of problems that can occur include intrusive interviewing, misquotation, and difficulties in protecting sensitive information. Psychiatrists should decline media interviews when it is not clear what will happen with the information to be offered, or when the information may not be helpful to the public or might even cause harm.

Conclusion

There is a need for mental health professionals to learn to play a role in communicating about risk, before, during or after a disaster, with their patients, their communities, and media representatives. With patients, it is essential for the mental health professional to respect their worries, fears, or confusion and to offer hope and direction regarding how they might reduce their fears and best care for themselves and their families, especially children and the elderly. With the public and the media, media training can help the mental health professional by providing practice in public speaking and by teaching how to select which points to convey and emphasize and how to avoid problems. In communicating about risk, it is helpful to provide information describing possible psychiatric consequences of disasters, including traumatic stress and depressive symptoms, and how to seek help.

■ Teaching Points

- When making decisions about their communications before, during, or after disasters, mental health professionals should review the recommendations of the Center for Mental Health Services (see Table 2–1).

- Mental health professionals should seek to
  - Receive media training.
  - Reduce counterproductive anxiety and psychosomatic symptoms.
  - Provide advice on how to remain safe or get help, including mental health resources, if needed.
  - Plan helpful information for leaders, first responders, medical personnel, the public, parents, and special populations.

Review Questions

2.1 The term *risk communication,* as used in disaster response planning, refers to effective exchange of information during or after a crisis with which of the following?

  A. Individuals (e.g., patients) and groups (e.g., schools).
  B. Businesses (e.g., those impacted or threatened).
  C. Public agencies (first responders such as police and fire departments).
  D. The news media (via Internet, radio, or TV).
  E. All of the above.

2.2 Important online resources for disaster mental health information include all of the following *except*

  A. American Psychiatric Association (APA).
  B. Substance Abuse and Mental Health Services Administration (SAMHSA).
  C. YouTube.
  D. National Child Traumatic Stress Network.
  E. American Academy of Child and Adolescent Psychiatry (AACAP).

2.3 The Center for Mental Health Services guidelines for public officials regarding how to provide public information following disasters include which of the following?

  A. Ease public concern.
  B. Give guidance on how to respond.
  C. Stay on message.
  D. Deliver accurate and timely information.
  E. All of the above.

2.4   Public communication may achieve outreach to underserved and vulnerable communities by identifying and communicating with community leaders, such as

    A. Trusted figures in the community.
    B. Supervisors.
    C. Primary care physicians.
    D. Religious leaders.
    E. All of the above.

2.5   Reasons for a psychiatrist to decline a media interview include

    A. The psychiatrist lacks media training.
    B. The information to be offered may not help the public.
    C. The information to be offered might cause harm.
    D. The information to be offered may be misquoted.
    E. All of the above.

References

American Academy of Child and Adolescent Psychiatry: Facts for Families, #70: Posttraumatic Stress Disorder. Washington, DC, American Academy of Child and Adolescent Psychiatry, 1999. Available at: http://www.aacap.org/cs/root/facts_for_families/posttraumatic_stress_disorder_ptsd. Accessed March 16, 2010.

American Academy of Child and Adolescent Psychiatry: Facts for Families, #67: Children and the News. Washington, DC, American Academy of Child and Adolescent Psychiatry, 2002. Available at: http://www.aacap.org/cs/root/facts_for_families/children_and_the_news. Accessed March 16, 2010.

American Academy of Child and Adolescent Psychiatry: Facts for Families, #87: Talking to Children About Terrorism and War. Washington, DC, American Academy of Child and Adolescent Psychiatry, 2008. Available at: http://www.aacap.org/cs/root/facts_for_families/talking_to_children_about_terrorism_and_war. Accessed March 16, 2010.

American Psychiatric Association: Disaster Psychiatry. Washington, DC, American Psychiatric Association, 2010. Available at: http://www.psych.org/Resources/DisasterPsychiatry.aspx. Accessed October 14, 2010.

Beard R, Kantor E: Managing the Message in Times of Crisis: Risk Communication and Mental Wellness in Disaster Health Care. Charlottesville, VA, University of Virginia Medical Reserve Corps, Public Relations Office, University of Virginia Health System, 2004

Bennett P, Coles D, McDonald A: Risk communication as a decision process, in Risk Communication and Public Health. Edited by Bennett P, Calman K. Oxford, UK, Oxford University Press, 1999, pp 207–221

Bills CB, Levy NAS, Sharma V, et al: Mental health of workers and volunteers responding to events of 9/11: review of the literature. Mt Sinai J Med 75:115–127, 2008

Center for Mental Health Services: Communicating in a Crisis: Risk Communication Guidelines for Public Officials. Rockville, MD, Substance Abuse and Mental Health Services Administration, 2002. Available at: http://www.riskcommunication.samhsa.gov. Accessed October 14, 2010.

Charney DS: Psychobiological mechanisms of resilience and vulnerability: implications for successful adaptation to extreme stress (review). Am J Psychiatry 161:195–216, 2004

Covello VT: Lessons learned from the front lines of risk and crisis communication: 21 guidelines for effective communication by leaders addressing high anxiety, high stress, or threatening situations. Presented as part of keynote address, U.S. Conference of Mayors Emergency, Safety, and Security Summit, Washington, DC, October 2001

DiGiovanni C: Pertinent psychological issues in the immediate management of a weapons of mass destruction event. Mil Med 166(suppl):59–60, 2001

Disaster Psychiatry Outreach: The Essentials of Disaster Psychiatry: A Training Course for Mental Health Professionals (Course Syllabus). New York, Disaster Psychiatry Outreach, 2008. Available as DPOCourseSyllabus_052108.pdf at: https://sites.google.com/a/disasterpsych.org/blog/File-Cabinet. Accessed December 28, 2009.

Fassler D: Talking to children about war and terrorism: tips for parents and teachers. American Psychiatric Association News Release, March 5, 2003. Available at: http://www.psych.org/Resources/DisasterPsychiatry/APADisasterPsychiatryResources/talkingtochildrenrewarterror.aspx. Accessed March 16, 2010.

Fremont WP: Childhood reactions to terrorism-induced trauma: a review of the past 10 years. J Am Acad Child Adolesc Psychiatry 43:381–392, 2004

Institute of Medicine: Preparing for the Psychological Consequences of Terrorism: A Public Health Strategy. Washington, DC, The National Academy of Sciences Institute of Medicine, 2003

MacGregor DG, Fleming R: Risk perception and symptom reporting. Risk Anal 16:773–783, 1996

Myers D, Zunin L: Phases of disaster, in Training Manual for Mental Health and Human Service Workers in Major Disasters, 2nd Edition (DHHS Publ No ADM 90–538). Edited by DeWolfe D. Washington, DC, U.S. Government Printing Office, 2000

National Child Traumatic Stress Network: National Center for Child Traumatic Stress Online Press Kit. Available at: http://www.nctsnet.org/nccts/nav.do?pid=ctr_aud_mdia_online_kit#q5. Accessed January 11, 2011.

Newman E, Franks RP: Child Clinicians and the Media: Guide for Therapists. New York, DART Center for Journalism and Trauma. Available at: http://dart-center.org/content/child-clinicians-media-2. Accessed March 16, 2010.

Newman E, Davis J, Kennedy SM: Journalism and the public during catastrophes, in 9/11: Mental Health in the Wake of Terrorist Attacks. Edited by Neria Y, Gross R, Marshall R, et al. Cambridge, UK, Cambridge University Press, 2006, pp 178–196

Nickell LA, Crighton EJ, Tracy CS, et al: Psychosocial effects of SARS on hospital staff: survey of a large tertiary care institution. CMAJ 170:793–798, 2004

Norris FH, Alegria M: Promoting disaster recovery in ethnic-minority individuals and communities, in Interventions Following Mass Violence and Disasters: Strategies for Mental Health Practice. Edited by Ritchie EC, Watson PJ, Friedman MJ. New York, Guilford, 2006, pp 319–342

Norris FH, Galea S, Friedman MJ, et al: Methods for Disaster Mental Health Research. New York, Guilford, 2006

North CS, Nixon SJ, Shariat S, et al: Psychiatric disorders among survivors of the Oklahoma City bombing. JAMA 282:755–762, 1999

Norwood AH, Sermons-Ward L, Blumenfeld M: Crisis communication: the role of psychiatric leaders in communicating with the media and government officials at the time of disaster, terrorism and other crises. Presented at the Speaker-Elect Forum, American Psychiatric Association, Washington, DC, November 10, 2005

Rauch PK: Talking With Children About Upsetting News Events. Boston, MA, Mass-General Hospital for Children, 2009. Available at: http://www.massgeneral.org/children/patientsandfamilies/familyhealth/talking_about_upsetting_events.aspx. Accessed March 16, 2009.

Reissman DB, Spencer S, Tanielian TL, et al: Integrating behavioral aspects into community preparedness and response systems. J Aggress Maltreat Trauma 10:707–720, 2005

Schlenger WE, Caddell JM, Ebert L, et al: Psychological reactions to terrorist attacks: findings from the national study of Americans' reactions to September 11. JAMA 288:581–588, 2002

Shalev A: Appraisal of terrorism: the media and the spectators. Presented at the Committee on Terrorism and Disasters, Group for Advancement of Psychiatry, Westchester, NY, March 16, 2004

Singer PA, Benatar SA, Berstein M, et al: Ethics and SARS: lessons from Toronto. Br J Med 327:1342–1345, 2003

Stoddard FJ: Book review: Intervention and Resilience After Mass Trauma, edited by Michael Blumenfield and Robert J. Ursano. Psychiatr Serv 60:997–998, 2009

Stoddard FJ, Menninger EW: Guidance for parents and other caretakers after disasters or terrorist attacks, in Disaster Psychiatry Handbook. Edited by Hall RCW, Ng AT, Norwood AE. Washington, DC, American Psychiatric Association, 2004, pp 44–56. Available at: http://www.psych.org/Resources/DisasterPsychiatry/APADisasterPsychiatryResources/DisasterPsychiatryHandbook.aspx. Accessed March 16, 2010.

Stoddard FJ, Katz CL, Kantor EM, et al: Risk communication, prevention and the media, in Hidden Impact: What You Need to Know for the Next Disaster. A Practical Mental Health Guide for Clinicians. Edited by Stoddard FK, Katz CL, Merlino JP. Sudbury, MA, Jones & Bartlett, 2010, pp 37–42

Teichroeb R: Covering Children and Trauma: A Guide for Journalism Professionals. New York, DART Center for Journalism and Trauma, 2006. Available at: http://dartcenter.org/files/covering_children_and_trauma_0.pdf. Accessed March 16, 2010.

Tinker TL, Vaughn E: Communicating the risks of bioterrorism, in Bioterrorism: Psychological and Public Health Interventions. Edited by Ursano RJ, Norwood AE, Fullerton CS. Cambridge, UK, Cambridge University Press, 2004, pp 308–329

2004 Indian Ocean earthquake and tsunami. Wikipedia, 2010. Available at: http://en.wikipedia.org/wiki/2004_Indian_Ocean_earthquake. Accessed July 7, 2010.

2010 Haiti earthquake. Wikipedia, 2010. Available at: http://en.wikipedia.org/wiki/2010_Haiti_earthquake. Accessed July 7, 2010.

Watson PJ, Ritchie EC, Demer J, et al: Improving resilience trajectories following mass violence and disasters, in Interventions Following Mass Violence and Disasters: Strategies for Mental Health Practice. Edited by Ritchie EC, Watson PJ, Friedman MJ. New York, Guilford, 2006, pp 37–53

Wray RJ, Becker SM, Henderson N, et al: Communicating with the public about emerging health threats: lessons from Pre-Event Message Development Project. Am J Public Health 98:2214–2222, 2008

Young BH, Ruzek JI, Wong M, et al: Disaster mental health training guidelines, considerations and recommendation, in Interventions Following Mass Violence and Disasters: Strategies for Mental Health Practice. Edited by Ritchie EC, Watson PJ, Friedman MJ. New York, Guilford, 2006, pp 16–34

3

Rescuing Ourselves

Self-Care in the Disaster Response Community

Joseph P. Merlino, M.D., M.P.A.

A New York–based physician working at Bellevue Hospital Center in 2001, witnessed responders mobilizing during the 9/11 attacks on the World Trade Center (Merlino 2004). A decade later, having relocated to Brooklyn's Kings County Hospital Center, he watched as colleagues left for Haiti after a devastating earthquake, a disaster that took 200,000–250,000 lives (Lacey 2010). Individuals acting selflessly responded quickly, perhaps impulsively, driven by altruistic motives and other personality characteristics. It seemed obvious to the physician then and now that "self-care" was not a priority for most of these responders, if it was a consideration at all. First responders rushed to New York's Ground Zero and worked hours to days without returning to their homes. Following the Haiti earthquake, response physicians and nurses insisted on traveling to the island with no preparation or disaster experience at all, against the recommendations of many (American Red Cross 2010).

In this chapter, I highlight core concepts in self-care for clinician responders and review the positive and negative impacts that disaster response can have at the individual level. I discuss some of the key issues in this important area, including personality characteristics of responders, the challenges of responding, vicarious traumatization, prevention of secondary trauma, and restoring normalcy.

Disaster responders cannot take care of others if they cannot take care of themselves. The ability to care for oneself is neither the solution to nor the source (Stamm 1999) of stress-related symptoms secondary to caring for those who are traumatized. Self-care does not imply that the person should keep the problem of stress-related symptoms from happening or that if such symptoms do happen, the person is at fault for not doing a good enough job.

Self-Awareness: Knowing One's Limits

Exactly who are the first responders to disaster settings, and what is known about their psychological makeup? The literature shows that the person with a so-called rescue personality (Mitchell and Bray 1990) is one who is "inner-directed, action oriented, obsessed with performance, traditional, socially conservative, easily bored, and highly dedicated" (p. 20); has difficulty saying no; is a risk taker; and can be addicted to trauma. Individuals who have enormous capacity for feeling and expressing empathy tend to be more at risk of compassion fatigue or secondary traumatic stress disorder (Figley 1995). Many of these characteristics also are found in people who pursue careers in medicine and health care (Gabbard 1985).

Although research does not uniformly support the rescue personality profile (Wagner et al. 2009), anecdotally many of these traits do appear in those clinicians who are first responders. To the extent that such a rescue personality does exist, it makes clear both why such individuals can perform emergency tasks well and why the issue of self-care must be a focus of disaster response planning at multiple levels, including the individual, organizational, and governmental levels. Also, using the ecological perspective of primary prevention of stress-related problems, the workplace must be seen as a health-promoting environment fostering the principles of self-care (Stamm 1999).

Important in self-care is being aware of one's own emotions and the effects of others' emotions on oneself. Much has been written about this topic, in particular the concept of *emotional intelligence* as "the ability to manage ourselves and our relationships effectively" (Goleman 2000, p. 6). The four major skills that make up emotional intelligence are self-awareness, self-management, social awareness, and relationship management.

Many authors writing in the field of secondary trauma prevention agree on two key pieces of advice for clinicians (Stamm 1999):

1. Do not do this work alone.
2. Monitor your responses to the work through your own careful attendance to your process and through supervision by your trusted colleagues.

The use of emotional intelligence concepts and training are helpful in this regard (Goleman 1998).

Just as there are many personal and professional benefits to being a disaster responder (Merlino 2010a), including the gratification that comes from using one's skills in helping fellow humans in need, there are also many reasons for *not* responding. In a brutally honest online commentary (Anonymous 2010), after a recently retired emergency physician listed many "excuses" for not responding to the 2010 Haiti earthquake, including not speaking French or Haitian Creole, not having disaster training, and not having all of his immunizations up to date, he finally acknowledged that "the real reasons" included the stresses and the Centers for Disease Control and Prevention's (CDC's) warnings of posttraumatic stress that can affect responders. "I had to admit to myself that I may not be up to that." He instead "cut some good-sized checks" to a variety of relief funds and organizations. That was indeed the advice given immediately after the Haiti earthquake, when people were told not to go but to send money instead. There are many ways to help during disasters. Physically mobilizing to the disaster site is an important response, but only one of many.

Self-Care Planning and Training

The CDC provides recommendations both for those who do respond by mobilizing (Centers for Disease and Prevention 2010b) and for all people (Centers for Disease Control and Prevention 2010a). The latter recommendations suggest that all individuals do the following:

1. Prepare a disaster emergency kit, including emergency food and water supplies as well as batteries and first aid materials.
2. Develop a family disaster plan.
3. Be informed: get one's questions answered by learning from experts in disaster preparedness, including those at the CDC and the American Red Cross.

Additionally, psychiatrists and other mental health clinicians who want to become directly involved as responders in a future disaster should receive adequate training from a recognized source, such as the Red Cross, the American Medical Association, or a local university or medical center (American Red Cross 2010).

An important part of preparation is the development of a self-care plan. This secondary prevention plan has several components, including the following (Yassen 1995):

- *Physical*—Maintaining the health of one's body through adequate diet, exercise, sleep, and rest is critical.

- *Psychological*—One should attempt to achieve an overall balance of work, outside interests, recreation, meditation/spirituality, and personal time.
- *Social/interpersonal*—Connection with others is restorative and involves educating social contacts of one's needs. Working with a team is an effective strategy to ensure positive social contacts.
- *Balance*—In determining how much and what kind of disaster work to do, one needs to set and maintain appropriate and realistic boundaries.
- *Getting help when needed*—Help can take the form of peer support, supervision, or consultation; personal therapy can be of benefit during or after one's disaster work experience.

Caring for Staff

In addition to preparing care plans for oneself and one's family, a clinician is advised to take the time to prepare a care plan for his or her clinical work setting, be it an office, clinic, or hospital (Merlino 2010b). The development of policies and procedures to respond to such a crisis is best undertaken *before* a disaster strikes. Staff buy-in is important, and staff should take an active role in the development of a workplace disaster plan. The planners should take into account issues as diverse as reduced work hours, provision of cash advances, and provision of day care for the children of staff.

As leadership pays more attention to staff morale and development, there is a corresponding growth in the knowledge of the cost *to caregivers* of caring, as well as the increasingly important need to develop social and professional support networks, administrative structures, and policies to support those workers in the affected caregiving fields (Rudolph and Stamm 1999). The following case vignette illustrates one hospital's efforts to reduce stress felt by staff.

> The leadership of a major inner-city hospital noted that staff members were experiencing increasing stress as a result of multiple pressures. Unable to remove the stresses or to increase compensation because of them, management put together a "wellness program," in which the hospital's therapeutic rehabilitation staff (creative arts therapists) conducted meditation groups, drumming circles, and dance/movement exercises. The hope was that this program would aid in reducing stress while building teamwork and increasing morale.

Being Prepared

The literature shows that those who are educated and trained about disaster response perform better in the field, experience lower levels of stress, are likely to be more resilient, and are likely to grow psychologically in response to the stress of disaster experience (Merlino 2010a). Because no two disasters are the same, the particulars of each, including the type of disaster (e.g., natural disaster, bioterrorism, accident) and the geographic setting (e.g., nearby urban center, rural impoverished distant site), will demand different things from those responding. The Haiti earthquake response of 2010 highlights this point. Because of the tremendous need for outside assistance, many responders, including psychiatrists, traveled to the island of Haiti to offer aid. Some of the unique requirements to ensure the health and safety of responders to the Haitian earthquake are listed in Table 3–1.

Stress and Reactions to It

Even with the best preparation, disaster responders will experience emotional challenges. The American Medical Association newspaper ran a story about physicians' reflections on their volunteer disaster efforts in Haiti (O'Reilly 2010). When physicians arrived in Haiti, the enormity of the catastrophe and the never-ending stream of patients took most aback. Many physicians said they struggled to rein in their emotions when confronted with the tremendous medical demands there. One said, "It really was about maintaining my sanity…the need was greater than we could physically provide." Another reported needing to frequently step away to collect himself, recalling, "It was just overwhelming. You've never seen anything like that."

TABLE 3–1.   Requirements for responder safety after the Haiti earthquake

---

Vaccines: measles/mumps/rubella, diphtheria/pertussis/tetanus, polio, seasonal and H1N1 flu, varicella, hepatitis A and B, and typhoid

Protection against insect-borne diseases, including malaria and dengue

Protection against other infections, including HIV, tuberculosis, and anthrax

Safe food and drink (e.g., avoid tap water and ice cubes, use bottled water when brushing teeth)

Protections against insects and other animals (use insect repellent; prevent animal bites and scratches to avoid rabies; if bitten or scratched, use povidone-iodine solution such as Betadine)

Special care to avoid injury due to severe structural damage and electrocution from downed power lines

Awareness and avoidance of exposure to human remains and infection by diarrhea-causing bacteria

---

Source.   Adapted from Centers for Disease Control and Prevention 2010b.

As noted by the CDC, "As a first responder or relief worker, you may encounter extremely stressful situations, such as witnessing a tremendous loss of life, serious injuries, missing and separated families, and destruction of whole areas. It is important to recognize that these experiences may cause you psychological or emotional difficulties" (Centers for Disease Control and Prevention 2010a).

In training of emergency department (ED) workers, Disaster Psychiatry Outreach (2004) points out the following:

- Disasters will have an emotional impact on ED personnel, especially if their work involves a potential health threat to themselves.
- The emotional impact of disasters may influence the clarity of their knowledge and clinical decision making.
- ED personnel should be aware of the potential tension between their disaster relief work and their family.

As discussed in detail in Chapter 5, "Psychiatric Evaluation," normal reactions to trauma and major stress may involve physical, emotional, and behavioral symptoms (Victim Support Act 2007), such as the following:

- *Physical*—headache, loss of appetite, sleep impairment, and nausea
- *Emotional*—irritability, anxiety, anger, guilt, and fear
- *Behavioral*—withdrawal, emotional outbursts, unwillingness to leave scene until work is done, and denying need for rest

As research into the field of trauma response grows, it is increasingly apparent that the effects of a traumatic event go well beyond the victims who immediately and directly experience the event. As stated above in "Self-Awareness: Knowing One's Limits," two of the key skills of emotional intelligence are self-awareness and self-management (Bradberry and Greaves 2009). Responding psychiatrists and other clinicians must monitor themselves for the listed stress and trauma reactions, even though these responses are normal, because such awareness is important in deciding what changes, if any, need to be made in their self-care plans. Changes can be as straightforward as getting more rest or exercise or talking to someone whom one respects and who is known to be supportive.

Secondary traumatic stress, compassion fatigue, and vicarious victimization—three overlapping concepts—are potential adverse consequences of disaster relief work. Developing and practicing a self-care plan provides some protection against these outcomes but does not always prevent them. Secondary traumatic stress and secondary traumatic stress disorder are conceptualized by Figley (1995) as akin to primary traumatic stress (acute stress reaction) and primary traumatic stress disorder. The secondary trauma reactions are experienced by another (e.g., a significant other or someone providing care to a directly traumatized individual), whereas the primary reactions are directly experienced by the traumatized person. Secondary traumatic stress is also referred to as secondary victimization, vicarious traumatization, or emotional contagion (Miller et al. 1988). Vicarious traumatization encompasses a cluster of responses similar to those experienced by survivors who are directly traumatized. In contrast, *compassion fatigue* implies that the responder is physically and/or emotionally "exhausted" from the efforts given thus far. Nevertheless, the term *compassion fatigue* is the most palatable to those affected, a fact that highlights the altruism of compassion instead of the pathology-implying terms of *victim, trauma,* or *contagion* (Stamm 1999). Although there is not a lot of research to quantify secondary traumatization, empirically many disaster responders have seen and experienced it. Efforts should be made to avoid any implications that this phenomenon is equivalent to the much better defined and much more disabling phenomenon of posttraumatic stress disorder, also referred to as primary traumatic stress disorder (Stamm 1999).

Countertransference and burnout are overlapping concepts often used in describing secondary stress reactions. More specifically, *countertransference* is defined as the complex of feelings a psychotherapist has toward a patient and applies more generally to working with people with all kinds of problems, not specifically trauma-related incidents. *Burnout* is a syndrome of physical, emotional, or attitudinal exhaustion characterized by impaired work performance; fatigue; insomnia; depression; increased susceptibility to physical illness; reliance on alcohol or other drugs of abuse for temporary relief, with a tendency toward escalation into physiological dependency; and, in some cases, suicide. The syndrome is generally considered to be a stress reaction to unrelenting performance and emotional demands stemming from one's occupation (Campbell 2009). Research indicates that general practitioners have the highest rate of burnout. In contrast to burnout, which emerges gradually and is the result of emotional exhaustion, compassion stress or fatigue can emerge suddenly without warning. Secondary traumatic stress, in contrast with burnout, more frequently evidences feelings of helplessness, confusion, and isolation. Secondary traumatic stress also has a faster recovery time (Figley 1995). Table 3–2 lists some symptoms of compassion fatigue. According to Figley, compassion fatigue symptoms lasting less than 1 month are considered normal, acute, crisis-related reactions; symptoms lasting longer than 1 month qualify for the disorder; and symptom onset 6 or more months after the traumatic event is considered a delayed onset.

TABLE 3–2. **Symptoms of compassion fatigue**

Apathy, lowered self-esteem, preoccupation with trauma

Anxiety, guilt, numbing, anger, sadness, hypersensitivity

Impatience, irritability, hypervigilance, moodiness

Hopelessness, anger at God, loss of purpose

Sweating, rapid heartbeat, dizziness, aches and pains

Negativity, low morale, poor work performance, withdrawal

Substance abuse, relationship conflicts

Source. Figley 2002.

The suggested treatment for compassion fatigue involves counseling the individual to help him or her cope with the symptoms of the disorder and find solutions for moving forward that will help the person to be a better caregiver. Treatment programs generally involve group or individual counseling. The focus is on the individual and his or her needs, and treatment emphasizes that the caregiver is deserving of care and that his or her needs are valid and important. Individual expressive therapy, such as art, music, and movement, has also been found to be helpful in centering responders and facilitating the reclaiming of their emotional lives (Myers and Wee 2002).

Success in convincing disaster responders that they can and should avail themselves of mental health care can be aided by "depsychologizing" their symptoms by relating to the individuals in a "medicalized" manner, normalizing their signs and symptoms as much as possible, and focusing on function rather than feelings (Katz 2010). One such intervention utilizes blood pressure screening as a way of engaging individuals concerned about their medical well-being; a dialogue can then develop about appropriate diet and fluid intake, getting adequate rest, and so forth. It may even be possible to administer simple mental health screens such as the Patient Health Questionnaire–2 (Kroenke et al. 2003) to screen for depression and the CAGE (Ewing 1984) to assess possible alcohol abuse. Responders should be encouraged to follow specific recommendations for self-care at disaster sites (Table 3–3).

Returning Home

Sooner or later, responders to a disaster will return home. The CDC estimates that approximately one-third of aid workers will report depression shortly after arriving home; in addition, more than half have reported predominantly negative emotions once home (Centers for Disease Control and Prevention 2010b). Responders who experience depressive symptoms without relief after settling home should seek professional guidance to help readjust to postdisaster life. Those who do not feel physically well should consult their primary care physician to screen for possible infections that may have been acquired while away. The CDC has listed recommendations to assist responders once they return home (Table 3–4).

TABLE 3–3. Recommendations for self-care at the disaster site

---

Pace yourself.

Take frequent rest breaks away from the area.

Watch out for each other.

Maintain as normal a schedule as possible.

Drink plenty of fluids (water and juices) and eat a variety of foods.

Accept what you cannot change.

Allow yourself to feel badly.

Stay in contact with loved ones at home as much as possible.

Source.   Centers for Disease Control and Prevention 2001.

TABLE 3–4. Recommendations for self-care after returning home

---

Reach out to friends, neighbors, and colleagues.

Reconnect with family, community, and spiritual supports.

Do not make any major life-altering decisions at this time.

Make smaller decisions to regain a sense of control.

Consider keeping a journal.

Spend time with others.

Accept that you may feel fearful for your family initially.

Maintain a sense of humor.

Get plenty of rest and exercise.

Eat well-balanced meals.

Avoid excessive use of alcohol, sedatives, or sleep medications.

Remember that getting back to "normal" takes time.

Source.   Centers for Disease Control and Prevention 2001.

Conclusion

Despite the risks and precautions described in this chapter, volunteer responders can gain tremendous benefit from disaster work. Post and Neimark (2008) found that people who are generous with their time and talents live longer, healthier, and happier lives. As expressed by the National Mental Health Information Center (U.S. Department of Health and Human Services 2005, p. 17):

> Despite the inevitable stresses and challenges associated with community crisis response, workers experience personal gratification by using their skills and training to assist fellow humans in need. Active engagement in the disaster response and "doing" for others can be an antidote for feelings of vulnerability, powerlessness, and outrage commonly experienced by non-impacted community members. Witnessing the courage and resilience of the human spirit and the power of human kindness can have profound and lasting effects.

Therefore, the recommendation is not to *avoid* disaster response work but rather to undertake it with an adequate plan for self-care and with sufficient introspection to monitor for distress and dysfunction.

■ Teaching Points

- Self-care for responders is critical to their ability to care for others and to reduce the negative consequences some experience during and after disaster work.
- Those who have enormous capacity for feeling and expressing empathy tend to be more at risk of compassion fatigue or secondary traumatic stress disorder.
- Important in self-care are one's awareness of one's emotions and the effects of others' emotions on oneself.
- Mental health clinicians who want to become directly involved as responders in a future disaster should receive adequate training from a recognized source such as the Red Cross, the American Medical Association, or a local university or medical center.
- There is growing knowledge of the cost *to caregivers* of caring, as well as an increasingly important need to develop social and professional support networks, administrative structures, and policies to support those workers in the affected caregiving fields.

- Secondary traumatic stress, compassion fatigue, and vicarious victimization—three overlapping concepts—are potential adverse consequences of disaster relief work. The recommendation is not to *avoid* disaster response but rather to engage in it with an adequate plan for self-care.

Review Questions

3.1 Self-care...

A. Means that it is up to each person to keep him- or herself free of stress-related symptoms.
B. Means that one's awareness of one's own emotions is important.
C. Means that if stress-related symptoms do appear, it is the person's fault for not doing a good enough job.
D. Implies putting one's own needs above those of everyone else.
E. Is a sign of pathological narcissism.

3.2 Focusing on the workplace as a health-promoting environment is an example of

A. Primary prevention of stress-related problems.
B. Tertiary prevention of stress-related problems.
C. Secondary prevention of stress-related problems.
D. An inconsistency with the mission and values of health care.
E. Displacement from the trauma at hand.

3.3 One of the major skills that make up emotional intelligence is

A. Auto-awareness.
B. Social avoidance.
C. Self-management.
D. Abstracting ability.
E. Judgment.

3.4 The development of a self-care plan includes

A. A psychological component, requiring overall balance of work and outside interests.
B. Use of moderate amounts of alcohol to induce sleep.
C. Venting of anger whenever it is felt.
D. Scheduling an off-duty shift every 8 hours.
E. Negotiating a fair salary for one's disaster work.

3.5   The CDC has made the following recommendations for self-care at the disaster site:

    A.   Push yourself.
    B.   Watch out for each other.
    C.   Resist experiencing bad feelings.
    D.   Be careful not to overconsume food and water.
    E.   All of the above.

3.6   After responders return home, the CDC recommends which of the following?

    A.   Reach out to friends, neighbors, and colleagues.
    B.   Consider making major life-altering decisions.
    C.   Utilize all remaining sick and vacation time at work to de-stress.
    D.   Consider early retirement.
    E.   Advocate for a salary increase based on one's new skills.

3.7   Symptoms of compassion fatigue include which of the following?

    A.   Apathy and low morale.
    B.   Delusional religiosity.
    C.   Inappropriate levity.
    D.   Psychotic rage.
    E.   Memory gaps.

References

American Red Cross: Take a Red Cross Course. Washington, DC, American Red Cross, 2010. Available at: http://www.redcross.org/flash/course01v01. Accessed December 26, 2010.

Anonymous: Why I didn't go to Haiti. The Central Line, January 24, 2010. Available at: http://thecentralline.org/?p=1080. Accessed April 24, 2010.

Bradberry T, Greaves J: Emotional Intelligence 2.0. New York, TalentSmart Publishers, 2009

Campbell RJ: Campbell's Psychiatric Dictionary, 9th Edition. New York, Oxford University Press, 2009

Centers for Disease Control and Prevention: Traumatic Incident Stress: Information for Emergency Response Workers. Atlanta, GA, Centers for Disease Control and Prevention, 2001. Available at: http://www.cepis.ops-oms.org/bvsacd/cd49/traumatic.pdf. Accessed April 24, 2010.

Centers for Disease Control and Prevention: Emergency Preparedness and Response: Coping With a Disaster or Traumatic Event. Atlanta, GA, Centers for Disease Control and Prevention, 2010a. Available at: http://www.bt.cdc.gov/mentalhealth. Accessed December 26, 2010.

Centers for Disease Control and Prevention: Guidance for Haiti Earthquake Response and Relief Workers. Atlanta, GA, Centers for Disease Control and Prevention, 2010b. Available at: http://wwwnc.cdc.gov/travel/content/news-announcements/relief-workers-haiti.aspx. Accessed December 26, 2010.

Disaster Psychiatry Outreach: Mental Health Consequences of Bioterrorism: A Disaster Preparedness Course for Hospital Emergency Department Staff. New York, Disaster Psychiatry Outreach, 2004. Available at: http://www.disasterpsych.org/home. Accessed April 25, 2010.

Ewing JA: Detecting alcoholism: the CAGE questionnaire. JAMA 252:1905–1907, 1984

Figley CR: Compassion fatigue as secondary stress disorder: an overview, in Compassion Fatigue: Coping With Secondary Traumatic Stress Disorder in Those Who Treat the Traumatized (Routledge Psychosocial Stress Series). Edited by Figley CR. New York, Routledge, 1995, pp 1–20

Figley CR (ed): Treating Compassion Fatigue (Routledge Psychosocial Stress Series). New York, Routledge, 2002

Gabbard GO: The role of compulsiveness in the normal physician. JAMA 254:2926–2929, 1985

Goleman D: Working With Emotional Intelligence. New York, Bantam Books, 1998

Goleman D: Leadership that gets results. Harvard Business Review (March–April):2–16, 2000

Katz CL: Understanding and helping responders, in Hidden Impact: What You Need to Know for the Next Disaster. A Practical Mental Health Guide for Clinicians. Edited by Stoddard FJ, Katz CL, Merlino JP. Sudbury, MA, Jones & Bartlett, 2010, pp 123–130

Kroenke K, Spitzer RL, Williams JB: The Patient Health Questionnaire–2: validity of a two-item depression screener. Med Care 41:1284–1292, 2003

Lacey M: Estimates of quake damage in Haiti increase by billions. New York Times, February 16, 2010, p. A6

Merlino JP: The other ground zero, in Disaster Psychiatry. Edited by Pandya A, Katz CL. Hillsdale, NJ, Analytic Press, 2004

Merlino JP: Self-care, in Hidden Impact: What You Need to Know for the Next Disaster. A Practical Mental Health Guide for Clinicians. Edited by Stoddard FJ, Katz CL, Merlino JP. Sudbury, MA, Jones & Bartlett, 2010a, pp 19–26

Merlino JP: Staff support, in Hidden Impact: What You Need to Know for the Next Disaster. A Practical Mental Health Guide for Clinicians. Edited by Stoddard FJ, Katz CL, Merlino JP. Sudbury, MA, Jones & Bartlett, 2010b, pp 171–178

Miller KI, Stiff JB, Ellis BH: Communication and empathy as precursors to burnout among human service workers. Commun Monogr 55:336–341, 1988

Mitchell JT, Bray GP: Emergency Services Stress: Guidelines for Preserving the Health and Careers of Emergency Services Personnel (Continuing Education Series). Upper Saddle River, NJ, Prentice Hall, 1990

Myers D, Wee DF: Strategies for managing disaster mental health worker stress, in Treating Compassion Fatigue (Routledge Psychosocial Stress Series). Edited by Figley CR. New York, Routledge, 2002, pp 181–212

O'Reilly KB: Helping Haiti: U.S. doctors reflect on crisis care experiences. American Medical News. February 15, 2010. Available at: http://www.ama-assn.org/amednews/2010/02/15/prl20215.htm. Accessed April 24, 2010

Post S, Neimark J: Why Good Things Happen to Good People. New York, Broadway Books, 2008

Rudolph JM, Stamm BH: Maximizing human capital: moderating secondary traumatic stress through administrative and policy action, in Secondary Traumatic Stress: Self-Care Issues for Clinicians, Researchers, and Educators, 2nd Edition. Edited by Stamm BH. Lutherville, MD, Sidran Press, 1999, pp 277–278

Stamm BH (ed): Secondary Traumatic Stress: Self-Care Issues for Clinicians, Researchers, and Educators, 2nd Edition. Lutherville, MD, Sidran Press, 1999

U.S. Department of Health and Human Services: Mental Health Response to Mass Violence and Terrorism: A Training Manual (DHHS Publ No SMA 4025). Washington, DC, U.S. Department of Health and Human Services, 2005

Victim Support Act, 2007. Available at: http://www.victimsupport.act.gov.au/res/File/normal%20reactions%20final%20final%20final.pdf. Accessed October 15, 2010.

Wagner SL, Martin CA, McFee JA: Investigating the "rescue personality." Traumatology 15:5–12, 2009

Yassen J: Preventing secondary stress disorder, in Compassion Fatigue: Coping With Secondary Traumatic Stress Disorder in Those Who Treat the Traumatized (Routledge Psychosocial Stress Series). Edited by Figley CR. New York, Routledge, 1995, pp 178–208

Needs Assessment

Craig L. Katz, M.D.

An assessment team consisting of two experienced disaster psychiatrists arrived in Sri Lanka just 1 month after the 2004 tsunami. Their intent was to partner with chapters of Rotary International to create a system of lay trauma counseling around the city of Colombo that would be staffed by Rotarians. However, multiple attempts to coordinate this plan with the Sri Lankan Ministry of Health failed because the government insisted it did not need outside help. Deciding it would be nearly impossible to obtain a large enough assessment of the disaster-related mental health needs of the region without the government's assistance, the assessment team decided to narrow its focus. They met with the head of a trauma counseling program in northeastern Sri Lanka that predated the tsunami and learned of their need to have their staff better trained in cognitive-behavioral psychotherapy and in working with traumatized children. They then focused their assessment and planning efforts on gauging the extent of this need and getting to know the program, its staff and patients, and the surrounding community.

If disaster constitutes a community-level trauma, then in many respects the disaster psychiatrist's "patient" is the community. Psychiatric care ultimately occurs at the level of individual disaster survivors, but disaster-related ministrations begin with the recognition that a community has been stricken. A cascade of activities eventually delivers the psychiatrist into the familiar details of an individual encounter with a patient. This cascade may unfold in both planned and unplanned ways, but disaster psychiatrists can be most effectively deployed when their response path begins with a community-level needs assessment.

Information gathering is the first step of planning any disaster psychiatric response (Disaster Psychiatry Outreach 2006). If the community is the patient, then it makes sense that any intervention begins with an evaluation of the community. In this chapter, I describe the type of information to be gathered in a needs assessment, review what existing disaster psychiatry response guidelines say about how to gather the information, and discuss the practical considerations involved in conducting a needs assessment.

This detailed consideration of the disaster psychiatry needs assessment will be of assistance to psychiatrists or other mental health professionals who will be involved in planning and conducting such an assessment and to administrators who are charged with translating the information that is gathered into subsequent clinical work. An understanding of the needs assessment is just as critical, however, for the clinically oriented disaster psychiatrist. As discussed in Chapter 1, "Preparation and Systems Issues," to maximize their impact, disaster psychiatrists should work as part of an organized and coordinated effort rather than strike out on their own. Before they are deployed on behalf of such an effort, however, they can be assured that it is indeed organized and coordinated by ascertaining the extent to which the response is founded on a needs assessment. Reliance on a needs assessment establishes a minimal level of credibility for a disaster psychiatric mission. Also, once in the field, clinicians can function more comfortably and confidently amid chaotic and fluid circumstances if they are able to refer to a written needs assessment to orient, and periodically reorient, themselves to the rationale for their designated role.

Figure 4–1 outlines the flow of the disaster psychiatry needs assessment and can serve as a guide for the detailed material to be discussed in this chapter. In reviewing this flowchart, the disaster psychiatrist can see that systems-level needs assessment and planning is integral to all phases of the response. The midline arrows create a visual sense of what the needs assessment truly is—the backbone of all phases of disaster response. Whether involved in information gathering and logistical planning, a needs assessment mission, or a clinical deployment, the disaster psychiatrist will either be working toward or from a needs assessment.

Information Relevant to a Disaster Psychiatric Response

Disaster psychiatrists require two broad areas of knowledge to effectively respond to a disaster. First, they need education, training, and, wherever possible, experience in clinical aspects of disaster psychiatry. Then, in the event of a disaster, they will fold their clinical knowledge into information specific to that event. Three essential categories of information about a given disaster are relevant to launching a disaster psychiatry response (Disaster Psychiatry Outreach 2006): 1) basic facts of the general disaster type, including relevant science as well as extant knowledge about its psychiatric

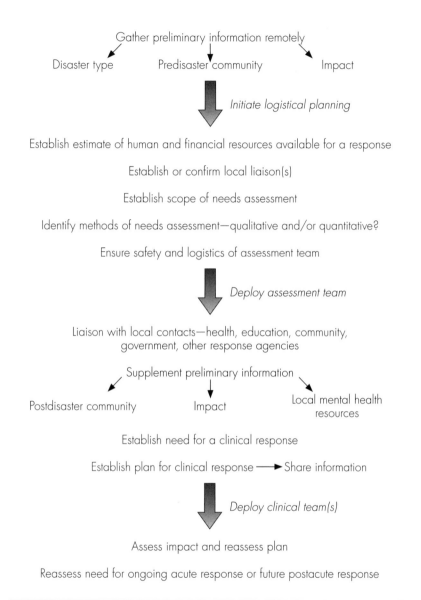

FIGURE 4–1.   Flowchart for conducting a disaster psychiatry needs assessment.

aspects; 2) information about the impact on the community; and 3) background information about the predisaster community.

Disaster Type

It is not clear whether types of disasters—considered broadly as human made versus natural or in more specific terms such as earthquakes versus aviation disasters—can be linked to particular types or extent of psychopathology (Disaster Psychiatry Outreach 2008). Common wisdom suggests that human-made events cause more psychiatric problems than do natural disasters, although careful review of the literature and clinical experience call this reasoning into question (Garakani et al. 2004). The disaster psychiatrist should therefore not approach any given disaster with a fixed preconception about whether it is likely be more or less distressing than other disasters, especially because a complex range of factors bear on this matter.

What is evident is that various types of disasters may engender very different reactions and concerns among survivors. For example, earthquakes involve a literal shake-up of one's entire world and raise such concerns as the unpredictability of nature, persistence through aftershocks, and even anger about man's role in assuring structural safety. Being armed with this information can help psychiatrists to anticipate what will be on people's minds.

Having this type of information is especially important when considering nuclear, biological, or chemical terrorist events, which will be unfamiliar to most survivors and responders because of their rarity (Disaster Psychiatry Outreach 2004). Biological terrorism may raise fears about an unseen, invisible agent. The invisibility of the agent may make it difficult to delineate a circumscribed disaster "site." Individuals may demonstrate a range of reactions to the need for quarantine or isolation. As was seen in the 1995 sarin gas attacks in the Tokyo subway, chemical events can engender large numbers of psychosomatic responses because the agents may cause physical reactions similar to anxiety responses (Kawana 2001). In nuclear attacks, concerns will arise regarding long-term consequences of exposure (e.g., birth defects), social stigma among the exposed, and the decontamination process (Disaster Psychiatry Outreach 2004).

In addition to the psychological themes common to a given disaster type, psychiatrists should have general information about the disaster for two reasons. First, they need to understand the areas of potential concern for their own involvement. For example, during the 2001 anthrax scare in New York City, psychiatrists were invited to assist staff at the headquarters of two television networks that were affected. Information on the spread of anthrax was obtained to reassure volunteer psychiatrists that it was safe to meet with potentially exposed staff because human-to-human spread does not occur.

Second, knowledge about disasters permits psychiatrists to be more effective mental health professionals. This is akin to the situation of consultation-liaison psychiatrists who, to be truly helpful, must understand the medical problems of the patients for whom they provide consultation. Excellent disaster preparedness fact sheets are available at the Web sites of the American Red Cross (www.redcross.org) and the Federal Emergency Management Agency (www.fema.gov).

Disaster psychiatrists can assess and assist with anxiety and fear only if they understand what should be fearsome. This is demonstrated in the following vignette.

> A team of American psychiatrists traveled to El Salvador in 2001 following a major earthquake. While working with survivors in a rural part of the country, they were confronted with frequent insomnia in the patients they saw. When they offered to provide short-term sleep medication from a supply they had brought, Salvadorans repeatedly refused, citing the need to be alert in case of a significant aftershock in the middle of the night. The psychiatrists decided to better educate themselves about basic earthquake safety and learned that people are advised to evacuate a structure or at least stand under a door frame in the event of a tremor. They then decided to lead group drills in how to respond to a tremor, practicing evacuations. This intervention seemed to have a calming effect on participants without the need to prescribe what could realistically have been overly sedating medication.

Disaster Impact

Having general information about a category of disaster can inform the types of questions the disaster psychiatrist ought to ask before responding to a specific occurrence. The particulars of an event supplement the broad outline of the facts. This category of information again pertains to personal safety and logistical issues, which need to be addressed before deciding to deploy. The first rule of disaster psychiatry dictates that psychiatrists should not expose themselves to excessive risk to their own safety or well-being.

Relevant information is best obtained via situation reports generated by disaster response agencies. Disaster psychiatrists who work within the disaster response system and in collaboration with emergency management agencies and other responders will have access to these reports, which provide regular updates on all facets of an event, sometimes several times per day during the acute phase. In the example of an intentional anthrax exposure via aerosolization, a situation report should provide information regarding where the exposure was found to have occurred or at least what areas public health authorities believe to be free of the agent or are working to sterilize. Logistical information can also be obtained in this manner, shaping how disaster psychiatrists can travel to the affected area and where they may work, remain in communication, and, if relevant, safely live.

Beyond providing safety and logistical information, detailed data about a disaster can also shape when it makes clinical sense to deploy. When the environment has not stabilized sufficiently to reduce some of the immediate stresses placed on survivors, the role of the psychiatrist is limited. When the stresses are too high, emphasis should be placed on resources that can reduce the intensity of the stresses rather than on assisting people with coping. As discussed in Chapter 12, "Psychological First Aid," meeting survivors' basic needs for safety and comfort is an essential early intervention that has physical and psychological benefit. In simple terms, peoples' feelings will be based on a wound needing medical attention, an empty stomach, or uncertainty regarding where they will sleep at night. During this acute phase, the psychiatrist should expect to function more as a humanitarian or physician than as a traditional psychiatrist.

Finally, determination of the magnitude of the mental health impact of a disaster lies at the core of the information needed by the disaster psychiatrist. This may involve a community-level assessment of symptoms or behavioral changes during the acute phase and of disorders during the postacute phase. This information helps to guide the size of an eventual clinical program.

Predisaster Community

The third pillar of information consists of background facts about the stricken community. Gathering information about the community's political, social, economic, and cultural history is comparable to obtaining a complete psychosocial history from an individual patient. The impact of an event on a community cannot be fully gauged without knowing about the strength and vitality that preceded it. As discussed in Chapter 5, "Psychiatric Evaluation," it is well established that preexisting psychosocial problems predispose a disaster survivor to a psychopathological reaction (Disaster Psychiatry Outreach 2008). If the problems are great before an event, it is to be expected that the risk will be worse afterward.

Knowledge about the predisaster community not only helps predict needs but also provides context for how the disaster psychiatrist will function. Working in an environment where there was a robust public health and mental health system before a disaster is entirely different from working in a situation where this was lacking. The difference influences the possibility of collaborations in the field and the ultimate goals of a disaster psychiatry mission: Will the disaster psychiatrists be able to partner with local mental health professionals, other health professionals, or others such as spiritual care providers or teachers? Will their goal be to help restore or supplement a previously functioning system of psychiatric care, or are they faced with the more daunting challenge of effectively having to create such a system?

The World Health Organization (WHO), an agency of the United Nations (UN) has created an instrument for establishing the nature and details of a local mental health system, the Assessment Instrument for Mental Health Systems (WHO-AIMS; World Health Organization 2005). This instrument has 156 items to be assessed across six different domains: legislative and policy framework; mental health services; mental health in primary care; human resources; public education and links with other sectors; and monitoring and research. The results provide a comprehensive picture of a local mental health system. The WHO-AIMS offers guidance with identifying sources of data for establishing these items, and WHO will even provide an Excel database into which these data can be entered and guidance for writing a summary report of the data.

Importantly, the purpose of the WHO-AIMS is to collect information with which to improve the mental health systems of countries or regions. It was not designed for use in the setting of disaster, where the aim would be to either restore or build a mental health system, and its breadth and depth might suggest why. Nonetheless, it is valuable for several reasons. First, it presents a framework for the kind of information the disaster psychiatrist would ideally have available when planning and implementing a disaster response. Second, the WHO-AIMS is available in a brief form (Table 4–1) that can be more practically completed in the pressurized disaster environment. Finally, WHO publishes findings from those countries it has surveyed with the WHO-AIMS, providing an invaluable platform from which the disaster psychiatrist can work (World Health Organization 2009). This information is currently available for 42 countries.

Disaster Psychiatry Guidelines

A number of authoritative guidelines have been published that provide varying levels of detail about how to provide psychiatric, or what tends to be called psychosocial, care in the disaster setting. These are wide-ranging documents meant to address all facets of care. I review them from the perspective of conducting a needs assessment.

TABLE 4–1.   Brief Version of Items for WHO-AIMS 2.2

Item code	Item title
B1–1.1.1	Last version of mental health policy
B2–1.1.3	Psychotropic medicines included on the essential medicines list
B3–1.2.1	Last version of the mental health plan
B4–1.3.1	Last version of mental health legislation
B5–1.4.2	Inspecting human rights in mental hospitals
B6–1.5.1	Mental health expenditures by the government health department
B7–1.5.2	Expenditures on mental hospitals
B8–1.5.4	Free access to essential psychotropic medicines
B9–2.1.1	Existence and functions of a national or regional "mental health authority"
B10–2.1.2	Organization of mental health services in terms of catchment areas/service areas
B11–2.2.1	Availability of mental health outpatient facilities
B12–2.2.2	Users treated through mental health outpatient facilities
B13–2.2.6	Children and adolescents treated through mental health outpatient facilities
B14–2.3.2	Users treated in day treatment facilities
B15–2.4.1	Availability of community-based psychiatric inpatient units
B16–2.4.2	Beds in community-based psychiatric inpatient units
B17–2.4.6	Time spent in community-based psychiatric inpatient units per discharge
B18–2.5.2	Beds/places in community residential facilities
B19–2.6.2	Availability of mental hospital beds
B20–2.6.3	Change in beds in mental hospitals
B21–2.6.6	Involuntary admissions to mental hospitals
B22–2.6.7	Long-stay patients in mental hospitals
B23–2.6.10	Physical restraint and seclusion in mental hospitals
B24–2.7.3	Long-stay patients in forensic units
B25–2.8.2	Number of beds/places in other residential facilities
B26–2.9.1	Availability of psychosocial interventions in mental hospitals
B27–2.9.3	Availability of psychosocial interventions in mental health outpatient facilities
B28–2.10.1	Availability of medicines in mental hospitals
B29–2.10.3	Availability of medicines in mental health outpatient facilities
B30–2.11.1	Psychiatry beds located in or near the largest city

TABLE 4–1. Brief Version of Items for WHO-AIMS 2.2 *(continued)*

Item code	Item title
B31–3.1.2	Refresher training programmes for primary health care doctors
B32–3.1.5	Interaction of primary health care doctors with mental health services
B33–3.1.7	Availability of medicines to primary health care patients in physician-based primary health care
B34–3.2.3	Refresher training programmes for primary health care nurses
B35–3.2.4	Refresher training programmes for nondoctor/nonnurse primary health care workers
B36–3.2.6	Mental health referrals between non-physician based primary health care to a higher level of care
B37–3.3.3	Interaction of mental health facilities with complementary/alternative/traditional practitioners
B38–4.1.1	Human resources in mental health facilities per capita
B39–4.1.4	Staff working in or for mental health outpatient facilities
B40–4.1.5	Staff working in community-based psychiatric inpatient units
B41–4.1.6	Staff working in mental hospitals
B42–4.2.2	Refresher training for mental health staff on the rational use of psychotropic drugs
B43–4.2.3	Refresher training for mental health staff in psychosocial (nonbiological) interventions
B44–4.4.1	User/consumer associations and mental health policies, plans or legislation
B45–4.4.2	Family associations involvement in mental health policies, plans or legislation
B46–4.4.8	Other nongovernmental organizations involved in community and individual assistance activities
B47–5.1.4	Professional groups targeted by specific education and awareness campaigns on mental health
B48–5.3.1	Provision of employment for people with serious mental disorders
B49–5.3.2	Primary and secondary schools with mental health professionals
B50–5.3.8	Mental health care of prisoners
B51–5.3.9	Social welfare benefits
B52–6.1.5	Data transmission from mental health facilities
B53–6.1.6	Report on mental health services by government health department
B54–6.2.2	Proportion of health research that is on mental health

Source. Reprinted from Brief Version of Items for WHO-AIMS 2.2, in World Health Organization Assessment Instrument for Mental Health Systems, Version 2.2 (WHO-AIMS 2.2), pp. 58–59. Geneva, Switzerland, World Health Organization, 2005. Used with permission.

Inter-Agency Standing Committee Guidelines

The Inter-Agency Standing Committee (IASC) was established in 1992 by the UN to coordinate the efforts and expertise of various UN and nongovernmental agencies involved in humanitarian assistance. In 2007, the IASC's Task Force on Mental Health and Psychosocial Support in Emergency Settings developed guidelines to help response agencies to "plan, establish and coordinate a set of minimum multisectoral responses to protect and improve people's mental health and psychosocial well-being in the midst of an emergency" (Inter-Agency Standing Committee 2007, p. 3). These guidelines delineate 11 major areas of intervention and describe minimal and comprehensive levels of response for each. One of these domains consists of assessment, monitoring, and evaluation.

The IASC guidelines specify six different types of information to be collected as part of a needs assessment (Table 4–2), and these are essentially an amplification of the three types of assessment information discussed in the previous section, "Information Relevant to a Disaster Psychiatric Response." Some important points are made in the guidelines concerning conducting of an assessment. First, the assessment determines not only how a response should look but also whether it is needed at all. A desire to help can sometimes erroneously translate into an assumption that psychiatric help is needed and perhaps even that help of a certain kind is needed. Although some form of postdisaster mental health assistance can be reasonably assumed necessary, by virtue of either heightened need or limited resources, there is a risk in assuming that a particular type of disaster psychiatric service offered by a response agency is needed.

Another point made in the IASC guidelines is that assessment needs to be done in a collaborative fashion with local stakeholders, governments, communities, and other relief agencies. Mental health responders coming from outside a stricken community should neither act nor appear to act as though they are expert diagnosticians who can paternalistically ascertain the local mental health needs. Deference should be given to local health providers and, where available, mental health agencies or providers. Deference should also extend to other local groups, such as educators and religious leaders. Responders should respect, as much as possible, when help may be needed but is not wanted or welcomed.

A third and related suggestion in the IASC guidelines is that needs assessments should be shared. Ideally, these needs assessments would be shared with a disaster psychiatry coordinating body that oversees mental health efforts in a disaster setting. This means that given the humanitarian implications of the situation, agencies should not try to maintain their assessments as proprietary. It also means that any given disaster psychiatry re-

TABLE 4–2. Inter-Agency Standing Committee Guidelines on Mental Health and Psychosocial Support in Emergency Settings: categories of information for assessment

Relevant demographic and contextual information

Experience of the emergency

Mental health and psychosocial problems

Existing sources of psychosocial well-being and mental health

Organizational capacities and activities

Programming needs and opportunities

Source. Inter-Agency Standing Committee 2007.

sponse team should research whether a mental health needs assessment has already been done and disseminated before launching into an assessment. Further assessment may not need to be done or perhaps could be done in a focused fashion.

Finally, the IASC recommends that a "rapid" assessment be completed within 1–2 weeks of a disaster, focusing on the experience of survivors. A more comprehensive evaluation of all six domains of information listed in Table 4–2 would follow later. This stepwise approach appears reasonable but may be overly optimistic. It may be problematic in at least two regards. First, limited disaster psychiatry resources may render it difficult to launch a response within 1–2 weeks. During this time, a more reasonable approach might be to research historical background on the affected community, much of which can be done prior to travel to the affected community. Second, mental health needs are likely to be especially fluid in the early days and weeks after a disaster, such that an evaluation done in the first 1–2 weeks may become rapidly outdated. Monitoring such shifts and targeting mental health resources appropriately may not be possible with limited resources, and a more pragmatic approach might be to conduct an initial assessment after several weeks to a month or more, when the initial stresses of impact have subsided and postdisaster life has assumed a relative rhythm.

World Health Organization Guidelines

In 2001, WHO released the Rapid Assessment of Mental Health Needs of Refugees, Displaced and Other Populations Affected by Conflict and Post-Conflict Situations (RAMH), which includes specific assessment guidelines for use in conflict or complex humanitarian emergencies triggered by conflict (World Health Organization 2001). Although focused on conflict situations, this tool may be tailored for assessing needs in any catastrophic situation. Similar to the IASC guidelines, the RAMH emphasizes collecting information across seven areas: information about the conflict; description of the affected populations; mental health needs; cultural, religious, socioeconomic, and political aspects of the affected communities; cultural responses to trauma; mental health resources; and recommendations. The RAMH includes a six-page tool that specifies the information to be collected within each of these seven domains. Unlike the IASC guidelines' focus on the initial 1–2 weeks, the RAMH suggests that an assessment be done once basic survival needs are addressed.

The RAMH's recommendations are more operationalized than the IASC guidelines. For example, the RAMH specifies the composition of the RAMH team. It suggests that the team be multidisciplinary, consisting of at least one mental health professional and both local and international members. Experts in crisis situations and refugee mental health are deemed essential. Of note, the RAMH allows for and even expects the inclusion of non–mental health professionals who can be trained as evaluators. This expectation arises from the reality that many situations lack sufficient mental health professionals but also suggests that even when more resources are available, psychiatrists may not need to be the evaluators of the affected community. This reflects a departure from how American psychiatrists usually expect to directly assess their "patients."

The RAMH also underscores that one or more agencies must invite the assessment. Although WHO may recommend the assessment, a government, another UN agency, a nongovernmental organization, or a funding source also may request it. This point highlights that disaster psychiatrists ought not to just show up and embark on assessing a situation for logistical, political, financial, and even clinical reasons. The information will have a much greater impact if it is collected collaboratively.

The RAMH also lays out three broad sources of information for the needs assessment. The RAMH team should contact *central and regional authorities,* which include ministries of health, education, and social welfare; *representatives of agencies, associations, services, and universities,* which span UN agencies in the affected country, nongovernmental organizations, churches, and even youth associations; and *intersectoral sectors,* which include health care providers, existing mental health care providers, teachers and professors, and law enforcement representatives. In the chaos of post-conflict or other disasters, having access to a list of potential contacts from each of these three categories can render a needs assessment much more organized and efficient.

Although the RAMH was developed in pilot form in 2001, information on its implementation and evaluation does not yet appear to be available.

Its authors indicated a plan to develop a subsequent Comprehensive Assessment of Mental Health, but this also does not yet appear to be available.

Disaster Psychiatry Outreach Guidelines

Tables 4–3 and 4–4 represent a suggested composite of information that should be gathered in any disaster psychiatry needs assessment (Disaster Psychiatry Outreach 2007). They are the product of both literature review and the clinical experience of Disaster Psychiatry Outreach. These templates highlight critical elements of the circumstances and the needs of affected populations. Although much less exhaustive than the WHO-AIMS, the IASC guidelines, or the RAMH guidelines, these guidelines are proposed as realistic and concise enough for most disaster mental health needs assessments.

Practical Considerations

In the remainder of this chapter, I focus on practical concerns in undertaking a needs assessment. The ranges of possible circumstances, disasters, and even resources render it difficult to lay out a "one-size-fits-all" approach to assessment. However, a number of issues apply across most possibilities.

Perhaps the foremost consideration in shaping a needs assessment is one of scope, which can be looked at in terms of time and space. Regarding time, does the eventual disaster psychiatry mission that will grow from an assessment have as its focus the acute or longer-term, postacute period (Disaster Psychiatry Outreach 2008)? To some degree the answer to this question lies in the ambitions or resources of the response agency. It is certainly easier to focus on the acute period, both in terms of information needed and eventual resources. On the other hand, there are circumstances that require a longer-term commitment, particularly international responses where building of partnerships with local counterparts is essential but labor intensive (Silove and Bryant 2006).

On the matter of space, disaster psychiatry planning requires consideration of the possible breadth of the efforts and the potential size of the mental health footprint. The "patient" requires identification. Will the needs of an entire country or region be the concern, or will the focus be much narrower, even limited to assisting one institution? For example, Calderon-Abbo (2008) described the efforts to reopen and even expand the inpatient mental health services offered by several New Orleans hospitals following Hurricane Katrina. Conceivably, a disaster psychiatry mission could meaningfully choose to focus on revitalizing and staffing the inpatient psychiatric services of just one hospital. The assessment around which this effort would

TABLE 4–3.   Assessment items regarding the relevant circumstances of a stricken community, according to time period

Assessment item	Predisaster	Acute disaster	Postacute disaster
Living conditions			
Travel			
Communication			
Government			
Educational system			
Emergency system			
Public health system			
Mental health system			
Religion			
Economy			

Source.   Disaster Psychiatry Outreach 2007.

be built would then be largely confined within the walls of the hospital, albeit informed by the potential demand from without. In the opening vignette of this chapter about Sri Lanka, the assessment team narrowed its focus to the counseling center that predated the tsunami in northeastern Sri Lanka.

The techniques of assessment can vary as well. Will the assessment or scouting team be conducting a scientifically rigorous study of mental health needs or relying more on an observational approach to assessment? Epidemiological studies of postdisaster mental health needs abound in the literature and have examined the mental health effects of an oil spill (Palinkas et al. 1993), maritime accidents (Lindal and Stefansson 2011), and Hurricane Katrina (Kessler et al. 2006). However, these studies take enormous planning and oversight due to the practical, ethical, and scientific challenges of working in a postdisaster environment (North et al. 2002). The immediacy of needing to forecast disaster-related needs and services may not afford the luxury of time required to address these challenges. Publication-quality scientific rigor may not be possible or necessary when clinical and service needs beckon.

Therefore, typically a disaster psychiatry assessment team relies on liaison with local professionals and community leaders, as well as its own clinical impressions, to assess need. For example, Humayun (2008) described a team consisting of a psychiatrist and three trainees that worked for 3 weeks at a 650-bed hospital following the 2005 Pakistan earthquake; the team

TABLE 4–4. Assessment items regarding the needs of specific populations, according to time period

Assessment item	Survivors	Bereaved	Responders	Economically impacted	Community at large
Acute disaster					
Safety needs					
Physical needs					
Medical needs					
Mental health needs					
Postacute disaster					
Safety needs					
Physical needs					
Medical needs					
Mental health needs					

Source.   Disaster Psychiatry Outreach 2007.

used clinical work as the medium for assessing need while ministering to what were deemed to be high-risk patients. There are many similar examples of several-person assessment teams that rely on what is essentially qualitative data gathering done amid clinical work (e.g., Choudhury et al. 2006; Math et al. 2006).

Even if needs assessments are unlikely to be epidemiological in quality, they do not need to rely solely on clinical impressions. Screening and assessment tools can be used to improve diagnostic accuracy, while also permitting reliance on non–mental health professionals to administer them in an effort to capture a larger sample (Connor et al. 2006). This practice requires identifying the posttraumatic mental health problems of interest, often posttraumatic stress disorder (PTSD), and selecting the proper instrument. The following vignette demonstrates such an effort.

> An assessment team of three psychiatrists who traveled to postearthquake El Salvador in 2001 took with them a self-report questionnaire about PTSD. They encountered a 6,000-tent camp of displaced Salvadorans. Although a mental health tent had been set up by another nongovernmental organization, few people were coming to the tent, and camp leaders expressed concern that there was considerable unidentified mental suffering in their camp. The psychiatrists decided to distribute the PTSD survey among camp residents but quickly realized that many people were not literate enough to read the survey. They proceeded to administer the survey themselves, only to find that this procedure was too time consuming. The psychiatrists then enlisted the help of a local school of social work and trained the students in how to administer the survey. Survey information from the hundreds of residents was then turned over to camp officials so that they could establish better resources.

One final consideration in conducting a disaster psychiatry needs assessment involves the resources available for responding. Researchers have calculated that providing full mental health services to populations affected by Hurricanes Katrina and Rita for up to 30 months after the disasters would have cost $1,133 per capita or $12.5 billion for the affected population (Schoenbaum et al. 2009). This estimate may indicate a scope far larger than most disaster psychiatry responses intend to assume, but it does lend some perspective to the magnitude of resources potentially needed to "do things right." This consideration is especially important because the IASC guidelines are explicit in discouraging, on ethical grounds, the collection of information that will not be used toward future services (Inter-Agency Standing Committee 2007). Ultimately, the information gathering should be proportionate to the capacity for future services.

Conclusion

Systems-level assessment lays the groundwork for an effective clinical response by disaster psychiatrists, enabling them to render maximal assistance without contributing to the chaos of the situation. In the inevitable rush to help a disaster-stricken community, psychiatrists can apply the principles of their usual practice by first assessing the "patient" or community before launching into interventions. A collaborative and methodical approach to systems-level assessment will yield the most useful information, especially when such an approach is guided by awareness of the potential resources and scope of the eventual clinical response.

■ Teaching Points

- Planning for a disaster psychiatry response requires both general and specific information about the disaster, as well as information about the predisaster community.

- Having general, nonpsychiatric information about disaster types will inform clinical work, just as knowing about medical problems informs consultation-liaison work.

- Knowing the likely impact of a specific disaster is helpful in planning for safe and timely deployment of a disaster psychiatry team.

- Learning about the predisaster community is akin to learning about the psychosocial history of an individual patient.

- A number of operational guidelines for disaster psychiatry are available that address various elements of how to conduct a needs assessment.

- Practical issues related to conducting a needs assessment include determining the scope of information needed, deciding on the scientific rigor of the information collection, and matching the assessment to available resources.

Review Questions

4.1 In deploying psychiatrists to assist after disaster,

   A. The urgency of the crisis often obviates the need to conduct a needs assessment.
   B. A needs assessment is not relevant during the acute phase.
   C. Needs should be reassessed as the situation evolves.

    D. Full scientific rigor is required for a needs assessment to be considered valid.

    E. All of the above.

4.2   Information essential to a disaster psychiatry needs assessment includes all of the following *except*

    A. General information about the type of disaster.

    B. Information about mental health dimensions of a given type of disaster.

    C. Knowledge about life in the community before the event.

    D. Specific information about the impact of the event.

    E. Structured mental health interviews of survivors.

4.3   Regarding the IASC's Task Force on Mental Health and Psychosocial Support in Emergency Settings recommendation that a rapid needs assessment be conducted within 1–2 weeks of the event,

    A. It should focus on the human experience of the disaster.

    B. It represents an internationally accepted standard.

    C. It may not always be realistic or relevant as the situation shifts.

    D. All of the above.

    E. A and C.

4.4   True or False: A needs assessment should be aimed at capturing the largest amount of information possible.

4.5   When staffing a needs assessment team,

    A. Only mental health professionals should be included.

    B. Non–mental health professionals may be included.

    C. Local professionals should not be included because they are too traumatized to be objective.

    D. All members should have a background in epidemiology.

    E. At least five members should be included.

References

Calderon-Abbo J: The long road home: rebuilding public inpatient psychiatric services in post-Katrina New Orleans. Psychiatr Serv 59:304–309, 2008

Choudhury WA, Quraishi FA, Haque Z: Mental health and psychosocial aspects of disaster preparedness in Bangladesh. Int Rev Psychiatry 18:529–535, 2006

Connor KM, Foa EB, Davidson JRT: Practical assessment and evaluation of mental health problems following a mass disaster. J Clin Psychiatry 67(suppl):26–33, 2006

Disaster Psychiatry Outreach: Mental Health Consequences of Bioterrorism: A Disaster Preparedness Course for Hospital Emergency Department Staff. New York, Disaster Psychiatry Outreach, 2004. Available at: http://www.disasterpsych.org/home. Accessed February 24, 2010.

Disaster Psychiatry Outreach: DPO Clinical Protocol. New York, Disaster Psychiatry Outreach, 2006. Available at: http://www.disasterpsych.org/downloads. Accessed February 24, 2010.

Disaster Psychiatry Outreach: DPO Assessment Team Protocol. New York, Disaster Psychiatry Outreach, 2007. Available at: http://www.disasterpsych.org/downloads. Accessed February 24, 2010.

Disaster Psychiatry Outreach: The Essentials of Disaster Psychiatry: A Training Course for Mental Health Professionals (Course Syllabus). New York, Disaster Psychiatry Outreach, 2008. Available as DPOCourseSyllabus_052108.pdf at: https://sites.google.com/a/disasterpsych.org/blog/File-Cabinet. Accessed December 21, 2009.

Garakani A, Hirschowitz J, Katz CL: General disaster psychiatry. Psychiatr Clin North Am 27:391–406, 2004

Humayun A: South Asian earthquake: psychiatric experience in a tertiary hospital. East Mediterr Health J 14:1205–1216, 2008

Inter-Agency Standing Committee: IASC Guidelines on Mental Health and Psychosocial Support in Emergency Settings. Geneva, Switzerland, Inter-Agency Standing Committee, 2007. Available at: http://www.who.int/mental_health/emergencies/guidelines_iasc_mental_health_psychosocial_june_2007.pdf. Accessed February 22, 2010.

Kawana N: Psycho-physiological effects of the terrorist sarin attack on the Tokyo subway system. Mil Med 166 (suppl):23–26, 2001

Kessler RC, Galea S, Jones RT, et al: Mental illness and suicidality after Hurricane Katrina. Bull World Health Organ 84:930–939, 2006

Lindal E, Stefansson JG: The long-term psychological effect of fatal accidents at sea on survivors: a cross-sectional study of North-Atlantic seamen. Soc Psychiatry Psychiatr Epidemiol 46:239–246, 2011

Math SB, Girimaji SC, Benegal V, et al: Tsunami: psychosocial aspects of Anandam and Nicobar islands. assessments and intervention in the early phase. Int Rev Psychiatry 18:233–239, 2006

North CS, Pfefferbaum B, Tucker P: Ethical and methodological issues in academic mental health research in populations affected by disasters: the Oklahoma City experience relevant to September 11, 2001. CNS Spectr 7:580–584, 2002

Palinkas LA, Petterson JS, Russell J, et al: Community patterns of psychiatric disorders after the Exxon Valdez oil spill. Am J Psychiatry 150:1517–1523, 1993

Schoenbaum M, Butler B, Kataoka S, et al: Promoting mental health recovery after Hurricanes Katrina and Rita. Arch Gen Psychiatry 66:906–914, 2009

Silove D, Bryant R: Rapid assessments of mental health needs after disasters. JAMA 296:576–578, 2006

World Health Organization: Rapid Assessment of Mental Health Needs of Refugees, Displaced and Other Populations Affected by Conflict and Post-Conflict Situations, and Available Resources. Geneva, Switzerland, World Health Organization, 2001

World Health Organization: WHO-AIMS Version 2.2—Assessment Instrument for Mental Health Systems. Geneva, Switzerland, World Health Organization, 2005

World Health Organization: Mental Health Systems in Selected Low- And Middle-Income Countries: a WHO-AIMS Cross National Analysis. Geneva, Switzerland, World Health Organization, 2009

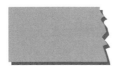

PART II

EVALUATION

Craig L. Katz, M.D., Section Editor

5

Psychiatric Evaluation

Craig L. Katz, M.D.

Mental health assistance to people affected by disasters begins with evaluation, first of the situation and the community and then of the affected people. Acute psychiatric evaluation of disaster survivors is distinguished from postacute evaluations that occur later in conventional psychiatric settings such as clinics or offices. Disaster blankets an affected community with a new chapter of human experience, creating a unique trajectory of evolving reactions and emerging diagnoses for the disaster psychiatrist to follow. In this chapter, I trace this trajectory and the clinical and logistical issues that shape it, and I lay out how to conduct general psychiatric evaluations of adults in the immediate wake of disasters. Other chapters include discussions of psychiatric evaluation in specific populations (Chapter 6, "Special Populations"; Chapter 17, "Child and Adolescent Psychiatry Interventions"; and Chapter 18, "Geriatric Psychiatry Interventions").

Psychological Consequences of Disaster

The Institute of Medicine has developed a useful framework for categorizing the psychological consequences of disaster (Goldfrank et al. 2003). As depicted in Figure 5–1, three broad categories of responses are posited: behavioral change, distress responses, and psychiatric illness. The end of what is essentially a spectrum of reactions consists of psychiatric illness, which is by definition of clinical significance. Short of that point lies a range of reactions that may be variably problematic, if at all.

Behavioral changes encompass a broad range of how people do things and go about their lives after disaster. When a community is turned upside

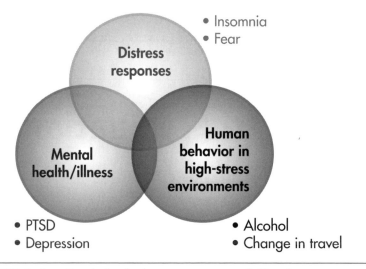

FIGURE 5–1.   Psychological consequences of disasters.

PTSD = posttraumatic stress disorder.
Source.   Reprinted from Ursano R: Terrorism and mental health: public health and primary care. Presentation at the Eighteenth Annual Rosalyn Carter Symposium on Mental Health Policy, November 6-7, 2002. Published in Status Report: Meeting the Mental Health Needs of the Country in the Wake of September 11, 2001 (http://www.cartercenter.org/documents/1441.pdf). Atlanta, GA, The Carter Center, 2002, pp 64–68. Used with permission.

down by disaster, people must act differently to adapt and survive. Although pitching a Red Cross tent so that one's family has shelter following the destruction of their home by a hurricane is not part of anyone's usual routine, it is necessary under the circumstances. Maladaptive behavior in response to disaster is demonstrated by those earthquake survivors who insist that the Red Cross accommodate them in a hotel as it might do with victims of a house fire, even though the extent of sudden homelessness and destruction make such accommodations impossible and potentially unsafe due to aftershocks. More common behavioral changes include reverting to regressive and potentially problematic behaviors, such as smoking cigarettes and drinking more alcohol (Vlahov et al. 2004). Sometimes, even a reduction in alcohol intake is found, such as following the 1995 Great Hanshin earthquake in Japan (Shimizu et al. 2000). This reduction was perhaps the result of a culturally based increase in self-discipline. Finally, a positive change in activity might be helping to organize a committee to reopen the local school.

Distress responses include all of the ways in which people experience a disaster. Again, these may or may not be abnormal or even maladaptive. These responses span cognitive, emotional, and physical reactions (Disaster Psychiatry Outreach 2008). Insomnia is a very common reaction that probably overlaps behavior and distress. Cognitive changes can include feeling confused or distracted. A range of thoughts about the event are possible, spanning disbelief to a sense of dependency to a decision to finally change one's career once things are back to normal. Emotional responses are as varied as the people involved but typically involve anxiety, fear, grief, and resignation. Positive emotions may also arise, including a heightened sense of community or spirituality.

Some people, especially those from certain cultures, may experience their distress in their bodies rather than their minds, even without having a disorder such as somatoform disorder or histrionic personality disorder (Van Moffaert 1998). Somatic reactions such as headaches or abdominal pain may lead survivors to seek medical care, even when there is no clear medical etiology. For example, a study of survivors of severe flooding and mudslides in Puerto Rico in 1985 showed that highly exposed individuals had significantly elevated rates of medically unexplained gastrointestinal symptoms (e.g., pain, vomiting, gas) and neurological symptoms (e.g., amnesia, paralysis, double vision) (Escobar et al. 1992). These reactions highlight the importance of collaboration between, including collocation of, disaster mental health professionals and medical providers or first aid stations.

Many people's reactions to disaster may be fluid and shifting, leading to a frequent experience of feeling that they are on an oft-described emotional roller coaster. At one moment survivors may feel inspired by the unity of their community's response to an event, whereas in the next instance they feel overwhelmed and paralyzed by the recovery tasks that lie ahead. Over time, the peaks and oscillations in behaviors or distress will subside for many or most people. If not, the problems begin to coalesce into psychiatric disorders. The most common postdisaster psychiatric disorders are posttraumatic stress disorder (PTSD), major depression, and alcohol use disorders (Disaster Psychiatry Outreach 2008).

The division between behavioral changes, distress, and disorders may be complicated in practice. Consider a study of the academic performance of Tulane School of Medicine medical students who had to be relocated from New Orleans to Houston to continue their studies after Hurricane Katrina in 2005 (Crawford et al. 2008). Their post-Katrina performance on nationally based examinations in several basic science courses (e.g., pathology, biochemistry) and clinical clerkships (e.g., medicine, psychiatry, pediatrics) was significantly worse than their pre-Katrina performance. Although this is a behavioral consequence of the event, it may be explained by countless factors that span distress and disorder. The investigators suggested that these factors could include grief, practical stresses involved in relocating, dealing with new faculty and schedules, or possible psychiatric disorders.

Psychological Consequences of Special Concern

Suicidality

Concerns about suicidality abound in disaster settings, at least in the popular imagination, but it is unclear whether an evidence base supports this concern. Among the few studies examining suicide, the findings have been conflicting. Investigators who initially reported finding elevated suicide rates following natural disasters in the United States between 1982 and 1989 ultimately published a retraction of this finding, wherein they clarified that they detected statistically significant increases in predisaster rates only in counties affected by two disasters (Krug et al. 1999). Examining regions of Louisiana, Alabama, and Mississippi affected by Hurricane Katrina 5–8 months and then 1 year later, researchers found increases in suicidal thinking and planning across the two time points (Kessler et al. 2008). On the other hand, a study of the community affected by the 1995 Great Hanshin earthquake in Japan found that suicide rates declined for the 2 years after the event (Nishio et al. 2009).

Given these varied findings, it is probably most accurate to say that with death and destruction literally and figuratively in the air of a disaster-stricken community, questions about the meaning and value of life will naturally arise (Hung 2010). It is natural and expectable that survivors will question how they could go on in life after suffering the loss of loved ones or the destruction of their life as they knew it. Survivors are confronted with valid spiritual and existential questions about life, but these thoughts do not equate with suicidality. On the other hand, even if such questioning is understandable, it does not preclude the presence of suicidality and should not falsely reassure the evaluating clinician. A disaster psychiatrist should therefore be sure to include a basic suicide assessment as a fundamental element of psychiatric assessment, especially when a survivor is questioning the ability or desirability of living the life he or she sees ahead.

Violence

Prevailing wisdom suggests that harmony and altruism reign in the immediate aftermath of disaster. A small body of research, however, indicates some potential for heightened violence, at least in the long term. A study of murder in post-Hurricane Katrina New Orleans revealed that murder rates in 2006 were approximately 50% higher than in 2005 and nearly two-thirds higher than in 2004 (Van Landingham 2007). Gender-based violence directed at women is assumed to be higher in disaster-affected populations, as seen in a study of internally displaced people living in trailer parks in Mississippi in the 2 years after Hurricane Katrina (Anastario et al. 2009). Meanwhile, inflicted traumatic brain injuries in children increased more than fivefold in North Carolina counties severely affected by Hurricane Floyd for 6 months following the disaster (Keenan et al. 2004).

Implications of these findings for psychiatric assessment are unclear. Generalizability is limited by the small number of studies. Psychiatrists' ability to predict violence under even normal circumstances is open to question. Also, violence probably springs from a number of sources beyond psychopathology. For example, the elevated murder rates in post-Katrina New Orleans could have resulted just as much from the socioeconomic stresses in a devastated city as from any discernible psychiatric condition.

Pending evidence to the contrary, disaster mental health professionals should not be distracted from a more balanced evaluation by the possibility of heightened violence in disasters in general. Even in situations of foreseeable violence, such as civil or military conflict, violence is not a psychiatric phenomenon but rather a political or social one. On the other hand, Phua (2008) suggested that the broader umbrella of "postdisaster victimization" may be an overlooked, although still not necessarily common, outcome of disasters; it includes not only violence but also such activities as exploitation of survivors, profiteering, theft/looting, and discrimination. Therefore, asking whether a survivor has been victimized in any way since (and before) a disaster provides a brief and potentially revealing glimpse into some of the secondary stresses that may be affecting him or her.

Psychosis

The intersection of psychosis and disasters has received little attention from researchers and especially epidemiologists (Katz et al. 2002). Although clinical lore has tended to suggest that patients with schizophrenia likely fare better than people who are healthy or have nonpsychotic conditions following a disaster, very limited evidence is available to support this speculation. In fact, psychotic episodes might become more common, as reflected in a postearthquake study in Taiwan, in which Tseng et al. (2010) found that incidence of hospitalizations for schizophrenia increased by 11.0% and 21.6%, respectively, in years 1 and 2 following the event. The topic of psychosis and people with serious mental illness is covered in depth in Chapter 7, "Serious Mental Illness."

Factors Relevant to Psychiatric Evaluation

Clinical Encounters

In usual clinical practice, psychiatrists and other mental health professionals have two main goals: evaluating and treating. Every other clinical activity occurs in the service of one of these overarching goals. This clarity of purpose and function becomes clouded in the disaster setting. The disaster mental health professional may engage in a range of functions that go beyond clinical care to include blanket distribution, needs assessments, and interagency liaison. Whereas professional exchanges with individuals always begin with a formal evaluation in the traditional clinical setting, this is not necessarily, or usually, the case in times of disaster. The following case vignette demonstrates a possible occurrence following a disaster.

> A psychiatrist staffing a family assistance center in the days after an airline crash is assigned to work in the dining area and attend to people in need. He accomplishes this by engaging people while they are having coffee, eating a meal, or perhaps just getting lost in thought. One person he encounters is an airline pilot who knew several of the employees on the doomed flight. After the psychiatrist and he introduce themselves, the pilot describes his devastation but says he cannot wait to get back in the cockpit as a way of maintaining the spirit of his friends and their joy of flying. After talking for 10 minutes, the psychiatrist wishes him well, lets the pilot know where he can find him if ever he wants to talk more, and moves on. He writes a two-sentence note describing the encounter but without the name of the pilot or other personal information, which he did not collect.

This so-called brief encounter, which is so named less for the brevity of the interaction and more for its anonymity and superficiality, is nevertheless an important psychiatric encounter. The psychiatrist is functioning as humanely as he is professionally, lending a compassionate ear to another person but also looking for indicators that the conversation should be extended into a "full encounter," in which a thorough psychiatric evaluation is conducted. As a rough rule, this transition occurs when the psychiatrist decides he or she needs to know the name of the person for a full encounter or when the person requests a more formal session. The largely heuristic process of deciding when to conduct a formal evaluation can be guided by a number of factors, as listed in Table 5–1.

Many, if not most, people with whom a disaster psychiatrist speaks in a disaster setting are not designated clients or patients. They remain survivors, and the psychiatrist is a humanitarian until he or she identifies the need for their roles to become that of patient and professional and has the resources and time to affect this transition.

TABLE 5–1.   Factors influencing the decision to conduct a full encounter with disaster survivor

---

How rested, cared for, and nourished the person looks

The degree of organization and focus the person exhibits in behavior and communication

Any mention of questioning life

Bizarre ideas or dysfunctional levels of denial (e.g., still holding out hope that a loved one survived a month after disappearing during flooding)

At the request of the person or of a family member, friend, or coworker

The psychiatrist's "gut feeling"

Availability of resources and time

Time Frame

One of the most helpful factors in guiding clinical assessment in the aftermath of disaster is timing (Disaster Psychiatry Outreach 2008, 2009). The determination of whether a reaction represents psychopathology is often dependent on the amount of time that has elapsed since the event. For example, losing sleep for the first few days after an earthquake is normal and possibly even adaptive. Sleeping lightly could be lifesaving in the event of a major aftershock in the middle of the night. However, losing sleep weeks or months after aftershocks subside suggests reason for clinical concern. The persistence of the problem suggests that it is pathological and possibly symptomatic of a larger disorder, such as PTSD or major depression.

The timeline of disasters is portrayed in Figure 5–2. In terms of response, the acute phase has been defined, by extrapolation from the definition of acute stress disorder, as the initial 2 months after the event (Katz et al. 2002). It begins with the immediate impact of the event, which can be defined as lasting as long as the first 48 hours of the acute phase (Disaster Psychiatry Outreach 2009). In practice, the acute phase is probably more fluid than these time parameters suggest. For example, when terrorists strike multiple times over a short span or when aftershocks rumble on following an earthquake, it is harder to circumscribe the time period of impact. Therefore, the acute phase can also be considered to be the time dating from the impact to days and weeks later (Disaster Psychiatry Outreach 2008). The impact itself encompasses the earliest initial minutes to hours of the event. The dust is literally or figuratively being "kicked" up during impact and settling during the acute phase.

In the acute period, evaluations are more likely to focus on subsyndromal symptoms, specifically distress and behavioral changes. During this

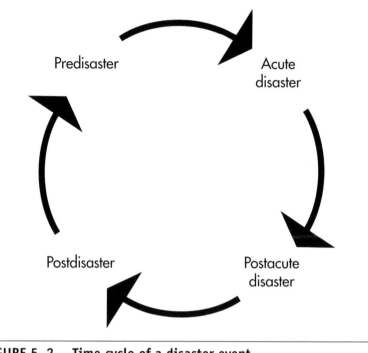

FIGURE 5–2.   Time cycle of a disaster event.

Source.   Disaster Psychiatry Outreach 2008, 2009.

time, reactions can be fluid and transient, which befits a stage wherein the dust is literally and figuratively settling but not settled. Disorders are not the focus, primarily because it often takes time for disorders to materialize. Definitions of psychiatric disorders have duration requirements. For example, it is not accurate to diagnose someone as having onset of PTSD 3 days after a catastrophic event. Instead, the person could have acute stress disorder, because its minimal duration is 2 days of PTSD-like symptoms plus dissociative symptoms (American Psychiatric Association 2000). Risk factors for future psychopathology and resilience factors can also be ascertained during this phase and may have great predictive value for how someone will do in the postacute period to follow. Acute evaluations inform the application of elements of Psychological First Aid as the primary intervention (see Chapter 12, "Psychological First Aid").

Biopsychosocial Needs

The psychiatric review of systems in the acute aftermath of disaster should be considered a biopsychosocial review of systems. When a community has literally been turned upside down, its members have a plethora of needs in order to right it again. To obtain a complete picture of a survivor, the disaster mental health professional must go beyond the individual's psychological responses to look at his or her broader biopsychosocial needs.

Specifically, the disaster mental health professional must assess four levels of need: safety needs, physical needs, medical needs, and mental health needs (Disaster Psychiatry Outreach 2008). In many ways, in the earliest days of the acute aftermath of a disaster, mental health needs arise directly from the other three. For example, if hurricane survivors have not had any food since the storm, it is superfluous and even misguided to ask how they are feeling until they are properly nourished. Indeed, it behooves the mental health professional to think and act in humanitarian terms and help get them food. Likewise, it is not useful to think of insomnia as an expression of inner distress when a disaster survivor has been unable to find shelter for the night. The following case vignette demonstrates how physical complaints must be thought of in medical terms and not just psychological ones.

> Several families are about to board a plane to fly to the site of an airplane crash to recover the remains of lost loved ones. A woman in her 70s whose daughter was a passenger on the fatal flight has been sobbing inconsolably but now begins to complain of chest pain. A nervous flight attendant beckons the disaster psychiatrist to evaluate her. As the only physician on the scene, he decides that the woman's cardiac history necessitates an electrocardiogram (ECG) before he can allow her to fly. The flight is held temporarily until he escorts the woman to the airport's first aid station, where her ECG is found to be normal. She is provided with some anxiolytic medication and rushed back to the flight.

Risk Factors

A number of well-studied psychosocial factors have been identified as placing disaster survivors at risk for having a psychopathological consequence from the trauma (Disaster Psychiatry Outreach 2009; Katz et al. 2002) (Table 5–2). Biological markers of risk remain under investigation and do not yet have sufficient evidence to support their becoming a part of routine clinical evaluations (Katz et al. 2002).

The most evident risk factor is the "dose" of exposure. A variety of studies provide support for the notion that greater exposure to a disaster increases the risk for developing PTSD (see Katz et al. 2002 for a review). For example, a survey of 8,487 firefighters following the 9/11 terrorist attacks revealed a much higher risk for those who responded on the day of the World Trade Center collapse compared with those who responded within 2 days, who in turn had a greater risk than the firefighters who arrived thereafter (Corrigan et al. 2009). In the end, however, trauma expo-

---

TABLE 5–2.   Psychosocial risk factors for psychopathology following disaster

---

"Dose" of exposure to the disaster

Prior exposure to trauma such as disaster

Prior psychiatric history

Problems of living prior to the disaster/low socioeconomic status

Lack of perceived or actual social supports after the event

Presence of "secondary stressors"

Female gender

Middle age

Ethnic minority

---

sure does not lend itself to quantification or clinical thresholds as does, say, exposure to radiation. What can be said is that exposure can encompass a range of items, both personal and economic (Table 5–3). It may come in the form of lives lost or livelihood lost, and it appears that the more exposed someone has been, the less protective it is to have few or no other risk factors.

Someone with other significant risk factors may only require what for others may be a small exposure to disaster to be tipped into psychopathology. Contrast an ironworker performing demolition at the World Trade Center for several months immediately following the 9/11 attacks with a volunteer who spent 12 hours the day after the attack handing out food and water to responders. Duration alone suggests a greater exposure for the ironworker, even though nothing in his background, such as past trauma or psychiatric history, would otherwise render him psychiatrically vulnerable; however, he does not go on to develop any psychiatric disorder and may even feel better for having worked at Ground Zero. The volunteer distributing food and water, who has past traumatic exposures and an associated psychiatric history (which may even have in some ways propelled her to spontaneously volunteer despite ill preparation), could be more likely to have recurrent or new psychiatric problems despite having been at Ground Zero only briefly.

Knowledge of psychosocial risk factors is a useful tool in acute phase evaluations. Irrespective of the level of acute reactions and symptoms, it can be predicted that among people exposed to the event, those with a greater quantity or severity of risk factors should be identified and followed longitudinally. At the least, they should be candidates for psychoeducation about their psychiatric risks. Unfortunately, this public health approach to

---

TABLE 5–3.   Elements of exposure to trauma and disaster

Scope of event

Proximity to event

Duration of event

Personal loss and injury

Extent of prior warning

Uncertainty

---

disaster psychiatry remains hampered by lack of study about how to best use these factors alone or together for stratifying risk. For now, in the absence of known algorithms or validated surveys for this purpose, clinical judgment must suffice.

Resilience

Resilience is a concept that has garnered significant interest in both scholarship and treatment of trauma, although definitions vary. It has been variously defined as those factors that promote a positive outcome or growth from trauma, enable people to be affected minimally by trauma, or allow survivors to bounce back entirely (Bonnano 2004; Disaster Psychiatry Outreach 2008). However the concept is defined, resilience certainly underscores how the Institute of Medicine's framework for psychological consequences of disaster reviewed earlier (Goldfrank et al. 2003; see Figure 5–1) are appropriately called "psychological consequences of concern," because there are other consequences that may be positive. Including resilience factors in the assessment of a disaster survivor will provide a more multidimensional portrait while ensuring that healthy coping is identified, validated, and promoted. Resilience is discussed in detail in Chapter 11, "Grief and Resilience."

Meaning

Another way in which acute phase psychiatric evaluations should extend beyond symptoms and diagnoses involves exploring the meaning of the disaster. Specifically, when someone has acute symptoms following exposure to disaster, these should be considered as common final pathways for layers of underlying personal meaning (Katz and Nathaniel 2002). As much as stress reactions are part of a biologically based "fight-or-flight" response, the biology/brain and the psychology/mind affect one another.

In practice, exploring the meaning of disaster translates into an approach that goes beyond quantifying symptoms to fully characterizing them. For example, when someone suffers from insomnia, in addition to pinpointing the nature, onset, and course of the problem, the disaster mental health professional can go further and ask about what goes through the person's mind when he or she lies awake at night. Such practice probably makes sense under any conditions, but especially in times of disaster and trauma. It is believed that trauma is particularly devastating because the sufferer cannot find the words to make sense of the experience and weave it into a personal narrative (van der Kolk 1994). Therefore, the more disaster survivors are supported in trying to articulate their thoughts and experiences in the acute aftermath of disaster, the more the trajectory of their recovery is presumably tilted in a healthy direction. This process begins with elucidating the meaning underlying symptomatic responses.

Naming the Problem

Psychiatric evaluations end with an assessment and diagnosis, usually within the multiaxial diagnostic framework of DSM-IV-TR (American Psychiatric Association 2000). The acute phase of disasters poses a challenge to this approach for at least two reasons. First (as referred to earlier), the symptomatic response may be fluid and transient, meeting neither duration nor symptom criteria of any diagnosis. Practitioners often approach this problem by labeling any reaction "PTSD," however ill-fitting and incorrect this label may be (Disaster Psychiatry Outreach 2009). Second, many responses to disaster may be normal and adaptive, rendering the idea of a diagnosis overly pathologizing. It benefits neither those being helped nor the field of psychiatry to pathologize what is normal.

There does not yet exist an appropriate nosology for the spectrum of acute psychological consequences of disaster. Such a nosology would need to distinguish clinical significance from pathology. For example, isolated insomnia occurring for several days after a disaster may be clinically significant and warrant intervention, but it does not rise to the level of pathology. Probably the best approximation is provided by the diagnosis of adjustment disorder from DSM-IV-TR. In practice, this diagnosis often seems imprecise; it may even be inaccurate, as its very name explicitly underscores the presence of a disorder when no pathology may be present. Figley and Nash (2007) have provided perhaps the best solution to date for this nosological challenge. Writing based on their experience in the military, these authors suggest labeling acute traumatic reactions as "stress injuries" and then differentiating these based on the causative agent. The three types of stress injuries are trauma, grief, and fatigue. This is a compelling approach, because the notion of an injury captures clinical significance without labeling the situation a disorder.

Figley and Nash's (2007) nosology cannot readily be recommended for use in the postdisaster setting because it has not been validated and has no place within the DSM framework. One working solution for the disaster mental health professional is to use the adjustment disorder diagnosis but to parenthetically qualify it as one of the three types of stress injuries (e.g., diagnosis: adjustment disorder, depressed ["stress injury due to grief"]). Perhaps the best recommendation of all is for the disaster mental health professional to be mindful of the limitations of the nosology of acute trauma.

Mental Health Surveys

Psychiatric evaluation in the setting of disaster can be supplemented by surveys, which may provide an efficient mechanism for identifying problems in a setting of potentially limited resources amid high need. A discussion of the psychometric properties and clinical use of specific mental health or trauma-related surveys is beyond the scope of this chapter and can be found elsewhere (Connor et al. 2006). Instead, potential strategies for utilizing surveys in the disaster setting are highlighted.

Surveys may be used as a screening tool, helping to identify people with clinically significant distress for referral to on-site disaster mental health professionals (Katz et al. 2002). Integrating a mental health survey into the general functioning of a disaster assistance center may help to elevate awareness about mental health problems. It could also help with planning and staffing ongoing mental health services for that center once the scope of need is apparent.

If a survey were implemented epidemiologically in the disaster-affected community rather than among people seeking help at a disaster center, then it could serve as a needs assessment for planning mental health services for the general community. Whether used for screening or needs assessment, the survey(s) selected could be targeted either at general psychiatric distress ("caseness") or toward a specific diagnosis such as PTSD or major depression. Resilience may also be surveyed (Connor and Davidson 2003), although the clinical relevance of such an approach remains to be elucidated.

Surveys may also help to address the problem of a shortage of psychiatric expertise in a disaster setting. If primary care professionals are staffing the scene, their divided attention may be more reliably drawn to mental health issues among their patients if all able patients complete a screening mental health survey before meeting with them. Alternatively, primary care professionals who have limited expertise in psychiatry, let alone in disaster psychiatry, may welcome the use of mental health surveys to supplement their clinical assessments of their patients.

Conclusion: The Three *Ws*—What, Who, and When

The three *Ws* are three questions that represent a suggested clinical framework for synthesizing the ideas of this chapter and cohesively applying them in the event of a disaster (Disaster Psychiatry Outreach 2004). These three questions, with related considerations, are as follows:

1. **What** is known about the event, including its scope, impact, and public health implications?
    - Impact of disaster—injured, dead, exposed, displaced, unemployed
    - Information about the affected community's *predisaster* public health/mental health, social, political, and economic functioning
    - Unique psychological theme for the type of event (e.g., earthquake, aviation disaster, terrorist event)

2. **Who** are the persons under consideration, including their personal, social, and psychological history, as well as their connection to the disaster?
    - Demographics—age, gender, marital status, employment, living situation
    - Psychological responses
    - Exposure
    - Role in the "disaster community"
    - Presence of other risk factors for psychological problems
    - Resources (e.g., family, friends, relatives)
    - Culture

3. **When** in the time course of the event are the persons being seen?
    - Impact—requires provision of basic empathy, support, orientation, accurate information, structure and direction to the experience
    - Acute phase—requires brief and full encounters, evaluating for biopsychosocial needs, distress responses, behavioral changes, risk factors, personal meaning, and resiliency
    - Postacute phase—requires full encounters, evaluating for psychiatric illness as well as biopsychosocial needs, risk factors, personal meaning and resiliency

Application of these three questions will help to create a three-dimensional view of each survivor under evaluation. The questions will also orient the disaster mental health practitioner to the time frame and the psychological consequences appropriate for consideration.

■ Teaching Points

- Psychological consequences of concern after disasters are behavioral changes, distress responses, and psychiatric disorder.
- Suicidality may not be as common a problem after disasters as are existential and spiritual questions about the meaning of life.
- Postdisaster violence assessment should occur in the context of broader questions about postdisaster victimization.
- Factors influencing psychological recovery from disasters include the extent of a survivor's biopsychosocial needs, his or her psychosocial risk factors, and his or her resilience.
- The nosology of acute responses to disaster remains imprecise.
- Considering the "three *Ws*"—what, who, and when—will help the disaster mental health professional to determine the essential questions to ask of a survivor.

Review Questions

5.1 According to the Institute of Medicine, which of the following is a psychological consequence of disaster?

A. Distress.
B. Behavioral change.
C. Psychiatric illness.
D. Violence.
E. A, B, and C.

5.2 Which of the following statements regarding postdisaster psychosis is *true*?

A. Postdisaster psychosis is infrequent.
B. Patients with psychotic illnesses fare better than others.
C. Postdisaster psychosis has received little attention in the research literature.
D. Postdisaster psychosis is associated with violence during civil conflicts.
E. Patients taking antipsychotic medication should have their dosages increased.

5.3   What are the three types of stress injuries?

    A. Fatigue, trauma, and grief.
    B. Acute, postacute, and chronic.
    C. Physical, mental, and idiopathic.
    D. First, second, and third degree.
    E. None of the above.

5.4   True or False: If someone has been sufficiently exposed to a disaster, then his or her resiliency is irrelevant to recovery.

5.5   Risk factors for postdisaster psychopathology include all of the following *except*

    A. "Dose" of exposure.
    B. Perceived or actual lack of social support.
    C. Prior psychiatric history.
    D. Presence of acute symptoms.
    E. Prior trauma.

References

American Psychiatric Association: Diagnostic and Statistical Manual of Mental Disorders, 4th Edition, Text Revision. Washington, DC, American Psychiatric Association, 2000

Anastario M, Shehab N, Lawry L: Increased gender-based violence among women internally displaced in Mississippi 2 years post-Hurricane Katrina. Disaster Med Public Health Prep 3:18–26, 2009

Bonnano GA: Loss, trauma, and human resilience: have we underestimated the human capacity to thrive after extremely aversive events? Am Psychol 59:20–28, 2004

Connor KM, Davidson J: Development of a new resilience scale: the Connor-Davidson Resilience Scale (CD-RISC). Depress Anxiety 18:76–82, 2003

Connor KM, Foa E, Davidson JR: Practical assessment and evaluation of mental health problems following a mass disaster. J Clin Psychiatry 67 (suppl 2):26–33, 2006

Corrigan M, McWilliams R, Kelly KJ, et al: A computerized, self-administered questionnaire to evaluate posttraumatic stress among firefighters after the World Trade Center collapse. Am J Public Health 99 (suppl):S702–S709, 2009

Crawford BE, Kahn MJ, Gibson JW, et al: Impact of Hurricane Katrina on medical student performance: the Tulane experience. Am J Med Sci 336:142–146, 2008

Disaster Psychiatry Outreach: Mental Health Consequences of Bioterrorism: A Disaster Preparedness Course for Hospital Emergency Department Staff. Health Resources and Services Administration Grant Number U3RMC01549–01, January to August 2004. New York, Disaster Psychiatry Outreach, 2004

Disaster Psychiatry Outreach: The Essentials of Disaster Psychiatry: A Training Course for Mental Health Professionals (Course Syllabus). New York, Disaster Psychiatry Outreach, 2008. Available as DPOCourseSyllabus_052108.pdf at: https://sites.google.com/a/disasterpsych.org/blog/File-Cabinet. Accessed December 21, 2009.

Disaster Psychiatry Outreach: A primer in disaster psychiatry. Presentation at the Cambridge Health Alliance Psychiatric Residency Retreat, Cambridge, MA, May 2009

Escobar JI, Canino G, Rubio-Stipec M, et al: Somatic symptoms after a natural disaster: a prospective study. Am J Psychiatry 149:965–967, 1992

Figley CR, Nash WP: Combat Stress Injury. New York, Brunner-Routledge, 2007

Goldfrank LR, Bulter AS, Panzer AM: Preparing for the Psychological Consequences of Terrorism: A Public Health Strategy. Washington, DC, National Academies Press, 2003

Hung E: Assessment and management of suicide after disasters, in Hidden Impact: What You Need to Know for the Next Disaster. A Practical Mental Health Guide for Clinicians. Edited by Stoddard FJ, Katz CL, Merlino JP. Sudbury, MA, Jones & Bartlett, 2010, pp 53–59

Katz CL, Nathaniel R: Disasters, psychiatry, and psychodynamics. J Am Acad Psychoanal 30:519–530, 2002

Katz CL, Pellegrino L, Pandya A, et al: Research on psychiatric outcomes subsequent to disasters: a review of the literature. Psychiatry Res 110:201–217, 2002

Keenan HT, Marshall SW, Nocera MA, et al: Increased incidence of inflicted traumatic brain injury in children after a natural disaster. Am J Prev Med 26:189–193, 2004

Kessler RC, Galea S, Gruber MJ, et al: Trends in mental illness and suicidality after Hurricane Katrina. Mol Psychiatry 13:374–384, 2008

Krug EG, Kresnow MJ, Peddicord JP, et al: Retraction: suicide after natural disasters. N Engl J Med 340:148–149, 1999

Nishio A, Akazawa K, Shibuya F, et al: Influence on the suicide rate two years after a devastating disaster: a report from the 1995 Great Hanshin-Awaji earthquake. Psychiatry Clin Neurosci 63:247–250, 2009

Phua K: Post-disaster victimization: how survivors of disasters can continue to suffer after the event. New Solut 18:221–231, 2008

Shimizu S, Aso K, Noda T, et al: Natural disasters and alcohol consumption in a cultural context: the Great Hanshin Earthquake in Japan. Addiction 95:529–536, 2000

Tseng KC, Hemenway D, Kawachi I, et al: The impact of the Chi-Chi earthquake on the incidence of hospitalizations for schizophrenia and on concomitant hospital choice. Community Ment Health J 46:93–101, 2010 van der Kolk BA: The body keeps the score: memory and the evolving psychobiology of posttraumatic stress. Harv Rev Psychiatry 1:253–265, 1994

Van Landingham MJ: Murder rates in New Orleans, La, 2004–2006. Am J Public Health 97:1614–1616, 2007

Van Moffaert M: Somatization patterns in Mediterranean migrants, in Clinical Methods in Transcultural Psychiatry. Edited by Okpaku SO. Washington, DC, American Psychiatric Press, 1998, pp 301–320

Vlahov D, Galea S, Ahern J, et al: Consumption of cigarettes, alcohol, and marijuana among New York City residents six months after the September 11 terrorist attacks. Am J Drug Alcohol Abuse 30:385–407, 2004

6

Special Populations

Frank G. Dowling, M.D.
Kristina Jones, M.D.

With a previous history of panic attacks and just recently divorced, Ms. D was still, 2 months after the attacks, having difficulty leaving her 12-year-old daughter alone for a few hours until she arrived home from working in New York City each day. Because Ms. D had been "lucky enough" to be off from work on 9/11, her friends and parents could not understand why she was unable to accept her good fortune and "get over" the guilt she experienced from knowing that a few friends and coworkers had died or were among the missing. Ms. D could not bear to tell them that she had gone for a breast biopsy on 9/11 and that the results were positive. Ironically, she actually felt guilty about having cancer. Ms. D was now suffering a recurrence of panic attacks, tearfulness, and excessive guilt about leaving her daughter to go to work. Part of her was wondering whether it might not have been better if she *had* gone to work on 9/11.

When disaster strikes, everyone in a community is affected. The psychiatrist who responds must keep in mind that both collective trauma and individual trauma occur in response to a disaster. In addition, individual members of a community are not affected equally. Both characteristics of the disaster itself and individual vulnerabilities play significant roles in the impact of a disaster on individuals (Somasundaram and van de Put 2006). Age, gender, and culture have an influence on the risk of developing postdisaster stress-related symptoms or clinical problems and have an influence on access to and acceptance, utilization, and effectiveness of psychosocial supports and treatments offered in the postdisaster setting. In addition, assumptions by disaster psychiatrists regarding other cultures' experience and presentation of distress can be inaccurate and may result in harm to an individual or group (Disaster Psychiatry Outreach 2008). Therefore, familiarity with the potential needs of special populations is essential for a psychiatrist to be effective and to reduce the possibility of doing harm in the disaster setting.

In this chapter, we discuss several populations that may have specific needs in the disaster setting. These include children and adolescents, elderly people, women, and people with physical disabilities. We also discuss ethnocultural issues.

Children and Adolescents

Many children who experience psychological trauma cannot adequately describe their symptoms to meet the specific diagnostic criteria of posttraumatic stress disorder (PTSD), depression, or anxiety disorders that are commonly seen after a disaster. Some children may be misdiagnosed with other disorders whose criteria are behaviorally focused, such as oppositional defiant disorder, attention-deficit/hyperactivity disorder (ADHD), or conduct disorder. In addition, children who have prior traumatic exposures or previously existing psychiatric disorders are particularly vulnerable in the disaster setting. The DSM-IV-TR (American Psychiatric Association 2000) diagnostic category of PTSD does not adequately account for the range of presentations and difficulties observed in children exposed to traumatic events (Cook et al. 2005). A child may be experiencing significant disturbance requiring clinical intervention yet might not meet clear diagnostic criteria for PTSD, or a child might simultaneously meet criteria for PTSD and other comorbid disorders. The National Child Traumatic Stress Network recommends that rather than focusing on DSM diagnostic categories, psychiatrists should use a comprehensive approach to assessment and intervention that takes into account the following seven domains of impairment seen in children and adolescents exposed to trauma: attachment, biology, affect regulation, dissociation, behavioral regulation, cognition, and self-concept (Cook et al. 2003).

Until recent years, the impact of disasters on children was not well studied, but some observations from the literature can be shared. Direct exposure to an event, proximity, loss of a family member, serious injury, younger age, and female gender have been found to have an association with post-disaster difficulties in children. In addition, previous psychiatric difficulties (particularly anxiety disorders) and parental posttraumatic stress symptoms have been correlated with posttraumatic stress in children (Hoven et al. 2003).

Interest in posttraumatic stress reactions in children after a disaster has increased since 9/11 in 2001. In a population-based study of New York City schoolchildren 6 months after 9/11 (Hoven et al. 2005), a wide range of psychiatric disorders were found to be elevated, including PTSD, agoraphobia, separation anxiety, and alcohol abuse (in older children). Over 28% of students were found to have one or more of six anxiety or depressive disorders. Risk factors that most strongly correlated with disorders included female gender, being in fourth or fifth grade, direct exposure, family exposure, prior trauma, and high media exposure. Interestingly, attendance at a Ground Zero–area school was inversely correlated with disorder, possibly the result of significant social supports and mental health interventions that were made available. Finally, exposure to prior trauma was a significant risk factor for postdisaster difficulties (Hoven et al. 2005). The available information suggests that children are particularly vulnerable to the negative impact of disaster, and that vulnerable children and families would benefit from psychosocial interventions and supports that are tailored to their vulnerabilities and needs.

In assessing a child, a disaster psychiatrist should begin by making sure that the child's essential needs for safety, food, water, clothing, and shelter are met. Although children need to be assessed directly, a parent or family member is needed to provide permission for the clinician to meet with a child and to share observations and answer questions that a child may not be able to answer. The mental health professional should ask the parents about the child's initial reaction to the event; previous emotional or learning difficulties; family members injured (physically or psychologically), missing, or deceased as a result of the event; any previous deaths or losses and how the child reacted to them; and family beliefs, traditions, or practices after a death or traumatic event. Parents need to be educated regarding normal bereavement or traumatic responses of children, because some of the common signs of distress seen in children postdisaster may be misinterpreted as illness. Common signs of distress seen in children experiencing traumatic stress or bereavement include fear for self, parents, or other close family; anxiety or separation anxiety; tantrums; changes in sleep and appetite; social withdrawal; refusal to follow usual routines or rules; and trust issues. An overview of age-related development and common responses seen in acute bereavement or after traumatic events appears in Table 6–1.

In assessment and early intervention with children, Psychological First Aid (PFA) is beneficial because it incorporates a series of strategies focusing on children, parents, and families, and it uses parents, teachers, and community resources to give basic psychological support for children and adolescents. Variations focus on how parents can help their children and how schoolteachers and administrators can support children at a time of disaster or crisis at school (Schreiber and Gurwitch 2006a, 2006b). Because most children will not need formal treatment but will benefit from assistance, a familiarity with PFA is useful. (For further information on PFA, see Chapter 17, "Child and Adolescent Psychiatry Interventions.")

In the wake of a disaster, the availability of formally trained child and adolescent psychiatrists will likely be very limited. Therefore, each psychi-

TABLE 6–1. Child development phase, developmental hallmarks, and common responses to trauma and loss

Developmental period	Age range (years)	Developmental hallmarks	Common trauma response
Infancy	0–2.5	Healthy attachment formation Development of separate individual identity Rapid growth in motor, language, cognitive areas	Irritability, excessive crying Excessive separation anxiety Failure to thrive, developmental delays Extreme sensitivity to parental, other stimuli
Preschool (exploration)	2.5–6	Egocentricity Magical thinking Perception of death as reversible	Regression—bedwetting, thumb sucking, clinging Inadequate verbal expression and comprehension (due to immature cognitive skills) Fear of separation from parents Extreme sensitivity to parental reactions Difficulty identifying feelings Nightmares, sleep disturbances Grief related to "abandonment" by caretaker
Elementary school age (mastery)	6–12	Mastery of skills, logical thinking Appreciation of others' viewpoints Increased awareness of actual danger Concretization of concept of *death*	Somatic complaints School refusal, performance decline Regression Irritability, temper outbursts, aggression Sleep disturbance, nightmares Social withdrawal, loss of interest Feelings of responsibility, guilt Close attention to parents' anxieties Reenactment play (can be upsetting, misunderstood by caretakers)

TABLE 6–1. Child development phase, developmental hallmarks, and common responses to trauma and loss *(continued)*

Developmental period	Age range (years)	Developmental hallmarks	Common trauma response
Adolescence	12–18	Abstract thinking Emphasis on autonomy and sexuality Effort to appear competent, independent, separate identity Physical attractiveness central to esteem Perception of death as final and inevitable Significance of peer group, interactions	Similar to those of adults (e.g., flashbacks, nightmares, avoidance, numbing, depression, substance misuse, social withdrawal) Somatic complaints Suicidal ideation Depression, guilt Sleep disturbance Anger and revenge fantasies that interfere with usual functioning Abrupt shifts in relationships Decline in school performance Trauma-driven acting out Accident proneness

Source. Adapted from Disaster Psychiatry Outreach 2008.

atrist who responds to a disaster should be prepared to screen, supply PFA, and determine when a child or adolescent may need a referral to a specialist. When talking to a parent, the psychiatrist needs to remember that one of the best predictors of how a child will fare after a traumatic event is how a parent or family is doing. In addition, when listening to a parent sharing history or observations of his or her child, the mental health provider needs to be aware that the parent might be projecting his or her own distress onto the child. In this situation, the psychiatrist should consider a referral for the parent, with the recommendation that the individual would benefit from further support so that he or she can be better able to assist his or her child.

As in work with adults, the psychiatrist can have difficulty determining when a child's reaction is normal or pathological, particularly when signs and symptoms of distress occur on a continuum with stress-related disorders. Although designed for the primary care provider, the Pediatric Symptom Checklist (Jellinek and Murphy 2003; Figure 6–1) also can be used by mental health providers; this instrument has been translated into several languages, has been tested and validated in many countries, and has established cutoff scores. Some items may correlate with a specific disorder, but the checklist is designed primarily to pick up impairment in a child's role or social functioning that may be suggestive of a more serious problem and not to make a specific diagnosis. Observation of a child's play and interactions is critical. An evaluation by a child psychiatrist is warranted if a child is not functioning reasonably well with others in school, play, or other usual activities; or if parents report significant changes in a child's behaviors or demeanor; or if a child is demonstrating significant signs of depression or anxiety, is having significant behavioral difficulties, or talks about suicide (Disaster Psychiatry Outreach 2008).

The psychiatrist who responds during the acute phase of a disaster should keep in mind that it is entirely possible, perhaps even likely, that schools will be closed and that many usual activities for children and families will be canceled. The psychiatrist may need to tailor screenings and interventions to adapt to the space and time that is available. It is important to reunite children with their parents as soon as reasonably possible and to minimize their time apart if some separation is needed during the provision of screening, support, or treatment. If parents and children are separated by the death, illness, or serious injury of a parent, then reuniting with other close family may be necessary. Flexibility is warranted.

When possible, the creation of a separate child-friendly play area or "kids' corner" (Disaster Psychiatry Outreach 2008) can be instrumental in 1) providing a break for parents impacted by an event, including time to address their own mental health needs, and 2) allowing children a place to play and to seek positive interactions and distractions. The intention of the

CHILD'S NAME:	DATE OF BIRTH:		TODAY'S DATE:	
RECORD NUMBER:	FILLED OUT BY:			
Please mark under the heading that best fits your child:	Never	Sometimes	Often	
1. Complains of aches and pains				
2. Spends more time alone				
3. Tires easily, has little energy				
4. Fidgety, unable to sit still				
5. Has trouble with teacher				
6. Less interested in school				
7. Acts as if driven by a motor				
8. Daydreams too much				
9. Distracted easily				
10. Is afraid of new situations				
11. Feels sad, unhappy				
12. Is irritable, angry				
13. Feels hopeless				
14. Has trouble concentrating				
15. Less interested in friends				
16. Fights with other children				
17. Absent from school				
18. School grades dropping				
19. Is down on him- or herself				
20. Visits the doctor with doctor finding nothing wrong				
21. Has trouble sleeping				
22. Worries a lot				
23. Wants to be with you more than before				
24. Feels he or she is bad				
25. Takes unnecessary risks				
26. Gets hurt frequently				
27. Seems to be having less fun				
28. Acts younger than children his or her age				
29. Does not listen to rules				
30. Does not show feelings				
31. Does not understand other people's feelings				
32. Teases others				
33. Blames others for his or her troubles				
34. Takes things that do not belong to him or her				
35. Refuses to share				
Other comments:				

FIGURE 6–1. Pediatric Symptom Checklist.

Source. Additional copies available at http://psc.partners.org/psc_english.pdf.
Copyright 1999, Michael Jellinek, M.D. Reprinted with permission.

kids' corner is to provide a brief respite and an oasis of normalcy for children whose families have been impacted by the disaster. The kids' corner can also be used for providing screening, PFA, and referrals for children when needed. Such an area should include supplies such as snacks and drinks, toys, art supplies, and educational materials for families and children. Staff should be available to observe, support, and assess in a location and through activities (i.e., play) that allow children to naturally express their thoughts or feelings about their experiences. More detailed information, particularly for child and adolescent psychiatrists, child mental health clinicians, and pediatric primary care clinicians, is available in Chapter 17, "Child and Adolescent Psychiatry Interventions."

Elderly People

Studies show mixed results about whether elderly people are at higher risk for posttraumatic stress, depression, or anxiety disorders after a disaster. Although some research has indicated that elderly people have a lower risk of psychiatric difficulties compared with other age groups, other research has shown increased risk for elderly people or similar risk across age groups (Galea et al. 2008). Risk of psychiatric sequelae after a disaster may differ based on cultural background. For example, increased risk for elderly Eastern Europeans and decreased risk for elderly Mexicans have been reported (Disaster Psychiatry Outreach 2008). Several studies have found an increased risk for middle-aged adults and lower risks for elderly people, younger adults, and children (Norris et al. 2002a). After Hurricane Katrina, adults ages 55 years and older experienced lower rates of PTSD (15%) compared with adults ages 35–54 years (23.4%) and adults ages 18–34 years (30%) (Galea et al. 2008). Among New York City residents after 9/11, the prevalence of PTSD and depression among adults ages 55 years and older was lower than that among younger groups (Tracy and Galea 2006). In reviewing the available evidence, one should consider that many studies categorize older adults as "over age 55" and that a category of "over age 65 (or 70)" might have different results. In addition, it is possible that the most vulnerable older adults are underrepresented in studies because they may have been in institutional settings such as nursing homes.

For some elderly individuals, life experiences may have a protective effect by providing some degree of stress inoculation (Sakauye et al. 2009). Having overcome prior adversities may be protective for other age groups as well. Although it seems intuitive that short-term memory impairments may be protective against traumatic stress, disaster itself has been found to cause or worsen memory impairments in the elderly (Sakauye et al. 2009), which may adversely affect their ability to care for themselves or to access postdisaster resources and supports. In addition, elderly persons with cognitive impairments are at risk for increased confusion and memory problems due to difficulties with overstimulation, new situations, and obstacles for caregivers in providing usual support in the face of disaster. Furthermore, "flashbulb memory" of traumatic events may lead to retention and incorporation of traumatic memories by elderly individuals with dementia (Sakauye et al. 2009).

The key risk factor for elderly persons after disaster may not be age itself but rather the common complications of age. A recent consensus guideline suggests the following risk factors for elderly persons to experience negative outcomes after a disaster: advanced age or frailty; cognitive impairment; severe and persistent mental illness or chronic disability due to mental illness; poor physical health, complex medical illness, or mobility problems; sensory impairments; and lack of close family caregivers and/or social supports (Sakauye et al. 2009).

Nearly 80% of adults older than 65 years have at least one chronic medical condition, and nearly half have two chronic medical conditions, such as hypertension, coronary artery disease, diabetes, arthritis, cancer, or cerebrovascular disease (Aldrich and Benson 2008). After Hurricane Katrina, 74% of deaths in New Orleans occurred in those older than 65 years, and about 50% were in those older than 70 years, although only about 15% of the population was over age 65. The majority of people who ended up stranded in the Astrodome with limited supports and supplies were seniors. Emergency departments in nearby states were flooded with evacuated seniors who had significant difficulties with prescription medication refills (Sakauye et al. 2009). Many elderly persons with lower physical reserves or less resilience are at increased risk for hypothermia or hyperthermia, dehydration, electrolyte disturbance, or malnourishment. In addition, elderly with limited, fixed incomes may not have the financial resources to meet their short-term or long-term needs in the postdisaster environment.

Because many elderly persons may be isolated or experience mobility difficulties, outreach is critical. Psychiatric assessment must include a screening for medical illness, current medications, sensory and mobility deficits, availability of family and other social supports, and access to postdisaster community resources. Clinicians should remain mindful that the suicide rate is highest in the elderly compared with other age groups, the risk is significantly higher for males than for females, and firearms are the most commonly used method of suicide in this group (Conwell 2009). Because cognitive difficulties increase with age and may significantly impact postdisaster recovery, a brief cognitive screening such as the Montreal Cognitive Assessment should be considered (Nasreddine et al. 2005). This assessment is available in several languages and can be downloaded from www.mocatest.org/default.asp. As for other age groups, assessment for both transient stress reactions and clinical disorders is important, as is being mindful of the various risk factors or vulnerabilities that may increase the risk of psychiatric difficulties. Despite the debate on risk of psychiatric difficulties postdisaster, elderly persons should be evaluated for PTSD, clinical depression, clinical anxiety, or substance use disorders. Because older adults may be less psychologically minded or introspective, they may report fewer symptoms or understate symptom severity, and they may have more somatization symptoms (Sakauye et al. 2009). More detailed information is available in Chapter 18, "Geriatric Psychiatry Interventions."

Women

Although lifetime exposure to traumatic events in general is roughly equal for men and women, the available evidence suggests that women are at higher risk for psychiatric difficulties after a disaster (Norris et al. 2002a). This increased risk is fairly consistent across ages and cultures, but there are some differences. Relative to other women, Mexican and non-English-speaking women have the highest risk, and African American women have the lowest risk (Norris et al. 2002a).

Several factors may account for increased risk of psychiatric difficulties in women after disaster. In the general population, women have higher rates of depression, anxiety disorders, and PTSD, and preexisting disorders are a significant risk factor for postdisaster difficulties. Although rates of exposure to trauma may be similar for men and women, the types of trauma and the risk of resulting psychiatric disorder vary. Men are more likely to experience a motor vehicle accident, which has lower risk, and women experience a significantly higher rate of sexual assault, which has the highest risk of leading to psychiatric difficulties (Frans et al. 2005). After 9/11, the lifetime prevalence of probable PTSD in New York City 6–9 months after the attacks was reported to be higher in women (17.2%) than in men (12.1%). Preexisting psychiatric difficulties, prior sexual assault, marital status, and perievent panic were believed to be significant factors that contributed to women's greater susceptibility to PTSD (Stuber et al. 2006).

Women also may have more difficulties accessing needed relief services or medical care following disaster. In addition, they may experience more difficult social and economic consequences during the postdisaster recovery period (Somasundaram and van de Put 2006). Because women are traditionally expected to care for people who are injured, ill, old, or young, all of whom may be suffering from high rates of psychiatric difficulties, women may have a higher emotional burden, which can be a significant stressor and may limit their ability to address personal needs. If men are injured, killed, or involved in rescue and recovery efforts, women may be forced to take on the dual role of primary caretaker and head of the household/main source of income, which in addition to being a greater burden, may be unfamiliar or even socially unacceptable in certain cultures (Somasundaram and van de Put 2006).

Finally, sometimes after a disaster, women are increasingly targeted as victims of violence, including sexual assault and rape. This is particularly true when disasters occur in areas stricken by combat or war. Too often, rape victims are stigmatized, and women may additionally suffer from either the stigma of rape or the necessity to hide the fact that they were sexually assaulted, which may prevent them from accessing treatment if it is available (Disaster Psychiatry Outreach 2008; Lorch and Mendenhall 2000). Because most victims have not reported or addressed these issues in treatment, and a history of previous sexual assault will increase the risk of postdisaster difficulties, the importance of screening for previous history of sexual assault or rape must be emphasized.

Psychiatrists should establish rapport before screening for a history of sexual assault. It may be helpful to avoid charged words such as *rape*. The U.S. Department of Veterans Affairs recommends asking every woman at a health screening or mental health screening two general screening questions, intended to use nonjudgmental wording: "Did you ever experience unwanted sexual attention, like verbal remarks, touching, or pressure for sexual favors? Did anyone ever use force or the threat of force to have sex with you against your will?" (Street and Stafford 2004, pp. 68–69). When asking such questions, the clinician should take care to assure privacy, which may be lacking in the disaster setting. If a positive answer is given, this revelation of sexual trauma should be acknowledged and addressed with care and empathy. Specifically, referral to address the sexual assault in addition to disaster stress should be strongly considered.

People With Physical Disabilities

Psychiatrists and other mental health professionals should consider people with physical disabilities as a group that is at risk of suffering disproportionately during and after a disaster. Although an extensive literature search has not yielded any data on rates of postdisaster stress-related symptoms or psychiatric disorders in this population, it can be expected that the risk of both medical and psychiatric difficulties is high. However, as with other vulnerable populations, such as the elderly or children, planning that addresses these needs may mitigate the risks.

To date, emergency preparedness planning and research regarding vulnerable populations has focused on other aspects of vulnerability, such as age, gender, ethnocultural characteristics, or chronic psychiatric disabilities, and people with physical disability due to special health care needs have been overlooked. However, more than 23 million U.S. residents (approximately 12% of the population ages 16–64 years) have special health care needs due to disability (U.S. Census 2006).

In the wake of Hurricanes Katrina and Rita, vulnerable people with special health care needs 1) were left stranded because evacuation teams could not get to them, did not know where they were, or were unaware that they needed help with transportation (or else evacuation vehicles did not have the necessary equipment—e.g., motorized wheelchair, oxygen, or ventilator—to address their specific needs); 2) were refused shelter because workers were unfamiliar with, unprepared for, or unable to address their specific health care needs; and 3) were unable to gain access to emergency services due their preexisting health conditions (National Council on Disability 2006; Nick et al. 2009). People with visual or hearing disabilities were not able to obtain critical information because communication systems, in violation of federal law, did not address these needs. The National Council on Disability (2006) concluded that people with disabilities were disproportionately affected by the hurricanes because their needs were too often either overlooked or completely disregarded. The organization cited examples of nationally known charitable agencies publicly stating that they would not or could not help people with certain physical disabilities (e.g., paraplegia, quadriplegia). Although some shelters were designed to assist persons with special medical or nursing care needs, the number of spaces available was woefully inadequate, and these shelters were inaccessible to most in need.

In an effort to address the gaps in disaster preparedness for people with special health care needs in the Boston area, over 800 community-based organizations and leaders in emergency management, public safety, public health and health care, and academia participated in a symposium (Nick et al. 2009). They identified three themes of concern, presented in Table 6–2. They recommended increased collaboration by community-based organizations, emergency management organizations, and public health agencies to conduct a comprehensive needs assessment; develop and implement education and training, including tabletop exercises and drills; foster cooperative working relationships immediately, not just in an emergency; and develop continuity plans to prepare staff before an emergency occurs (Nick et al. 2009).

Ethnocultural Issues

Responders to a disaster should remain mindful that disasters are events that can be integrative, divisive, or both to a community. If psychiatrists

---

TABLE 6–2.   Areas of concern for disaster survivors with special health care needs

Risk communications—need for a diverse range of communication modalities tailored to specific disabilities and needs in populations of concern (e.g., visual communications for those with hearing deficits)

Evacuation decisions and procedures—burdens placed on people with special health care needs and their families/caregivers; confusion regarding privacy regulations and sharing of privileged health information in a crisis; need for evacuation routes and transportation services to account for the varying navigation abilities of persons with special health care needs

Continuity of services—provision of necessities (e.g., food, water, and medication) during emergencies; recommendations that community-based organizations train volunteers to facilitate individual preparedness by developing kits with specific individual information (e.g., about medical conditions, allergies, medications, and emergency contacts)

Source.   Adapted from Nick et al. 2009.

---

wish to be effective in helping those affected by disasters, then they must have some understanding and appreciation of how those directly affected by the disaster perceive and understand the following: the event itself, the meaning of distress and seeking or accepting of assistance, their needs as a result of the event, and the helpers or responders to the event. In a comprehensive overview and discussion of cultural issues, Marsella and Christopher (2004) define culture as "shared, learned behaviors and meanings that are transmitted socially, often across generations, for purposes of sustaining or promoting adaptation, adjustment, and development" (p. 529). They point out that culture has external representations, such as artifacts, roles, and institutions, and internal representations, such as values, attitudes and beliefs, and patterns of consciousness. They also discuss how culture becomes a template for reality among different groups of people, or "bifocals" through which a disaster and postdisaster events and interactions are seen and experienced.

One aspect of disasters is that each one results in a complex mixing of cultures, including victims, the local community, and outside responders, and that therefore an evolving and temporary disaster culture is created. When varying cultures converge, this disaster culture can be a source of support or a source of stress that can undo the good intentions of disaster responders. Awareness of cultural differences may reduce this stress and enhance a responder's effectiveness (Marsella and Christopher 2004).

When examining cultural variations, one should consider both quantitative and qualitative differences (Disaster Psychiatry Outreach 2008).

Quantitative differences refers to the understanding that different minority or cultural groups are at varying risk for poor outcomes after a disaster. *Qualitative differences* refers to the idea that minority or cultural groups may respond differently to a disaster. Different groups may apply different understanding or meaning to the event itself, experience different symptoms or signs of distress, and react differently to helpers, particularly outsiders who respond to the event. In addition, acculturative stress (uneasiness that develops when a person of one culture encounters another culture) may have a significant influence on postdisaster outcomes (Disaster Psychiatry Outreach 2008; Marsella and Christopher 2004).

The following are some important observations regarding quantitative differences in PTSD or other adverse outcomes after disaster:

- Several studies have found that Hispanic groups fare worse than African Americans, who fare worse than whites (Neria et al. 2008). Reasons for differences include both differential exposure and differential vulnerabilities.
- Variations within a culture or group that may be mistakenly seen as homogeneous are often present. In addition, varied symptom patterns may be observed. For example, after Hurricane Andrew, English-preferring Latinos experienced lower rates of posttraumatic stress than did Spanish-preferring Latinos. In addition, more intrusive symptoms were seen in Spanish-preferring groups (Perilla et al. 2002).
- Depression, PTSD, and anxiety disorders are common across cultures and ethnicities after disaster. However, significant variations exist in symptoms and how distress or disorders are identified. For example, ethnic minorities often present with more somatic complaints and may have familial or cultural beliefs that can be mistaken for delusions (Marsella and Christopher 2004).

There are various ways that qualitative differences contribute to cultural variations after a disaster. Some minority groups may place different meanings on an event compared with nonminority groups. For example, Latino cultures, including less acculturated Latino groups in North America, tend to view events with a high degree of fatalism (belief in an external control). On the other hand, non-Hispanic Western cultures tend to believe in instrumentalism, a belief system whereby the individual is considered responsible for both the occurrence of significant events and the recovery from such events (Disaster Psychiatry Outreach 2008; Marsella and Christopher 2004).

There are important differences between domestic minorities and foreign cultures in their reactions to disasters. For domestic minorities, the degree of acculturation may have more influence on outcomes (less acculturated individuals having more difficulties), whereas in foreign cultures, sociopolitical factors, government and medical structures, and access to and quality of care are more significant. Although disasters, particularly natural disasters, do not discriminate, persons who reside in poor countries are at increased risk for suffering from severe adversities after a disaster. The devastation seen after the recent earthquake in Haiti underscores this point (Disaster Psychiatry Outreach 2008; Marsella and Christopher 2004).

Lower socioeconomic status itself is a significant risk factor for death or other adverse outcomes following disaster. In an article about poverty and disasters, McMahon (2007) discusses several relevant factors:

- *Geography and environment*—Economically disadvantaged people disproportionately live in more vulnerable areas, such as low-lying land impacted by tsunamis or floods.
- *Limited personal resources*—Economically disadvantaged people lack emergency supplies, means or transportation to evacuate, and insurance/funds or other means to repair or rebuild.
- *Infrastructure*—Inexpensive construction is often more vulnerable to damage or destruction. Roads, bridges, utilities and telecommunications, hospitals, and other public services or institutions that are often inadequate predisaster are more vulnerable to damage or destruction, and resources for repair are often lacking. Health and mental health resources may be unavailable or inadequate.
- *Political instability*—Many poor countries are politically unstable, at war, or at risk for war, which often leads to displacement into camps or communities where work and resources are scarce, leaving many vulnerable to victimization and with no route to leave the impoverished area.

In responding to disaster, a psychiatrist should first learn about the culture or cultures found at the location of the event, including the ways that people within each culture may view the disaster or traumatic event, possible historical animosities between his or her own culture and that of the victims, the people's perceptions of symptoms and the meaning of distress, and the way they feel about asking for help or accepting assistance. An understanding of variations in help-seeking behaviors, the issue of humiliation and embarrassment, and feelings about loss of face is critical. A lack of understanding can lead to further harm of victims, and to frustration or demoralization in disaster workers themselves. Partnering with local people or others who are familiar with the culture (i.e., "culture brokers" or "cultural ambassadors," or indigenous healers) and, when possible, incorporating local healing rituals, religious ceremonies or practices, and community traditions can improve chances of success (Disaster Psychiatry Outreach 2008; Marsella and Christopher 2004). With individuals, the intent of PFA is to help victims by using and building on their natural strengths. The same goal is necessary when helping a community.

An awareness of culture-bound syndromes may be helpful for the mental health professional who responds to disaster. In DSM-IV-TR, *culture-bound syndromes* is defined as "recurrent, locality-specific patterns of aberrant behavior and troubling experience that may or may not be linked to a particular DSM-IV diagnostic category" (American Psychiatric Association 2000, p. 898). Many of these syndromes have local names and are seen as medical illnesses or may be seen as nonpathological by local people. Although culture-bound syndromes may originate in a specific locale and culture, they may be seen within cultures or groups that have relocated within Western or industrialized areas. Examples from Latino culture include *ataque de nervios* (a term for distress whose symptoms may include uncontrollable shouting, crying, trembling, dissociative episodes, fainting, aggression, and suicide attempts), which often occurs after a catastrophic event to a family member, and *susto* (a term meaning "fright" or "soul loss"), which is believed to be caused by a frightening event that causes the soul to leave the body; can result in sadness, nightmares, amotivation, and generalized somatic complaints; and is sometimes believed to result in death. Several other examples from around the globe are described in Appendix I ("Outline for Cultural Formulation and Glossary of Culture-Bound Syndromes") of DSM-IV-TR.

It is impossible to anticipate all cultures and ethnocultural issues that a psychiatrist may encounter when responding to a disaster. However, disaster responders must have an approach or mindset that remains sensitive to the needs of those who are impacted by disaster, particularly in light of ethnocultural differences that may have a significant impact on how survivors respond to the event over the short and long terms. Giger and Davidhizar's (1999) transcultural assessment and intervention model, a commonly cited framework for addressing cultural issues in health care, has been adapted and applied to disaster counseling (U.S. Department of Health and Human Services 2003). Their model was originally developed to assist in the provision of transcultural nursing care. It is currently used by several other health and human services professions. The model identifies five issues that can affect the interactions of providers and service recipients. These issues, adapted in Table 6–3 to apply to disaster crisis counseling, illustrate the importance of acknowledging culture and of respecting diversity. A complete description of the model can be found in *Transcultural Nursing: Assessment and Intervention* (Giger and Davidhizar 1999).

TABLE 6–3. Important considerations when interacting with people of other cultures

Communication	Both verbal and nonverbal communication can be barriers to providing effective disaster crisis counseling when survivors and workers are from different cultures. Culture influences how many people express their feelings, as well as what feelings are appropriate to express, in a given situation. The inability to communicate can make both parties feel alienated and helpless.
Personal space	"Personal space" is the area that immediately surrounds a person, including the objects within that space. Although spatial requirements may vary from person to person, they tend to be similar among people in a given cultural group (Watson 1980). A person from one subculture might touch or move closer to another as a friendly gesture, whereas someone from a different culture might consider such behavior invasive. Disaster crisis counselors must look for clues to a survivor's need for space. Such clues may include, for example, moving the chair back or stepping closer.
Social organization	Beliefs, values, and attitudes are learned and reinforced through social organizations, such as family, kinships, tribes, and political, economic, and religious groups. Understanding these influences will enable the disaster crisis counselor to more accurately assess a survivor's reaction to disaster. A survivor's answers to seemingly trivial questions about hobbies and social activities can lead to insight into his or her life before the disaster.
Time	An understanding of how people from different cultures view time can help avoid misunderstandings and miscommunication. In addition to having different interpretations of the overall concept of time, members of different cultures view "clock time"—that is, intervals and specific durations—differently. Social time may be measured in terms of "dinner time," "worship time," and "harvest time." Time perceptions may be altered during a disaster. Crisis counselors acting with a sense of urgency may be tempted to set time frames that are not meaningful or realistic to a survivor. The result may be frustration for both parties.
Environmental control	A belief that events occur because of some external factor—luck, chance, fate, will of God, or the control of others—may affect the way in which a survivor responds to disaster and the types of assistance needed. Survivors who feel that events and recovery are out of their control may be pessimistic regarding counseling efforts. In contrast, individuals who perceive that their own behavior can affect events may be more willing to act (Rotter 1966). Disaster crisis counselors need to understand beliefs related to environmental control because such beliefs will affect survivors' behavior.

Source. U.S. Department of Health and Human Services 2003.

Conclusion

Certain groups or special populations are particularly vulnerable to difficulties in the aftermath of disaster. Effective postdisaster assistance and treatment must take into account the needs of these various groups. Although most children will recover, clinicians need to adjust PFA, screening, and interventions to be able to assist children and their families in a child- and family-friendly fashion, and should keep in mind that children generally fare as well or as poorly as do their parents or family system. For several reasons, women are more vulnerable than men to postdisaster difficulties, including having increased rates of PTSD and depression, and increased risk of victimization. Despite debates regarding whether elderly persons are at increased or decreased risk after a disaster, several factors, including comorbid medical problems, separation from families or social supports, potential cognitive decline, and mobility problems, need to be considered because there are subsets of elderly with several of these risk factors. Similarly, people with physical disabilities may face postdisaster difficulties with receiving communication updates, mobility difficulties and evacuation challenges, and need for continuity of critical medical services that may be disrupted in the postdisaster setting. Finally, people from various cultures or ethnic backgrounds may present with different symptom patterns and may have different perspectives on the disaster itself, on signs or symptoms of distress that they may be experiencing, and about those who have responded to assist them. Therefore, psychiatrists must remain mindful of the needs of special populations and approach those in need of assistance with tremendous care and flexibility.

■ Teaching Points

- Common problems in children during the acute period following a disaster include regression; separation anxiety; fears for the safety of parents, siblings, or themselves; impulsivity; and occasionally aggression. Psychiatrists are advised to use caution in diagnosing behavioral disorders in children during this time period.

- During the acute phase period, elderly persons are at increased risk for memory problems, which may be reversible and not a sign of dementia.

- Factors that increase risks for elderly persons in the postdisaster period include preexisting psychiatric and medical illness, mobility difficulties, separation or distance from family and natural supports, and cognitive or sensory impairments.

- Psychiatrists should be mindful of the fact that women are at increased risk for victimization, including sexual assault, after a disaster.
- People with special health care needs due to physical disability may face difficulties in receiving emergency communications; evacuating; and accessing postdisaster supports and treatment, including treatment for preexisting conditions.
- To help people from different ethnic or cultural backgrounds, the psychiatrist must understand how they may view the event itself, how they may view or express distress, and how they perceive helpers or responders, particularly when they are coming from another country or culture.
- Psychiatrists should keep in mind that there are varying vulnerabilities to trauma and loss even within the same culture or ethnic group. They should be careful to avoid making or acting on assumptions that could result in further harm to those already affected by a disaster.
- The best way to understand how someone from a vulnerable group views an event is to ask and to listen to their response.

Review Questions

6.1 Which of the following statements regarding postdisaster difficulties among children and adolescents is *true*?

A. Children generally fare worse than their parents after a disaster.
B. Illicit substance use is uncommon in adolescents.
C. Common problems observed in school-age children include somatic complaints, regression, and school refusal.
D. When evaluating children, a psychiatrist does not need a parent's permission or observation.
E. Children rarely worry about their parents or siblings after a disaster.

6.2 Variables found to be associated with worse postdisaster outcomes in children include all of the following *except*

A. Loss of a family member.
B. Serious injury.
C. Direct exposure to the event.
D. Male gender.
E. Younger age.

6.3   Factors that may contribute to the increased vulnerability of women in the aftermath of disaster include all of the following *except*

   A.   Higher rates of predisaster depression and anxiety.
   B.   Increased burden associated with the traditional expectations of the caretaker role.
   C.   Difficulties accessing postdisaster supports and medical care.
   D.   Low risk of violence or sexual assault in the postdisaster period.
   E.   More difficult economic consequences after a disaster.

6.4   Which of the following statements regarding cultural variations in response to disasters is generally *true?*

   A.   African Americans generally fare worse than Hispanic Americans after disasters.
   B.   Responses to a disaster are fairly homogeneous within a specific culture.
   C.   Less acculturated minorities generally experience fewer postdisaster difficulties.
   D.   Postdisaster assistance that includes partnerships with community "culture brokers" and incorporation of local healing rituals is more likely to worsen outcomes than to improve them.
   E.   Posttraumatic stress disorder, depression, and anxiety are common consequences of disasters across cultures and ethnicities.

6.5   Psychiatric evaluation of the elderly after disaster should include screening for

   A.   Medical illness.
   B.   Sensory and mobility deficits.
   C.   Availability of family or other social supports.
   D.   Medications.
   E.   All of the above.

References

Aldrich N, Benson WF: Disaster preparedness and the chronic disease needs of vulnerable older adults. Prev Chronic Dis 5:1–7, 2008. Available at: http://www.cdc.gov/pcd//issues/2008/jan/07_0135.htm. Accessed March 19, 2010.

American Psychiatric Association: Diagnostic and Statistical Manual of Mental Disorders, 4th Edition, Text Revision. Washington, DC, American Psychiatric Association, 2000

Conwell Y: Suicide prevention in later life: a glass half full or a glass half empty. Am J Psychiatry 166:845–848, 2009

Cook A, Blaustein M, Spinazzola J, et al (eds): Complex Trauma in Children and Adolescents: White Paper From the National Child Traumatic Stress Network Complex Trauma Task Force. Los Angeles, CA, National Child Traumatic Stress Network, 2003. Available at: http://www.nctsnet.org/nccts/nav.do?pid=typ_ct. Accessed March 3, 2010.

Cook A, Spinazzola J, Ford J, et al: Complex trauma in children and adolescents. Psychiatr Ann 35:390–398, 2005

Disaster Psychiatry Outreach: The Essentials of Disaster Psychiatry: A Training Course for Mental Health Professionals (Course Syllabus). New York, Disaster Psychiatry Outreach, 2008. Available as DPOCourseSyllabus_052108.pdf at: https://sites.google.com/a/disasterpsych.org/blog/File-Cabinet. Accessed December 28, 2009.

Frans O, Rimmö PA, Aberg L, et al: Trauma exposure and post-traumatic stress disorder in the general population. Acta Psychiatr Scand 111:291–299, 2005

Galea S, Tracy M, Norris F, et al: Financial and social circumstances and the incidence and course of PTSD in Mississippi during the first two years after Hurricane Katrina. J Trauma Stress 21:357–368, 2008

Giger JN, Davidhizar RE: Transcultural Nursing: Assessment and Intervention, 3rd Edition. St. Louis, MO, CV Mosby, 1999

Hoven CW, Duarte SD, Mandell DJ: Children's mental health after disasters: the impact of the World Trade Center Attack. Curr Psychiatry Rep 5:101–107, 2003

Hoven CW, Duarte CS, Lucas CP, et al: Psychopathology among New York City public school children 6 months after September 11. Arch Gen Psychiatry 62:545–552, 2005

Jellinek MS, Murphy JM: Pediatric Symptom Checklist for Screening of Psychiatric Disorders in Children. Boston, Massachusetts General Hospital, 2003. Available at: http://psc.partners.org/psc_english.PDF. Accessed March 16, 2010.

Lorch D, Mendenhall P: A war's hidden tragedy. Newsweek 136:35–37, 2000

Marsella AJ, Christopher MA: Ethnocultural considerations in disasters: an overview of research, issues and directions. Psychiatr Clin North Am 27:521–539, 2004

McMahon M: Disasters and poverty. Disaster Manag Response 4:9–75, 2007

Nasreddine ZS, Phillips NA, Bedirian V, et al: The Montreal Cognitive Assessment, MoCA: a brief screening tool for mild cognitive impairment. J Am Geriatr Soc 53:695–699, 2005. Available at: http://www.mocatest.org/default.asp. Accessed March 19, 2010.

National Council on Disability: The Impact of Hurricanes Katrina and Rita on People With Disabilities: A Look Back and Remaining Challenges. Washington, DC, National Council on Disability, 2006. Available at: http://www.ncd.gov/newsroom/publications/2006/pdf/hurricanes_impact.pdf. Accessed March 20, 2009.

Neria Y, Nandi A, Galea S: Post-traumatic stress disorder following disasters: a systematic review. Psychol Med 38:467–480, 2008

Nick GA, Savioa E, Elqura L et al: Emergency preparedness for vulnerable populations: people with special health-care needs. Public Health Rep 124:338–343,
2009

Norris F, Friedman MJ, Watson PJ, et al: 60,000 disaster victims speak, part I: an
empirical review of the empirical literature, 1981–2001. Psychiatry 65:207–
239, 2002a

Norris F, Friedman M, Watson P: 60,000 disaster victims speak, part II: summary
and implications of the disaster mental health research. Psychiatry 65:240–260,
2002b

Perilla JP, Norris FH, Lavizzo EA: Ethnicity, culture and disaster response: identifying and explaining ethnic differences in PTSD six months after Hurricane Andrew. J Soc Clin Psychol 21:20–45, 2002

Rotter JB: Generalized expectancies for internal versus external control of reinforcement. Psychological Monographs 80(1):1–28, 1966

Sakauye KM, Streiam JE, Kennedy GJ, et al: American Association of Geriatric Psychiatry position statement: disaster preparedness for older Americans: critical issues for the preservation of mental health. Am J Geriatr Psychiatry 17:916–
924, 2009

Schreiber M, Gurwitch R: Listen, Protect, and Connect—Model and Teach: Psychological First Aid for Students and Teachers. Washington, DC, Ready Campaign, 2006a. Available at: http://www.ready.gov/kids/_downloads/PFA_
SchoolCrisis.pdf. Accessed March 19, 2010.

Schreiber M, Gurwitch R: Listen, Protect, and Connect: Psychological First Aid for
Children and Parents. Washington, DC, Ready Campaign, 2006b. Available at:
http://www.ready.gov/kids/_downloads/PFA_Parents.pdf. Accessed March
19, 2010.

Somasundaram DJ, van de Put WACM: Management of trauma in special populations after disaster. J Clin Psychiatry 7 (suppl):64–73, 2006

Street A, Stafford J: Military sexual trauma: issues in caring for veterans, in Iraq War
Clinician Guide, 2nd Edition. Washington, DC, National Center for PTSD and
Walter Reed Army Medical Center, 2004, pp 66–70. Available at: http://www.
ptsd.va.gov/professional/manuals/manual-pdf/iwcgiraq_clinician_guide_v2.
pdf. Accessed August 29, 2009.

Stuber J, Resnick H, Galea S: Gender disparities in post-traumatic stress disorder after mass trauma. Gend Med 3:54–67, 2006

Tracy M, Galea S: Post-traumatic stress disorder and depression among older adults
after a disaster: the role of ongoing trauma and stressors. Public Policy Aging
Rep 16:16–19, 2006

U.S. Department of Health and Human Services: Developing Cultural Competence
in Disaster Mental Health Programs: Guiding Principles and Recommendations
(DHHS Publ No SMA 3828). Rockville, MD, Center for Mental Health Services, Substance Abuse and Mental Health Services Administration, 2003

Watson OM: Proxemic Behavior: A Cross-Cultural Study. The Hague, The Netherlands, Mouton, 1980

7

Serious Mental Illness

Anand Pandya, M.D.

Mr. B, a 35-year-old man who lived in New Orleans prior to Hurricane Katrina, has schizophrenia but is fortunate because he has a supportive family that helps him get to appointments, ensures that he gets his medication from the pharmacy, and pays for a small apartment to prevent him from becoming homeless. These supports were insufficient, however, when the notice for evacuation came shortly before the hurricane. Although Mr. B did not have the gross disorganization or persecutory delusions that could interfere with his ability to comprehend or believe that a hurricane was coming, he did have negative symptoms that made him reluctant to answer the telephone or door. Although his parents could generally overcome this barrier on weekends when they would check that he had enough food and reloaded his pillbox, they sometimes spent several minutes talking to their son through the door before he would build up enough trust to let them in. While preparing for their own evacuation, the family had very little time to go to Mr. B's apartment and coax him into evacuating. Mr. B's rigid thought process and his chronic ambivalence ate up much of the remaining time and, in frustration, the family realized that they would need to activate the local mental health system to force him to leave his apartment. Unfortunately, they were unable to get a quick enough response from Mr. B's case manager, and the emergency management services that would usually take Mr. B to the hospital when necessary had other priorities. Even if available, their ambulance service was intended to transport individuals the short distance to the nearest emergency department, not to take someone against their will all the way to a different town. Eventually, his family had to leave Mr. B behind.

Although Mr. B survived the flooding, he had no way to get food, and when his family was finally able to get disaster responders to check on him, they took food to Mr. B but could not find an open pharmacy for many miles to obtain his medication. The collective stress finally led Mr. B to get increasingly perseverative and agitated. The relief workers knew that he needed to be taken to treatment—against his will, if necessary. But where could they take him, with the clinics closed and the hospitals focused on the physically ill?

111

As this vignette shows, individuals with serious mental illness (SMI) are at increased risk for exposure to trauma in disasters because they may not be adequately responsive to predisaster public health interventions that can reduce risk. This decreased responsiveness could be a direct result of symptoms or an indirect effect of stigma that results in greater impoverishment and social isolation.

Many psychiatrists, when they think of disaster psychiatry, may exclusively envision the need to treat survivors and first responders for posttraumatic stress disorder (PTSD) and bereavement; however, the treatment of serious mental illnesses, such as schizophrenia and bipolar disorder, can also be necessary. Disasters are associated with new onsets of PTSD as well as other anxiety and depressive disorders (Pandya 2009). The evaluation and treatment of patients with these disorders are covered in many of this volume's chapters, including Chapter 5, "Psychiatric Evaluation," which opens the current section on evaluation, as well as the psychopharmacology and psychotherapy chapters in Part III, "Intervention." Because consideration of these disorders is important, I use "SMI" in this chapter to refer to SMIs other than anxiety disorders (including PTSD) and major depressive disorder, despite the fact that anxiety and depressive disorders are often referred to as SMIs in the disaster mental health literature (Kessler et al. 2008; Staugh 2009).

Broadly speaking, the postdisaster care of individuals with predisaster SMIs can be divided into the treatment of the predisaster SMI and the treatment of new diagnoses that are a consequence of the disaster. In Mr. B's case, introduced above, a psychiatrist or other mental health professional would want to consider how to treat Mr. B's schizophrenia in the chaos after the hurricane and to screen him for PTSD, depression, and other anxiety disorders that may have developed as a consequence of the hurricane. Although most psychiatrists and other mental health professionals will be familiar with the standard treatment of SMIs, disaster psychiatrists should be aware of the effect of the disaster on the course of SMIs and the systems issues that can complicate the treatment of SMIs.

Pathways to Postdisaster Decompensation of Serious Mental Illness

Despite the lack of literature to suggest that disasters cause the new onset of SMIs other than major depressive disorder, PTSD, and some other anxiety disorders, several studies have looked at the impact of disasters on those with preexisting SMI. Although findings have varied, studies suggest that at least some individuals with SMI are at risk for worsening of their symptoms (Staugh 2009; Tseng et al. 2010).

After a disaster, individuals with SMI may be at risk for a variety of disruptions that are associated with increased risk for decompensation. These may include decreased availability of medication; disruption of psychiatric care; and loss of psychosocial supports, including traditional supports such as friends and family who may be separated after a disaster as well as targeted psychosocial support for this population, such as local affiliates of the National Alliance on Mental Illness, case management services, support groups, and clubhouses. Furthermore, individuals with bipolar disorder may be especially vulnerable to disruption of sleep cycles, which can lead to decompensation. This disruption can extend beyond the impact phase for those individuals with SMI who are placed in shelters or become involved in disaster response. As with the general population, it is normal for individuals with SMI to want to help with the disaster response. The psychiatrists of Disaster Psychiatry Outreach have encountered many individuals with SMI among first responders and have been called upon to treat many such responders. The culture of first responders poses a variety of challenges for individuals with SMI. They may be pressured to engage in long hours of stressful work that does not encourage self-care. First responders also may engage in coping strategies that are especially problematic for individuals with SMI, such as bonding with other responders while drinking alcohol at the end of the day. Finally, it should be noted that a study of hospitalized psychiatric patients at Bellevue Hospital after the 9/11 attacks suggested that individuals with schizophrenia spectrum disorders fared worse after a disaster than individuals with affective spectrum disorders (DeLisi et al. 2004).

New Diagnoses After a Disaster

Despite a study after the Three Mile Island accident, in which Bromet et al. (1982) reported that psychiatric patients may not be more distressed by a disaster than the general population, a body of more recent work supports greater vulnerability after a disaster for individuals with SMI. As noted in Chapter 5, "Psychiatric Evaluation," PTSD and major depressive disorder are the two most common new-onset diagnoses after a disaster. In this chapter, I do not focus on the treatment of depression based on the assumption that it is one of the most commonly treated psychiatric diagnoses and is treated routinely when it is a comorbid diagnosis with another SMI.

PTSD, however, is underdiagnosed in people with SMI (Mueser et al. 1998). Aside from having higher rates of PTSD, individuals with SMI also have high rates of some of the risk factors for developing PTSD after a disaster, including high rates of past-year victimization (Teplin et al. 2005), substance-related diagnoses (Jané-Llopis and Matytsina 2006), and lifetime trauma (Mueser et al. 1998). A variety of beliefs have been identified that contribute to the underrecognition and undertreatment of PTSD in this population, including beliefs that a focus on trauma conflicts with the treatment of other diagnoses that should take precedence (Cusack et al. 2007). However, some of this underdiagnosis may also result from the similarity between some symptoms of PTSD and symptoms of SMI (Pandya and Weiden 2001). For example, numbing and avoiding symptoms, such as the markedly diminished interest or participation in activities and the restricted range of affect, may be misinterpreted as symptoms of depression or the negative symptoms of schizophrenia; some hypervigilance symptoms, such as irritability or outbursts of anger, may be misinterpreted as signs of mania if a clinician does not focus sufficiently on the longitudinal course; and signs and symptoms such as hypervigilance and reexperiencing phenomena may be written off simply as psychosis. Table 7–1 provides a comparison of similar symptoms in PTSD, schizophrenia, and depression.

Systems Interventions

Optimally, disaster psychiatrists need to ensure that there is a focused strategy to provide effective risk communication to individuals with SMI in case of a future disaster. Important issues to consider include impoverishment (e.g., What media is effective in communicating to a population that may or may not have regular access to a television, radio, or computer?), social isolation associated with SMI (e.g., Where will the disaster psychiatrist go to have a dialogue with a population that may not be well connected to neighbors or neighborhood institutions?), mobility, and medical comorbidities associated with SMI (e.g., How will the disaster psychiatrist ensure timely communication about the need to evacuate or to get supplies when individuals with SMI also have metabolic syndrome, diabetes, tardive dyskinesia, or cardiac disease that may greatly slow their ability to leave their homes?). To be effective, this predisaster planning should include individuals from this target population (National Council on Disability 2006). Although this planning may seem unrealistic to some psychiatrists, consumer input has been incorporated into the planning and monitoring of a variety of services for adults with SMI in a variety of states (Aron et al. 2009). At this time, individuals with SMI are less prepared for disasters than the general public, even when one controls for sociodemographic variables and general health (Eisenman et al. 2009).

Disaster psychiatrists also need to plan for a full range of nonpsychiatric as well as psychiatric services that target individuals with SMI. The plan must address disruptions to family and community supports, the loss of targeted psychosocial services, and such fundamental issues as shelter and

TABLE 7–1. Comparison of common symptom presentations in PTSD, schizophrenia, and depression

Symptom type	PTSD	Schizophrenia	Depression
Reexperiencing	Intrusive recollections	Perseveration	Ruminations
	Distressing dreams and flashbacks	Hallucinations, delusions	SSRI-induced vivid dreams
	Intense distress about cues that symbolize or resemble the trauma	Referentiality, paranoia	Depressed mood
Numbing and avoidance	Avoiding thoughts, feelings, activities, places, people	Alogia, paranoia, disorganized speech, disorganized behavior	Paucity of speech, decreased concentration, anhedonia, comorbid anxiety
	Inability to recall important aspects of the trauma	Disorganized speech	Pseudodementia
	Diminished interest in activities, feelings of detachment and estrangement	Avolition, paranoid avoidance	Anhedonia
	Restricted range of affect	Negative symptoms (flat affect), antipsychotic-induced	Constricted affect
	Foreshortened sense of future	Parkinsonism	Hopelessness, suicidality
Hyperarousal	Difficulty falling or staying asleep	Paranoia, antipsychotic-induced akathisia	Insomnia, usually early morning awakening
	Irritability	Inappropriate affect, paranoia	Dysphoria, agitated depression
	Difficulty concentrating	Cognitive impairment, distraction from positive symptoms	Impaired concentration
	Hypervigilance and exaggerated startle response	Paranoia	

Note. PTSD=posttraumatic stress disorder; SSRI=selective serotonin reuptake inhibitor.

Source. Reprinted from Pandya A, Weiden PJ: "Trauma and Disaster in Psychiatrically Vulnerable Populations." *Journal of Psychiatric Practice* 7:426–431, 2001. Copyright © 2001, Wolters Kluwer Health. Used with permission.

evacuation (National Council on Disability 2006). At the most basic level, psychiatrists need to ensure the continuity of psychiatric care, including medication. One relatively simple approach is to set up a psychiatric clinic in a location that is easy to access for disaster survivors. A more comprehensive approach might include assisting predisaster providers to systematically follow up on their patients to ensure that they receive continuity of care. Although ensuring shelter for individuals with SMI may seem to be such a fundamental issue that a psychiatrist may be inclined to assume that it will be managed by agencies such as the Red Cross, it is unfortunately the case that individuals with SMI were excluded from some shelters after Hurricane Katrina (National Council on Disability 2006).

Individual Evaluation and Treatment

The evaluation of individuals with SMI during the acute phase is essentially the same as that for the general population, covered in Chapter 5, "Psychiatric Evaluation." This procedure includes taking a detailed history of the patient's experience during the trauma. Although the clinician must remain attuned to signs that an individual does not want to discuss this issue, it is incorrect to presume that asking about a trauma will lead to a decompensation of the individual's more apparent SMI (Cusack et al. 2007). In situations where disaster survivors are evacuated, psychiatrists should inquire whether patients still have their medication (National Council on Disability 2006). Because many individuals with SMI in the United States are covered by Medicaid, which is a state-based program, individuals who are displaced across state lines may have a more difficult time getting prescriptions filled.

As noted in Chapter 14, "Psychotherapies," cognitive-behavioral therapy (CBT) has been studied extensively in the treatment of PTSD, but much less research has been done on the use of CBT in individuals with SMI. Preliminary data (Frueh et al. 2009; Mueser et al. 2007; Rosenberg et al. 2001), including one randomized controlled trial (Mueser et al. 2008), suggest that a variety of cognitive-behavioral techniques can be adapted for the treatment of PTSD in individuals with SMI. These techniques have been employed in both individual and group settings. The interventions described in the literature all lasted 12 weeks or longer. Education about PTSD was included in all of these SMI groups, and most interventions included homework. Completion of homework was predictive of response (Mueser et al. 2008). Other CBT strategies that have been described for the treatment of PTSD in individuals with SMI include breathing techniques, cognitive restructuring (Mueser et al. 2007), and exposure therapy (Frueh et al. 2009). Clinicians experienced in the treatment of this population have suggested that CBT for treatment of PTSD in individuals with SMI requires particular attention to the development of trust and rapport before therapy, a focus on safety plans before the exposure component of therapy, and an awareness of the cognitive deficits that may limit the effectiveness of CBT (Frueh et al. 2006).

Conclusion

Although empirical studies are limited, there is a strong theoretical basis for believing that individuals with SMI are at elevated risk for worsening of their predisaster diagnoses and for developing postdisaster PTSD. This includes evidence that they are less prepared for disasters and that they have high rates of predisaster trauma and PTSD, as well as experiences after Hurricane Katrina in which the disaster response community did not adequately consider issues such as housing for this population. The few studies of treatment for PTSD in people with SMI suggest that CBT techniques such as exposure therapy and breathing techniques can be adapted to this population, in a context of an adequate therapeutic alliance. As with other populations, expectations of the efficacy of CBT will need to be adjusted when cognitive deficits are present. Despite these caveats, disaster psychiatrists may be able to have a substantial impact, given that PTSD is generally overlooked and undertreated in this population.

▮Teaching Points

- Individuals with SMI may be especially vulnerable to disasters because much predisaster planning does not consider their special needs. Disaster psychiatrists may need to advocate for such basic needs as shelter for this population.

- Disaster psychiatrists should ensure that individuals with SMI receive continuity of treatment by ensuring access to their medications and to psychosocial structure and support.

- Disaster psychiatrists may encounter individuals with SMI among both disaster survivors and disaster responders.

- Individuals with SMI have high rates of trauma and PTSD, independent of disasters. This high rate of trauma and PTSD is often not addressed by the existing mental health system.

- Exposure therapy may be effective for the treatment of PTSD in this population, with some minor alterations to attend to issues of trust, safety, and cognitive limitations.

Review Questions

7.1   Symptoms of PTSD can be mistaken for signs of

    A. Mania.
    B. Depression.
    C. Negative symptoms of schizophrenia.
    D. Positive symptoms of schizophrenia.
    E. All of the above.

7.2   Which of the following interventions is *least* helpful when working with individuals with SMI after a disaster?

    A. Advocating for special attention to this population's need for housing and evacuation.
    B. Reducing the risk of retraumatization by waiting for individuals with SMI to bring up the subject of their traumas.
    C. Minimizing sleep cycle changes.
    D. Assessing whether the patient has stopped prior medications.
    E. Reestablishing psychosocial supports.

7.3   Which of the following interventions has been best studied for the treatment of PTSD in individuals with SMI?

    A. Cognitive-behavioral therapy.
    B. Eye movement desensitization and reprocessing (EMDR).
    C. Psychological debriefing.
    D. Antipsychotic medications.
    E. Antidepressant medications.

7.4   Compared with the general population, individuals with SMI have

    A. Lower rates of trauma and lower rates of PTSD.
    B. Higher rates of trauma and higher rates of PTSD.
    C. Lower rates of trauma but higher rates of PTSD.
    D. Approximately the same rates of PTSD and trauma.
    E. Higher rates of trauma but lower rates of PTSD.

7.5   Which of the following statements regarding individuals with SMI is *true*?

    A. Studies show that they fare much better than the general population after a disaster.
    B. Studies show that their social isolation places them at lower risk for postdisaster victimization.
    C. They are less prepared for disasters than the general population.

D. They are usually treated simultaneously for PTSD and their other mental illness, although best practice suggests a stepwise approach.

E. None of the above.

References

Aron L, Honberg R, Duckworth K, et al: Grading the States 2009: A Report on America's Health Care System for Adults With Serious Mental Illness. Arlington, VA, National Alliance on Mental Illness, 2009

Bromet E, Schulberg HC, Dunn L: Reactions of psychiatric patients to the Three Mile Island nuclear accident. Arch Gen Psychiatry 39:725–730, 1982

Cusack KJ, Wells CB, Grubaugh AL, et al: An update on the South Carolina Trauma Initiative. Psychiatr Serv 58:708–710, 2007

DeLisi LE, Cohen TH, Maurizio AM: Hospitalized psychiatric patients view the World Trade Center disaster. Psychiatry Res 129:201–207, 2004

Eisenman DP, Zhou Q, Ong M, et al: Variations in disaster preparedness by mental health, perceived general health, and disability status. Disaster Med Public Health Prep 3:33–41, 2009

Frueh BC, Cusack KJ, Grubaugh AL, et al: Clinicians' perspectives on cognitive-behavioral treatment for PTSD among persons with severe mental illness. Psychiatr Serv 57:1027–1031, 2006

Frueh BC, Grubaugh AL, Cusack KJ, et al: Exposure-based cognitive-behavioral treatment of PTSD in adults with schizophrenia or schizoaffective disorder: a pilot study. J Anxiety Disord 23:665–675, 2009

Jané-Llopis E, Matytsina I: Mental health and alcohol, drugs and tobacco: a review of the comorbidity between mental disorders and the use of alcohol, tobacco and illicit drugs. Drug Alcohol Rev 25:515–536, 2006

Kessler RC, Galea S, Gruber MJ, et al: Trends in mental illness and suicidality after Hurricane Katrina. Mol Psychiatry 13:374–384, 2008

Mueser K, Goodman L, Trumbetta S, et al: Trauma and posttraumatic stress disorder in severe mental illness. J Consult Clin Psychol 66:493–499, 1998

Mueser K, Bolton E, Carty P, et al: The Trauma Recovery Group: a cognitive-behavioral program for post-traumatic stress disorder in persons with severe mental illness. Community Ment Health J 43:281–304, 2007

Mueser K, Rosenberg S, Xie H, et al: A randomized controlled trial of cognitive behavioral treatment of posttraumatic stress disorder in severe mental illness. J Consult Clin Psychol 76:259–271, 2008

National Council on Disability: The Needs of People with Psychiatric Disabilities During and After Hurricanes Katrina and Rita: Position Paper and Recommendations. Washington, DC, National Council on Disability, 2006

Pandya A: Adult disaster psychiatry. Focus 7:155–159, 2009

Pandya A, Weiden PJ: Trauma and disaster in psychiatrically vulnerable populations. J Psychiatr Pract 7:426–431, 2001

Rosenberg SD, Mueser KT, Friedman MJ, et al: Developing effective treatments for posttraumatic disorders among people with severe mental illness. Psychiatr Serv 52:1453–1461, 2001

Staugh LM: The effects of disaster on the mental health of individuals with disabilities, in Mental Health and Disasters. Edited by Neria Y, Galea S, Norris FH. New York, Cambridge University Press, 2009, pp 264–276

Teplin LA, McClelland GM, Abram KM, et al: Crime victimization in adults with severe mental illness: comparison with the National Crime Victimization Survey. Arch Gen Psychiatry 62:911–921, 2005

Tseng K-C, Hemenway D, Kawachi I, et al: The impact of the Chi-Chi earthquake on the incidence of hospitalizations for schizophrenia and on concomitant hospital choice. Community Ment Health J 46:93–101, 2010

8

Substance Abuse

David J. Mysels, M.D., M.B.A.
Maria A. Sullivan, M.D., Ph.D.
Frank G. Dowling, M.D.

Disasters are by their nature highly stressful and calamitous events. In the wake of a disaster, one may expect an exacerbation of psychopathology, including substance use disorders, in the affected population. To date, few studies have been carried out examining substance use patterns in the context of publicized recent disasters, and results are mixed concerning the impact of such events on substance abuse. Although several studies indicate that substance use does increase after disasters, other investigations fail to demonstrate this effect, or even suggest a protective effect associated with disasters for general population samples. However, certain factors appear to increase the probability of substance use among victims of disasters, including a prior history of substance use disorders and certain comorbid psychiatric conditions, such as posttraumatic stress disorder (PTSD), major depressive disorder (MDD), and panic attacks. Other risk factors include proximity to the disaster, young age, and loss of resources. In this chapter, we review the current literature regarding patterns of substance use risk among victims of a wide array of recent disasters.

In addition, we seek to provide guidelines on performing efficient and effective screening of alcohol and substance use disorders, consistent with DSM-IV-TR (American Psychiatric Association 2000) diagnoses, in the setting of mental health response to a community disaster. We also consider treatment strategies that allow for intervention in a timely manner, by mental health professionals as well as by community workers and others who come into direct contact with individuals affected by a disaster.

Epidemiological Findings on Substance Use After Disasters

In the context of disaster survival, substance use disorders pose significant risks to individuals, including accidents and spread of infectious disease. In the wake of a disaster, when emergency and health care services are often compromised, the ramifications of substance use may be magnified considerably. Therefore, the study of substance use in the wake of disasters may provide a significant public health benefit, and more research in this area is needed. A meta-analysis of 52 studies concerning psychopathology following disasters included six involving alcohol abuse and three addressing drug abuse (nonexclusive categories). Taken together, the studies examining alcohol use among disaster victims ($N=712$) found that 35.5% of the victims ($N=253$) demonstrated increased consumption after the disaster. In the three studies exploring drug use ($N=630$), 144 disaster victims (22.9%) demonstrated increased use (Rubonis and Bickman 1991). These data suggest that disasters pose a risk for alcohol and substance use consumption.

Hurricane Agnes and its resulting floods caused significant loss of life and property damage in the Wyoming Valley of Pennsylvania in 1972. Increased consumption of alcohol among survivors of the hurricane was documented as early as 3 months after the storm (Okura 1975). Also, the consequences of postdisaster alcohol use may be long lasting. In a survey conducted 5 years after Hurricane Agnes, more than 50% of flood survivors reported that alcohol was useful for coping with stress, whereas respondents in only 16% of locales not affected by the flooding said the same ($P=0.001$) (Logue et al. 1979). Similarly, 1 year after the 1995 bombing in Oklahoma City, a twofold increase in alcohol and tobacco use was demonstrated in adults in the metropolitan area (D.W. Smith et al. 1999). Thus, patterns of at-risk drinking may persist or become evident only at some temporal distance from the precipitating event.

Alcohol is not the only drug that is consumed more following a cataclysmic event. In 1987, the ferry MS *Herald of Free Enterprise* capsized in the English Channel, killing 193 individuals. A survey of survivors revealed increased consumption of alcohol, tobacco, sleeping pills, and tranquilizers at 6 and 30 months after the event (Joseph et al. 1993). A more complex picture emerged after the eruption of Mount St. Helens in Washington State in 1980. Although police Breathalyzer tests and driving while intoxicated (DWI) arrests and court cases decreased, other alcohol-related court cases, referrals to the Community Alcohol Center, and police arrests for violation of liquor laws all significantly increased (Adams and Adams 1984). Thus, an overall net increase in alcohol-related violations was observed. The authors speculated that the ash fall from the eruption impeded driving, thereby resulting in fewer motor vehicle–related arrests and cases. However, a limitation of these studies is that subjects were not stratified by criteria relevant to substance abuse risk, such as history of alcohol or substance use, comorbid psychopathology, or demographic information.

Although several studies demonstrate a direct link between disaster survival and increased alcohol and substance consumption, other studies fail to replicate this finding. Analyses of survivors 2 and 14 years after the 1972 Buffalo Creek dam collapse found no associated increase in alcohol use (Green et al. 1990). In 1985, massive storms battered Puerto Rico, resulting in considerable flooding and destructive mudslides that left scores dead and thousands living in public shelters for months after losing their homes. Surveys conducted in 1987 yielded an association of alcohol consumption in survivors with "severe disaster exposure" (defined as considerable loss of property or threat to the life of oneself or one's family) compared with those who had no exposure to the disaster. On the other hand, further analyses demonstrated that survivors who had "severe" exposure to the disaster also had significantly more alcohol use pathology prior to the disaster. In the end, the authors were unable to find any clear association between disaster exposure and alcohol consumption (Bravo et al. 1990). In 1987, a plane crashed into a hotel in Indianapolis, Indiana. Among hotel employees who survived the crash, alcohol use disorders decreased by more than 50%, compared with their rate prior to the disaster (E.M. Smith et al. 1990). Although drug and alcohol use decreased among survivors of a 1991 mass shooting in a Killeen, Texas, cafeteria that resulted in 23 fatalities, 15% of the survivors endorsed using alcohol to cope with postdisaster stress. By contrast, much larger percentages reported using friends and family (88%), counselors and physicians (50%), or medications (27%) to cope (North et al. 1994).

No conclusive evidence is available to suggest that exposure to a disaster is an independent predictor of increased alcohol or substance use. However, studies have demonstrated that the combination of other independent variables, in conjunction with disaster exposure, tends to be significantly associated with increased alcohol and substance use (Vlahov et al. 2002, 2004). Among these factors are predisaster alcohol and substance use history, postdisaster psychopathology, proximity to the disaster, resource loss, young age, and single marital status (Table 8–1). The presence of these factors warrants particular attention for the risk of a new-onset alcohol or substance use disorder. Following a disaster, identification of at-risk individuals may be greatly enhanced by the use of brief screening measures (see "Screening and Assessment Tools" later in this chapter).

Predisaster history of alcohol or substance use represents a risk factor for increased use after a disaster. In the 1987 Indianapolis plane crash de-

---

TABLE 8–1.   Factors that may contribute to the development of alcohol and substance use pathology in the wake of a disaster

Presence of major depressive disorder or panic attacks at the time of the disaster

Prior history of alcohol or substance use disorder

Younger age, especially when combined with a disrupted support network

Serving as a rescue worker during the disaster

Perceived loss of considerable resources

---

scribed above, half of the hotel employees with alcohol use pathology after the crash had such pathology prior to the disaster (E. M. Smith et al. 1990). Furthermore, the vast majority of victims of the Puerto Rican floods and mudslides of 1985 who increased their alcohol consumption had also been drinking excessively before the storms (Bravo et al. 1990). Not only was there a decrease in substance use in the wake of the Oklahoma City bombing in 1995, but there were no new incident cases described in a survey of 182 survivors (North et al. 1999). Thus, assessing for past history of alcohol or substance use disorders is an important strategy for identifying victims of disasters who may be at current risk for relapse.

Posttraumatic Stress Disorder and Other Risk Factors

Although PTSD does not typically appear until the postacute period, a recurrence of prior PTSD may occur in the weeks immediately after a disaster. Epidemiological studies consistently show high prevalence rates of PTSD and substance use disorders (Shore et al. 1989; Stewart 1996). Individuals exposed to trauma differ in their vulnerability to PTSD and addictive disorders. Psychologically resilient trauma victims engage in significantly less tobacco and marijuana use than individuals described as mildly or moderately traumatized, as well as those with diagnosable PTSD (Bonanno et al. 2007). In a study of nearly 900 members of a Michigan health maintenance organization, PTSD was associated with increased drug and tobacco use, and a history of trauma without PTSD demonstrated no correlation with increased substance and alcohol use (Breslau et al. 2003). Generally, PTSD tends to precede alcohol abuse (Stewart 1996). PTSD and alcohol or substance use may be linked through a self-medication mechanism, whereas sedatives, such as benzodiazepines, are used to treat intolerable anxiety symptoms (Jacobsen et al. 2001). Furthermore, withdrawal from sedatives or from alcohol can exacerbate anxiety symptoms, leading to increased use of these substances (Jacobsen et al. 2001).

In terms of disaster exposure, 32% of survivors of the Oklahoma City bombing in 1995 with co-occurring PTSD or an affective disorder endorsed drinking alcohol to cope with stress, compared with 5.6% of survivors without those diagnoses (North et al. 1999). In the wake of the 2004 Indian Ocean tsunami, among nearly 2,000 Swiss survivors, severity of PTSD symptoms was independently associated with increased substance use (Vetter et al. 2008). A study of the Oklahoma City bombing survivors demonstrated that current grief and PTSD symptoms were significantly more predictive of increased alcohol consumption than was actual injury from the disaster (Pfefferbaum and Doughty 2001).

After the 9/11 terrorist attacks in New York City in 2001, there was a significant rise in alcohol, tobacco, and marijuana consumption in the exposed population. These increases occurred predominantly among individuals who had been using those substances prior to the disaster, especially those with comorbid PTSD or MDD diagnosed after the attack (Marshall and Galea 2001; Vlahov et al. 2002, 2004). However, other variables were also associated with increased alcohol and substance use in the wake of 9/11. The following findings are based on the responses of 988 New Yorkers who lived below 110th Street in Manhattan to a telephone survey conducted 5–8 weeks after the terrorist attacks. Regarding increased alcohol, tobacco, and marijuana use, multivariate analysis demonstrated a range of specific risk factors, including proximity to the attack (tobacco), life stresses present 12 months prior to the attack (tobacco), perievent panic attacks (tobacco, marijuana), and increased media exposure (alcohol). Protective factors associated with less marijuana use were older age, being married, and total household income less than $20,000 versus over $100,000 (Vlahov et al. 2002). If household income can be used to approximate potential resource loss in a disaster, the New York data are consistent with those demonstrated among survivors of Hurricane Katrina, which devastated New Orleans in 2005. In addition to the association between PTSD symptoms and increased drug and alcohol use described in a surveyed sample of students, staff and faculty at Louisiana State University perceived that loss of resources was associated particularly with alcohol dependence (Kishore et al. 2008).

Concerning the effect of age on risk for substance use disorders, data from 9/11 demonstrate that older age was protective against increased substance use following the disaster. Youth may be particularly vulnerable to alcohol and substance use in the wake of a disaster because of undeveloped coping skills, as well as the potential loss of caretakers and supports (Rowe and Liddle 2008). Living in homeless and emergency shelters is associated with significant substance use in adolescents (Thompson 2004) and among the teens' parents (Parker et al. 1991). It has been noted that PTSD is more likely in substance-abusing adolescents than in general community samples

(Deykin and Buka 1997; Giaconia et al. 2000). Substance use disorders precede the trauma and PTSD diagnoses in about half of adolescents with comorbid PTSD and substance use disorder (Giaconia et al. 2000). Thus, obtaining a thorough substance use history may help predict development of PTSD in adolescent disaster victims. Another important implication of these findings is that adolescent trauma victims manifesting symptoms of PTSD should be carefully watched for the emergence of substance use pathology. Efforts to screen for developing addiction disorders should include a particular focus on the adolescents and teens, as well as their parents.

Rescue workers represent a cohort particularly vulnerable to excessive alcohol consumption associated with disaster exposure. Firefighters who had responded to the Oklahoma City bombing were found to have a 47% lifetime prevalence of alcohol use disorder, more than twice that of civilian victims after the bombing (North et al. 2002b). Firefighters with postdisaster alcohol use disorder reported poorer job satisfaction and higher rates of functional interference from PTSD symptoms than did firefighters without a diagnosable alcohol use disorder (North et al. 2002a). Similarly, 2 years after the Beverly Hills Supper Club fire of 1977 in Southgate, Kentucky, having participated in the recovery of bodies was significantly associated with the development of substance abuse (Green et al. 1985). These findings highlight the importance of follow-up mental health care, including addiction risk assessment, in rescue workers who have been involved in a disaster response.

In summary, PTSD and alcohol or substance use disorders frequently co-occur following a disaster trauma. Certain demographic factors, including older age and being married, appear to offer some protection against addiction. On the other hand, adolescents, single individuals, and those who have suffered severe loss of resources appear especially at risk for developing an addictive disorder. Early postdisaster efforts directed at emerging PTSD pathology may represent an effective strategy for reducing individuals' risk of developing alcohol or substance use disorders. Thus, it is essential for treatment programs for postdisaster victims to address concurrently the dual risks of PTSD and addictive disorders.

The following vignette illustrates many of the principles we have reviewed, including risk factors that heighten vulnerability to an alcohol use disorder following a disaster.

> Mr. N, a 25-year-old single firefighter, has been referred for treatment of insomnia. He states that 2 months ago he was involved in a complicated rescue effort of dozens of people trapped in an illegal sweatshop during a fire. Because of the poor working conditions and multiple fire code violations, there were many fatalities. At one point during the rescue, Mr. N felt short of breath, and his heart started racing so uncomfortably that he believed he would die. Since the rescue, Mr. N has had recurrent nightmares of being trapped in the

inferno, seeing the deformed bodies and hearing the screams of people he simply could not rescue in time. Recently, these visions have begun to intrude on his daytime activities in the form of flashbacks. In the past month, Mr. N has taken several sick days because of fatigue and lack of motivation to go to work. He reports that the sound of sirens makes him anxious, and he is "jumpier" in the street. On further questioning, Mr. N states that the only way he has been able to get even a few hours of sleep nightly is by drinking a couple shots of whiskey and smoking "a bowl or two" of marijuana before bed. For several years, he has used marijuana or alcohol for occasional insomnia, but never with this regularity. For the past few days, Mr. N has needed a shot of whiskey first thing in the morning to steady his nerves in order to get to work. His coworkers have started gibing him about his unkempt appearance and the smell of whiskey on his breath. He punched a coworker in the nose yesterday for calling him a "wino." In fact, Mr. N confesses, he needed to go to a bar and have a few beers to muster the strength to come to this interview.

Mr. N in the preceding vignette evidences significant risk factors for development of a substance use disorder following survival of a disaster. He is a rescue worker who was intimately involved in the rescue effort and came in contact with the horrors of the disaster. He is in a high-risk group, because he is single and relatively young and is a rescue worker with a prior history of substance use. He is also manifesting several symptoms of PTSD, including nightmares, hypervigilance, and avoidance. He would score two positive items on the CAGE questionnaire (Table 8–2): **A**nnoyance at others who criticize his drinking and needing an **E**ye-opener to steady his nerves in the morning.

At-Risk Drinking

Just as in the general adult population, in which the prevalence of risky drinking is higher than that for alcohol abuse or dependence, it is expected that following a disaster many more individuals will engage in problematic drinking patterns than will meet formal criteria for an alcohol use disorder. Current U.S. guidelines for unsafe drinking are more than 4 drinks per day or 14 per week for men, and more than 3 drinks per day or 7 per week for women (Dawson et al. 2005). Drinking excessively may cause or increase the risk for depression and anxiety. In addition, heavy drinkers have an increased risk of a range of medical issues, including hypertension; hemorrhagic stroke; gastrointestinal bleeding; cirrhosis; cancers of the liver, breast, oropharynx, and esophagus; and sleep disorders (Rehm et al. 2003). Thus, the global burden of disease represented by at-risk drinking is considerable. At-risk drinking is often underdiagnosed by both primary care physicians and psychiatrists. Unless specific interview questions or structured assessments are employed to identify individuals with at-risk patterns of drinking,

---

TABLE 8–2.   CAGE Questionnaire

Two "yes" responses indicate that the respondent should be assessed further.

1.   Have you ever felt you needed to Cut down on your drinking?
2.   Have people Annoyed you by criticizing your drinking?
3.   Have you ever felt Guilty about drinking?
4.   Have you ever felt you needed a drink first thing in the morning (Eye-opener) to steady your nerves or to get rid of a hangover?

Source.   Ewing 1984.

---

this problem will likely be missed by many clinicians responding to a disaster; however, it is precisely at this time that risky drinking is likely to either develop or progress to alcohol abuse or dependence.

According to guidelines published by the National Institute on Alcohol Abuse and Alcoholism (NIAAA), the appropriate clinical response to at-risk drinking, once detected, is a brief intervention consisting of two parts: 1) advise (state conclusion and recommendation clearly) and 2) assist (gauge patient's readiness to change drinking habits). For instance, a physician or other relief worker could state, "You're drinking more than is medically safe. I strongly recommend that you cut down (or quit), and I'm willing to help." This recommendation should be followed with a direct question about readiness to change, such as, "Are you willing to consider making changes in your drinking?" (U.S. Department of Health and Human Services 2005). The patient should also be given a follow-up appointment for continued support.

Such follow-up care is essential whether or not the patient makes any change in his or her drinking. For the patient who has not been able to effect change, the clinician can support efforts to cut down while making it clear that abstinence is the goal. In addition, it is important to relate drinking problems to current medical, psychological, or social problems, as well as to address these concurrent problems. Other strategies to increase motivation include engaging significant others or recommending 12-step or other mutual-help groups. For the patient who has been able to meet the drinking goal, it is equally important to reinforce and support continued adherence and to coordinate care with an addiction specialist if the patient has accepted such a referral. In both cases, clinicians should remain vigilant for the need to treat coexisting medical and psychiatric disorders.

Screening and Assessment Tools

From the standpoint of disaster response, there are several addiction-related diagnoses that are important to make as early as possible for individuals to receive adequate medical care in a timely manner and thus prevent untoward consequences. Foremost among these are alcohol withdrawal and opiate withdrawal. A disaster of sufficient destructive magnitude may disrupt the infrastructures both for health care (e.g., hospitals, clinics, private offices, pharmacies) and for alcohol or substance distribution (e.g., liquor stores, drug-dealing operations). Patients with acute or emerging alcohol or sedative (benzodiazepine, barbiturate) withdrawal will appear anxious, be sweating, and have elevated heart rates and blood pressures as symptoms worsen. Many of these symptoms are also present in patients undergoing opioid withdrawal, which also might involve tearing, sweating or hot/cold flashes, abdominal cramps, and myalgias.

In disaster conditions, when triage capacity has been reached or exceeded, questions about alcohol and substance use may be overlooked or omitted in a medical history, and patients frequently do not volunteer such information unless directly asked. Therefore, use of a structured and validated instrument is recommended in triage settings as a general screening measure. Tables 8–2 through 8–4 present examples of commonly used screening and assessment tools.

Assessment tools are useful in determining the severity of an alcohol use disorder and, therefore, in identifying individuals who are physiologically dependent. The syndrome of alcohol withdrawal may begin at 6–12 hours after the last drink. It is vitally important to diagnose and treat alcohol withdrawal quickly so as to avoid morbidities such as seizures (with possible head injury), delirium, and death. In the aftermath of a disaster, access to alcohol may be suddenly interrupted, and alcohol-dependent individuals may begin to experience moderate or severe alcohol withdrawal symptoms (e.g., hypertension, tachycardia, sweating, nausea/vomiting, insomnia, agitation, elevated temperature). If untreated, these may progress within 12–24 hours to alcoholic hallucinosis, involving visual, auditory, or tactile hallucinations. The risk of withdrawal seizures, which are generalized tonic-clonic seizures, is greatest from 24–72 hours postwithdrawal, and the risk of alcohol withdrawal delirium—consisting of disorientation, agitation, tachycardia and hypertension, sweating, and predominantly visual hallucinations—peaks at 48–72 hours.

In the context of a disaster, an interruption in the supply of methadone at methadone clinics could result in a large number of methadone-maintained patients seeking opiates from emergency department doctors. These patients should be able to provide identification proving their enrollment in such a program. Illicit opiate users whose street supply of opiates has been interrupted may also appear with various pain complaints, desiring prescription opiates to stave off withdrawal symptoms, including elevated pulse, sweating, restlessness, constricted pupils, bone or joint aches, runny

TABLE 8–3. Screening and assessment instruments for substance use disorders

Instrument	Substance assessed	Description	Validation
AUDIT	Alcohol	Performs well across broad age range; 10 items	Bohn et al. 1995; Donovan et al. 2006; Saunders et al. 1993
CAGE	Alcohol	4 items: Cutting down, Annoyance by criticism of drinking, Guilt, use as Eye-opener (see Table 8–2)	Ewing 1984; Liskow et al. 1995
CIWA-Ar	Alcohol	Most widely used for alcohol withdrawal	Sullivan et al. 1989
COWS	Opiate withdrawal	11 most common signs/symptoms, including pulse, sweating, pupil size, GI upset, myalgias, aches, tremor, anxiety	Wesson and Ling 2003
CRAFFT	Alcohol, drugs	For use in adolescents and teens; 6 items	Cook et al. 2005; Knight et al. 2002
RAPS	Alcohol	High sensitivity for heavy drinking	Cherpitel 1995
RDPS	Drugs	Lower sensitivity for females	Cherpitel and Borges 2004

Note. AUDIT=Alcohol Use Disorders Identification Test (see Table 8–4); CIWA=Clinical Institute Withdrawal Assessment for Alcohol, Revised; COWS= Clinical Opiate Withdrawal Scale; CRAFFT=acronym for pattern of use: Car (driver or passenger), Relax, Alone, Forget (blackouts), Friends (advise cutting down), Trouble; GI=gastrointestinal; RAPS=Rapid Alcohol Problems Screen; RDPS=Rapid Drug Problems Screen.

nose or tearing, gastrointestinal upset, tremor, yawning, anxiety or irritability, gooseflesh, and hot/cold flashes.

Diagnosing alcohol and opioid dependence may be useful in that early intervention may prevent future cases of withdrawal. The DSM-IV-TR diagnostic criteria for substance or alcohol abuse require at least a 12-month period during which regular substance use is associated with negative social, legal, or physical consequences at work, school, or home, with continued use despite awareness of these consequences. By contrast, the diagnosis of alcohol or substance dependence requires that patients manifest physiological (bodily) changes resulting from chronic use (tolerance, withdrawal), and experience loss of control over use, as demonstrated by inability to decrease amount used, or use for longer periods than intended, with possible sacrifice of important personal, social, or occupational resources in order to continue the alcohol or drug use (Table 8–5). In the case of alcohol dependence, the presence of a tremor the day following drinking indicates moderate withdrawal, and any history of a withdrawal seizure confirms significant physiological dependence. For those addicted to opioids, whether heroin or prescription opioids, dependence results in the onset of moderate withdrawal symptoms, including muscle aches and abdominal cramping, if the next dose is delayed.

A more complicated issue is the identification of those individuals with potential alcohol or substance use disorders who have either no known prior histories of such or are not part of any particular risk group. Clinicians and other providers should become comfortable asking patients about addiction disorders, and be familiar with criteria for making such diagnoses. Sometimes, patients will openly bring these concerns to the forefront during the interview, or they may be observed to be intoxicated. Patients may express concerns about worsening mood, anxiety, or irritability; may be preoccupied with somatic issues, such as insomnia, exhaustion, or feeling unsteady; or may endorse cognitive problems, such as impaired concentration or memory. Clinicians may initiate a substance use assessment by suggesting that these symptoms are commonplace upon surviving a disaster, and that people sometimes self-medicate these symptoms with alcohol and drugs. Some patients may attempt to treat anxiety, irritability, or insomnia with sedatives such as alcohol or benzodiazepines, or to treat fatigue with stimulants, such as cocaine or amphetamines. Unfortunately, the very symptoms that patients are attempting to medicate with substances of abuse often return more acutely when these individuals are withdrawing from those substances. Anxiety and insomnia are common symptoms of sedative or alcohol withdrawal, whereas fatigue naturally occurs while "crashing" from stimulants, such as cocaine and amphetamines.

TABLE 8–4.   Alcohol Use Disorders Identification Test (AUDIT): Interview Version

Questions	0	1	2	3	4
1. How often do you have a drink containing alcohol? [Skip to Qs 9–10 if 0 (Never)]	Never	Monthly or less	2–4 times a month	2–3 times a week	4 or more times a week
2. How many drinks containing alcohol do you have on a typical day when you are drinking?	1 or 2	3 or 4	5 or 6	7–9	10 or more
3. How often do you have 6 or more drinks on one occasion? [Skip to Qs 9–10 if total score for Qs 2 and 3 is 0]	Never	Less than monthly	Monthly	Weekly	Daily or almost daily
4. How often during the last year have you found that you were not able to stop drinking once you had started?	Never	Less than monthly	Monthly	Weekly	Daily or almost daily
5. How often during the last year have you failed to do what was normally expected from you because of drinking?	Never	Less than monthly	Monthly	Weekly	Daily or almost daily
6. How often during the last year have you needed a first drink in the morning to get yourself going after a heavy drinking session?	Never	Less than monthly	Monthly	Weekly	Daily or almost daily
7. How often during the last year have you had a feeling of guilt or remorse after drinking?	Never	Less than monthly	Monthly	Weekly	Daily or almost daily
8. How often during the last year have you been unable to remember what happened the night before because you had been drinking?	Never	Less than monthly	Monthly	Weekly	Daily or almost daily
9. Have you or someone else been injured as a result of your drinking?	No		Yes, but not in the last year		Yes, during the last year
10. Has a relative, friend, doctor, or other health care worker been concerned about your drinking or suggested that you cut down?	No		Yes, but not in the last year		Yes, during the last year

TABLE 8–4. Alcohol Use Disorders Identification Test (AUDIT): Interview Version *(continued)*

Note. Read questions as written. Record answers carefully. Begin the AUDIT by saying "Now I am going to ask you some questions about your use of alcoholic beverages during this past year." Explain what is meant by "alcoholic beverages" by using local examples of beer, wine, vodka, etc. Code answers in terms of "standard drinks." The minimum score (for nondrinkers) is 0, and the maximum possible score is 40. A score of 8 is indicative of hazardous and harmful alcohol use and possibly of alcohol dependence. Scores of 8–15 indicate a medium level, and scores of 16 and above indicate a high level of alcohol problems.

Source. Adapted with permission from Babor TF, Biddle-Higgins JC, Saunders JB, et al.: *AUDIT: The Alcohol Use Disorders Identification Test: Guidelines for Use in Primary Health Care* (WHO/MSD/MSB/01.6a). Geneva, Switzerland, World Health Organization Department of Mental Health and Substance Dependence, 2001. Copyright 2001, World Health Organization.

TABLE 8–5.   DSM-IV-TR substance abuse and dependence criteria

DSM-IV-TR substance abuse criteria

A.   A maladaptive pattern of substance use leading to clinically significant impairment or distress, as manifested by one (or more) of the following, occurring within a 12-month period:

(1)   recurrent substance use resulting in a failure to fulfill major role obligations at work, school, or home (e.g., repeated absences or poor work performance related to substance use; substance-related absences, suspensions, or expulsions from school; neglect of children or household)

(2)   recurrent substance use in situations in which it is physically hazardous (e.g., driving an automobile or operating a machine when impaired by substance use)

(3)   recurrent substance-related legal problems (e.g., arrests for substance-related disorderly conduct)

(4)   continued substance use despite having persistent or recurrent social or interpersonal problems caused or exacerbated by the effects of the substance (e.g., arguments with spouse about consequences of intoxication, physical fights).

B.   The symptoms have never met the criteria for substance dependence for this class of substance.

DSM-IV-TR substance dependence criteria

A maladaptive pattern of substance use, leading to clinically significant impairment or distress, as manifested by three (or more) of the following, occurring at any time in the same 12-month period:

(1)   Tolerance, as defined by either of the following:

(a)   a need for markedly increased amounts of the substance to achieve intoxication or the desired effect

(b)   markedly diminished effect with continued use of the same amount of the substance

(2)   Withdrawal, as manifested by either of the following:

(a)   the characteristic withdrawal syndrome for the substance

(b)   the same (or a closely related) substance is taken to relieve or avoid withdrawal symptoms

(3)   The substance is often taken in larger amounts or over a longer period than was intended

(4)   There is a persistent desire or unsuccessful efforts to cut down or control substance use

(5)   A great deal of time is spent in activities necessary to obtain the substance…, use the substance…, or recover from its effects

(6)   Important social, occupational, or recreational activities are given up or reduced because of substance use

(7)   The substance use is continued despite knowledge of having a persistent or recurrent physical or psychological problem that is likely to have been caused or exacerbated by the substance

Source.   Reprinted from the *Diagnostic and Statistical Manual of Mental Disorders,* 4th Edition, Text Revision. Washington, DC, American Psychiatric Association, 2000, pp. 197, 199. Copyright © 2000, American Psychiatric Association.

Pharmacological and Treatment Interventions

The initial assessment of a patient at risk for alcohol withdrawal should consist of a complete history and physical examination. Laboratory tests are often indicated. Before administering dextrose-containing solutions, a 100-mg dose of thiamine hydrochloride should be given by intramuscular or intravenous injection. The next consideration is to select a treatment setting for the detoxification to be carried out. Although patients with mild to moderate alcohol withdrawal can be safely detoxified on an outpatient basis, inpatient detoxification is indicated for patients with history of severe withdrawal symptoms, history of withdrawal seizures or delirium tremens, multiple previous detoxifications, concomitant psychiatric or medical illness, recent high levels of alcohol consumption, pregnancy, or lack of a reliable support network (Myrick and Anton 1998).

The pharmacological treatment of alcohol withdrawal involves the use of medications that are cross-tolerant with alcohol. The standard treatment for alcohol or sedative withdrawal is the administration of benzodiazepines. Typically, the long-acting benzodiazepines diazepam and chlordiazepoxide are used on either a fixed or a symptom-driven schedule. The standard treatment often consists of a fixed schedule with additional as-needed doses (Saitz 1995). A typical fixed schedule would be as follows: chlordiazepoxide 50 mg every 6 hours for 24 hours, then 25 mg every 6 hours for 48 hours. An alternative symptom-triggered regimen would consist of hourly assessments with the Clinical Institute Withdrawal Assessment of Alcohol Scale, Revised (CIWA-Ar; Sullivan et al. 1989), and administration of diazepam 10–20 mg when the CIWA-Ar score is at least 8–10. The long half-life of these medications makes for a smoother course of detoxification, because it less likely that rebound withdrawal symptoms will occur.

In patients with mild to moderate alcohol withdrawal symptoms, carbamazepine may be an effective alternative to benzodiazepines (Stuppaeck et al. 1990). The advantages of carbamazepine are that it is not sedating and has little potential for abuse. Carbamazepine is used extensively in Europe, but its use in the United States has been limited by concerns that it does not prevent seizures and delirium (Bayard et al. 2004). Barbiturates, β-blockers, and antipsychotics can be used in some instances but are not generally recommended as first-line therapy. When patients fail other supportive therapy, benzodiazepines should be used to manage the more severe alcohol withdrawal syndromes. It is conceivable that the standard medications to treat alcohol withdrawal, described above, may not be available, especially in rural areas. Ethanol itself, in both oral and intravenous forms, has been used successfully to treat alcohol withdrawal (Funderburk et al. 1978; Hodges and Mazur 2004; Mayo-Smith 1997). Patients dependent on barbiturates require barbiturate administration to treat their withdrawal, which is generally unresponsive to benzodiazepine management.

Individuals experiencing opioid withdrawal for whom continued opioid maintenance is a realistic option should be restarted on a daily dosage of their previous opioid agonist (i.e., methadone or buprenorphine), if available. If a methadone dose cannot be verified, it is necessary to restart the patient on a low dose (20–30 mg) and observe for signs of sedation, so as not to risk inducing respiratory depression. If opioid withdrawal symptoms emerge, an additional small dose (5–10 mg) may be given and the patient observed for 4–6 hours. Because methadone has a very long half-life of up to 190 hours, doses can accumulate over the first few days of dosing and ultimately lead to an unintentional overdose if due caution is not taken with initial dosing.

On the other hand, if an individual is going through detoxification from street opioids or the previously prescribed opioids are not available, it is possible to carry out an opioid detoxification procedure over several days. It is even possible that methadone may be appropriated for management of clinical pain if opiate supplies dwindle in the pharmacies of hospitals or clinics. The clinical standard for opioid detoxification in the United States at present involves a 7-day taper from a long-acting opioid such as methadone. An opioid antagonist such as naltrexone is an option that requires close monitoring by nurses and physicians. Patients seeking detoxification are in a state of autonomic hyperactivity, which can best be managed with the use of an α_2-adrenergic agonist such as clonidine, combined with a benzodiazepine such as clonazepam to address myalgias and anxiety. Specific complaints such as diarrhea can be treated with loperamide. Insomnia should also be addressed promptly with medication management, because sleep disturbances are a significant barrier to the successful completion of detoxification. Fluids should be encouraged, because dehydration is a concern during opioid detoxification. Several medications useful in the treatment of alcohol, sedative, or opiate withdrawal are found in the World Health Organization's (2010) "WHO Model List of Essential Medicines, 16th Edition (Updated)" and should therefore be available in most medical settings worldwide (Table 8–6).

Treatment of alcohol or opiate withdrawal should be followed by treatment to address the underlying drug dependence. Patients completing detoxification should be referred to outpatient settings that offer either abstinence-based treatment or agonist maintenance with relapse prevention counseling. It is also important to warn patients that their tolerance is reduced by undergoing opiate detoxification. Thus, the risk of postdetoxification accidental overdose is high, and clinicians must take care to inform patients of this risk.

TABLE 8-6. WHO Model List of Essential Medicines: medications useful in treatment of alcohol/sedative and opiate withdrawal

Alcohol/sedative withdrawal: diazepam, lorazepam, phenobarbital, carbamazepine, valproic acid, ethanol (disinfectant)

Opiate withdrawal: methadone, morphine

Other treatments: nicotine replacement patches, parenteral fluids, antiemetics, antidiarrheals (codeine)

Source. World Health Organization 2010.

Because a shortage or absence of addiction specialists is possible, a psychiatrist who responds to a disaster during the postacute period may need to consider prescribing medications for alcohol dependence. More detailed information and recommendations regarding these medications are available from the National Institute on Alcohol Abuse and Alcoholism (2008) and are briefly summarized here. Evidence has shown that these medications may increase the duration of abstinence periods and decrease the amount of alcohol usage during a setback, both of which allow more opportunity to address posttraumatic stress difficulties. Fortunately, the medications available are generally tolerated well in healthy adults and pose significantly less risk than alcohol itself in patients with medical or psychiatric comorbidities.

Oral and long-acting injectable forms of naltrexone, which blocks opioid receptors related to the reward effects of alcohol and may lessen cravings, are available. Acamprosate, which acts on γ-aminobutyric acid (GABA) and glutamate systems and is thought to reduce prolonged abstinence symptoms (e.g., insomnia, restlessness, dysphoria, anxiety), may be considered. Finally, controlled studies show that topiramate, which is believed to increase inhibitory GABA receptors and to decrease excitatory glutamate receptor transmission, may be used effectively. Disulfiram, which interferes with the metabolism of alcohol, causing a buildup of acetaldehyde and resulting in a toxic reaction, including sweats, nausea, flushing, and palpitations, is often ineffective due to poor compliance. In addition, disulfiram presents some risk of liver toxicity, particularly in alcoholic patients with severe liver disease. Thus, disulfiram is less likely to be considered than the other options noted.

Dosing information, contraindications, and common side effects of these medications are listed in Table 8–7. For clinicians inexperienced with prescribing these medications, additional reading and/or discussion with an addiction specialist is advised. Further information is available from the National Institute on Alcohol Abuse and Alcoholism (2008).

TABLE 8–7.   Medications for treating alcohol dependence

	Oral naltrexone	Injectable naltrexone (extended release)	Acamprosate	Disulfiram	Topiramate
Usual dosing	50 mg qd	380 mg im monthly	666 mg tid	250 mg qd	25 mg qhs titrating slowly to 200 mg qhs
Contraindications	Recent opiate used, need 7–10 days abstinence	Same as oral naltrexone; rash or infection at injection site; lack of muscle mass for deep injection	Severe renal impairment	Metronidazole, alcohol or alcohol-containing medications; CAD or severe myocardial disease; hypersensitivity to rubber derivatives	History of hypersensitivity to topiramate
Common side effects	Anorexia, nausea, vomiting, fatigue, headache, dizziness, anxiety	Same as oral naltrexone; joint pain, muscle aches, or cramps, reaction at injection site	Diarrhea, somnolence	Metallic aftertaste, dermatitis, usually transient mild drowsiness	Paresthesias; altered taste; anorexia; somnolence, cognitive side effects

Note.   CAD=coronary artery disease; im=intramuscularly; qd=every day; qhs=every night; tid=three times a day.

Source.   Adapted from National Institute on Alcohol Abuse and Alcoholism 2008.

Comorbidity Issues in Treatment

Special consideration should be paid to the treatment of alcohol or substance use pathology in patients with comorbid MDD or PTSD. As described earlier in this chapter, the presence of MDD or PTSD is significantly associated with increased alcohol and drug consumption among survivors of disasters. Although we found no literature describing the efficacy of alcohol or substance abuse treatment in disaster survivors, we have gathered data from studies of general trauma survivors with comorbid substance and mood or anxiety disorders.

Overall, the outcomes were mixed, with no treatment showing clear benefit for both depression and alcohol use (Tiet and Mausbauch 2007). In terms of PTSD treatment, cognitive-behavioral therapy (CBT) models are preferred over exposure therapy in patients with comorbid alcohol or substance use pathology (Foa et al. 1999). Seeking Safety is a standard CBT protocol employed to treat trauma victims with comorbid PTSD and substance use disorder symptoms. This modality of therapy incorporates cognitive, supportive, and interpersonal styles, with an aim of prioritizing safety and insight into personal well-being and self-worth. Improved mood and substance use symptoms have been shown immediately following treatment, and even at 3-month follow-up (Najavitz et al. 1998). However, relapse prevention therapy to address substance use pathology has been found to outperform Seeking Safety at 9-month follow-up (Hien et al. 2004). This finding is consistent with the post-9/11 literature that documents diminishing PTSD and MDD symptoms by 6 months after the attack, but alcohol and substance use levels that remained increased and stable compared with immediately after the attack (Vlahov et al. 2004). A placebo-controlled study found no significant difference in symptom improvement among patients with PTSD and alcohol dependence treated with weekly CBT alone or with the selective serotonin reuptake inhibitor (SSRI) antidepressant sertraline (Labbate et al. 2004). In summary, treatment of PTSD does not replace the need for direct treatment of substance abuse, and no compelling evidence suggests that augmentation of effective psychotherapeutic modalities with antidepressant or anxiolytic medications provides added benefit for substance use symptom domains.

Conclusion

In the aftermath of a disaster, mental health resources in general are limited, and there are likely to be few health professionals who can focus on substance abuse issues. Thus, consideration must be given to addressing only those substance abuse issues that are critical in the immediate postdisaster period. From a clinical perspective, the most time-sensitive substance treatment issue is that of alcohol and sedative-hypnotic withdrawal. Alcohol-dependent individuals left untreated are at high risk for disorientation and seizures; alcohol withdrawal may be life threatening and is associated with a variety of medical complications. Opiate withdrawal, although physically quite uncomfortable, is not considered a life-threatening condition. Thus, if there is time to assess only one substance abuse–related issue in individuals affected by a disaster, identifying those who are heavily alcohol dependent and at risk for severe withdrawal is a critically important function for rescue workers to perform. A brief screening instrument, such as the Alcohol Use Disorders Identification Test (Saunders et al. 1993) or CIWA-Ar (Sullivan et al. 1989), allows for rapid assessment of withdrawal risk in a large number of individuals seeking medical attention.

Disaster exposure poses a significant risk for the development of alcohol and substance use pathology, although available evidence suggests that such exposure alone is not sufficient to predict the development of these problems. Relatively few studies to date, however, have sought to examine systematically the specific risk factors, both baseline and environmental, that raise the likelihood of new-onset or relapsing alcohol or substance use disorders in the wake of such traumatic life events. The onset of PTSD after a disaster has been shown to significantly increase the likelihood of developing an alcohol or substance use disorder. Other factors that may contribute to the development of alcohol and substance use pathology in the wake of a disaster were listed earlier in Table 8–1.

Several questions have yet to be answered regarding the association between surviving a disaster and substance use pathology. In the wake of a disaster, when mental health and medical health care delivery systems might be significantly disrupted, do the incidences of relapse and clinical withdrawal increase significantly in the affected population? Relapse and the development of new pathology can conceivably exacerbate social outcomes after a disaster by increasing the probability of accidents, crime, and the diversion of resources away from rescue efforts, food, and shelter and toward fueling an addictive disorder. For example, a sudden surge in law enforcement actions led to an acute heroin shortage in Australia in early 2001. This "heroin drought" was associated with a statistically significant surge in robbery, as well as breaking and entering arrests (Weatherburn et al. 2003). Does the treatment of emergent pain caused by injuries in the wake of a disaster lead to a significant increase in opioid dependence in the affected population? Does the treatment of emergent anxiety disorders, especially PTSD, with benzodiazepines lead to significant increases in the prevalence of sedative dependence in the affected population? Does the incidence of cocaine and stimulant pathology increase in these contexts, perhaps among rescue workers toiling endlessly in the midst of limited resources? Patterns of emergence of alcohol and substance use disorders in the context of disasters represent fertile areas for further research.

In this chapter, we have sought to provide guidelines for efficient and effective screening of alcohol and substance use disorders, consistent with DSM-IV-TR diagnostic criteria, in the setting of community disaster response. We have considered treatment strategies that permit timely interventions and suggested the need to prioritize such treatments, with first consideration being given to addressing potentially life-threatening alcohol and substance issues, such as alcohol withdrawal. The prognostic importance of PTSD or MDD symptoms for the later emergence of substance use disorders has been reviewed. Finally, we have suggested strategies for employing pharmacotherapies with proven efficacy for the treatment of alcohol and opioid withdrawal syndromes.

■ Teaching Points

- Disaster exposure is not in itself directly associated with increased substance and alcohol use.
- Disaster exposure for someone with a prior history of substance or alcohol use is associated with increased use postdisaster.
- Disaster exposure with resultant PTSD and/or MDD is associated with increased substance or alcohol use.
- In addition to those with substance use disorders prior to disaster exposure, vulnerable populations include youth (especially in shelters) and rescue workers.
- A good medical or psychiatric history can be augmented with several standardized screening and assessment tools to evaluate alcohol or substance dependence or withdrawal.
- Untreated alcohol, sedative, or opiate withdrawal can result in significant morbidity (and mortality in the case of alcohol or sedative withdrawal).
- Once recognized, withdrawal can be treated with readily available pharmacotherapies.
- Once patients are medically stable, psychotherapies and pharmacotherapies are available to treat diagnosed substance or alcohol use disorders upon referral to an expert.

Review Questions

8.1   Which of the following has *not* been found to be associated with increased drug or alcohol use in the wake of a disaster?

   A.   Having a prior history of drug use.
   B.   Being currently married.
   C.   Having posttraumatic stress disorder.
   D.   Having a history of panic attacks.
   E.   Being a rescue worker at the scene of the disaster.

8.2   Which of the following factors was protective against developing marijuana abuse after 9/11?

   A.   Single status.
   B.   Older age.
   C.   Annual household income greater than $100,000.
   D.   Peridisaster panic attack.
   E.   Predisaster marijuana abuse.

8.3   Agents from WHO's Model List of Essential Medicines available for treatment of alcohol withdrawal include all of the following *except*

   A.   Diazepam.
   B.   Morphine.
   C.   Carbamazepine.
   D.   Ethanol.
   E.   Lorazepam.

8.4   The CRAFFT assesses which of the following?

   A.   Alcohol intoxication severity.
   B.   Opioid withdrawal symptoms.
   C.   Alcohol withdrawal.
   D.   Adolescent drug and alcohol problems.
   E.   Posttraumatic stress disorder symptom severity.

8.5   The risk for alcohol withdrawal seizures begins to peak at how long following last alcohol ingestion?

   A.   6 hours.
   B.   12 hours.
   C.   24 hours.
   D.   48 hours.
   E.   1 week.

References

Adams PR, Adams GR: Mount Saint Helens's ashfall: evidence for a disaster stress reaction. Am Psychol 39:252–260, 1984

American Psychiatric Association: Diagnostic and Statistical Manual of Mental Disorders, 4th Edition, Text Revision. Washington, DC, American Psychiatric Association, 2000

Bayard M, McIntyre J, Hill KR, et al: Alcohol withdrawal syndrome. Am Fam Physician 69:1443–1450, 2004

Bohn MJ, Babor TF, Kranzler HR: The Alcohol Use Disorders Identification Test (AUDIT): validation of a screening instrument for use in medical settings. J Stud Alcohol 56:423–432, 1995

Bonanno GA, Galea S, Bucciarelli A, et al: What predicts psychological resilience after disaster? The role of demographics, resources, and life stress. J Consult Clin Psychol 75:671–682, 2007

Bravo M, Rubio-Stipec M, Canino GJ, et al: The psychological sequelae of disaster stress prospectively and retrospectively evaluated. Am J Community Psychol 18:661–680, 1990

Breslau N, Davis GC, Schultz LR: Posttraumatic stress disorder and the incidence of nicotine, alcohol, and other drug disorders in persons who have experienced trauma. Arch Gen Psychiatry 60:289–294, 2003

Cherpitel CJ: Screening for alcohol problems in the emergency room: a rapid alcohol problems screen. Drug Alcohol Depend 40:133–137, 1995

Cherpitel CJ, Borges G: Screening for drug use disorders in the emergency department: performance of the rapid drug problems screen (RDPS). Drug Alcohol Depend 74:171–175, 2004

Cook RL, Chung T, Kelly TM, et al: Alcohol screening in young persons attending a sexually transmitted disease clinic: comparison of AUDIT, CRAFFT, and CAGE instruments. J Gen Intern Med 20:1–6, 2005

Dawson DA, Grant BF, Ruan WJ: The association between stress and drinking: modifying effects of gender and vulnerability. Alcohol Alcohol 40:453–460, 2005

Deykin EY, Buka SL: Prevalence and risk factors for posttraumatic stress disorder among chemically dependent adolescents. Am J Psychiatry 154:752–757, 1997

Donovan DM, Kivlahan DR, Doyle SR, et al: Concurrent validity of the Alcohol Use Disorders Identification Test (AUDIT) and AUDIT zones in defining levels of severity among out-patients with alcohol dependence in the COMBINE study. Addiction 101:1696–1704, 2006

Ewing JA: Detecting alcoholism: the CAGE questionnaire. JAMA 252:1905–1907, 1984

Foa EB, Dancu CV, Hembree EA, et al: A comparison of exposure therapy, stress inoculation training, and their combination for reducing post-traumatic stress disorder in female assault victims. J Consult Clin Psychol 67:194–200, 1999

Funderburk FR, Allen RP, Wagman AMI: Residual effects of ethanol and chlordiazepoxide treatments for alcohol withdrawal. J Nerv Ment Dis 166:195–203, 1978

Giaconia RM, Reinherz HZ, Hauz AC, et al: Comorbidity of substance use and post-traumatic stress disorders in a community sample of adolescents. Am J Orthopsychiatry 70:253–262, 2000

Green BL, Grace MA, Gleser GC: Identifying survivors at risk: long-term impairment following the Beverly Hills Supper Club fire. J Consult Clin Psychol 53:672–678, 1985

Green BL, Lindy JD, Grace MC, et al: Buffalo Creek survivors in the second decade: stability of stress symptoms. Am J Orthopsychiatry 60:43–54, 1990

Hien DA, Cohen LR, Miele GM, et al: Promising treatments for women with comorbid PTSD and substance use disorders. Am J Psychiatry 161:1426–1432, 2004

Hodges B, Mazur JE: Intravenous ethanol for the treatment of alcohol withdrawal syndrome in critically ill patients. Pharmacotherapy 24:1578–1585, 2004

Jacobsen LK, Southwick SM, Kosten TR: Substance use disorders in patients with posttraumatic stress disorder: a review of the literature. Am J Psychiatry 158:1184–1190, 2001

Joseph S, Yule W, Williams R, et al: Increased substance use in survivors of the Herald Free Enterprise disaster. Br J Med Psychol 66:185–191, 1993

Kishore V, Theall KP, Robinson W, et al: Resource loss, coping, alcohol use, and posttraumatic stress symptoms among survivors of Hurricane Katrina: a cross-sectional study. Am J Disaster Med 3:345–357, 2008

Knight JR, Sherritt L, Shrier LA, et al: Validity of the "CRAFFT" substance abuse screening test among general adolescent clinic outpatients. Arch Pediatr Adolesc Med 156:607–614, 2002

Labbate LA, Sonne SC, Randal CL, et al: Does comorbid anxiety or depression affect clinical outcomes in patients with post-traumatic stress disorder and alcohol use disorders? J Compr Psychiatry 45:304–310, 2004

Liskow B, Campbell J, Nickel EJ, et al: Validity of the CAGE questionnaire in screening for alcohol dependence in a walk-in (triage) clinic. J Stud Alcohol 56:277–281, 1995

Logue JN, Hansen H, Struening E: Emotional and physical distress following Hurricane Agnes in Wyoming Valley of Pennsylvania. Public Health Rep 94:495–502, 1979

Marshall RD, Galea S: Science for the community: assessing mental health after 9/11. J Clin Psychiatry 65(suppl):37–43, 2001

Mayo-Smith MF: Pharmacological management of alcohol withdrawal. JAMA 278:144–151, 1997

Myrick H, Anton RF: Treatment of alcohol withdrawal. Alcohol Health Res World 22:38–43, 1998

Najavitz LM, Weiss RD, Shaw SR, et al: "Seeking Safety": outcome of a new cognitive-behavioral psychotherapy for women with post-traumatic stress disorder and substance dependence. J Trauma Stress 11:437–456, 1998

National Institute on Alcohol Abuse and Alcoholism: Helping Patients Who Drink Too Much: A Clinician's Guide (NIH Publication 07-3769). Washington, D.C., U.S. Department of Health and Human Services, October 2008

North CS, Smith EM, Spitznagel EL: Posttraumatic stress disorder in survivors of a mass shooting. Am J Psychiatry 1515:82–88, 1994

North CS, Nixon SJ, Shariat S, et al: Psychiatric disorders among survivors of the Oklahoma City bombing. JAMA 282:755–762, 1999

North CS, Tivis L, McMillen CJ, et al: Coping, functioning and adjusting of rescue workers after the Oklahoma City bombing. J Trauma Stress 15:171–175, 2002a

North CS, Tivis L, McMillen JC, et al: Psychiatric disorders in rescue workers after the Oklahoma City bombing. Am J Psychiatry 159:857–859, 2002b

Okura KP: Mobilizing in response to a major disaster. Community Ment Health J 11:136–144, 1975

Parker RM, Rescorla LA, Finkelstein JA, et al: A survey of the health of homeless children in Philadelphia Shelters. Am J Dis Child 145:520–526, 1991

Pfefferbaum B, Doughty DE: Increased alcohol use in a treatment sample of Oklahoma City bombing victims. Psychiatry 64:296–303, 2001

Rehm J, Gmel G, Sempos CT, et al: Alcohol-related morbidity and mortality. Alcohol Res Health 27:39–51, 2003

Rowe CL, Liddle HA: When the levee breaks: treating adolescents and families in the aftermath of Hurricane Katrina. J Marital Family Ther 34:132–148, 2008

Rubonis AV, Bickman L: Psychological impairment in the wake of disaster: the disaster-psychopathology relationship. Psychol Bull 109:384–399, 1991

Saitz R: Recognition and management of occult alcohol withdrawal. Hosp Pract (Minneap) 30:49–54, 56–58, 1995

Saunders JB, Aasland OG, Babor TF, et al: Development of the Alcohol Use Disorders Identification Test (AUDIT): WHO collaborative project on early detection of persons with harmful alcohol consumption. Addiction 88:791–804, 1993

Shore JH, Vollmer WM, Tatum EL: Community patterns of posttraumatic stress disorders. J Nerv Ment Dis 177:681–685, 1989

Smith DW, Christiansen EH, Vincent R, et al: Population effects of the bombing of Oklahoma City. J Okla State Med Assoc 92:193–198, 1999

Smith EM, North CS, McCool RE, et al: Acute post disaster psychiatric disorders: identification of persons at risk. Am J Psychiatry 147:202–206, 1990

Stewart SH: Alcohol abuse in individuals exposed to trauma: a critical review. Psychol Bull 120:83–112, 1996

Stuppaeck CH, Barnas C, Hackenberg K, et al: Carbamazepine monotherapy in the treatment of alcohol withdrawal. Int Clin Psychopharmacol 5:273–278, 1990

Sullivan JT, Sykora K, Schneiderman J, et al: Assessment of alcohol withdrawal: the revised Clinical Institute Withdrawal Assessment for Alcohol scale (CIWA-Ar). Br J Addict 84:1353–1357, 1989

Thompson SJ: Risk/protective factors associated with substance use among runaway/homeless youth utilizing emergency shelter services nationwide. Subst Abuse 25:13–26, 2004

Tiet QQ, Mausbauch B: Treatments for patients with dual diagnosis: a review. Alcohol Clin Exp Res 31:513–536, 2007

U.S. Department of Health and Human Services: Helping Patients Who Drink Too Much: A Clinician's Guide (NIH Publ No 05-3769). Bethesda, MD, National Institute on Alcohol Abuse and Alcoholism, 2005

Vetter S, Rossegger A, Rossler W, et al: Exposure to the tsunami disaster, PTSD symptoms and increased substance use: an Internet based survey of male and female residents of Switzerland. BMC Public Health 8:92, 2008

Vlahov D, Galea S, Resnick H, et al: Increased use of cigarettes, alcohol, and marijuana among Manhattan, New York, residents after the September 11th terrorist attacks. Am J Epidemiol 155:988–996, 2002

Vlahov D, Galea S, Ahern J, et al: Consumption of cigarettes, alcohol, and marijuana among New York City residents 6 months after the September 11 terrorist attacks. Am J Drug Alcohol Abuse 30:385–407, 2004

Weatherburn D, Jones C, Freeman K, et al: Supply control and harm reduction: lessons from the Australian heroin drought. Addiction 98:83–91, 2003

Wesson DR, Ling W: The Clinical Opiate Withdrawal Scale (COWS). J Psychoactive Drugs 35:253–259, 2003

World Health Organization: WHO Model List of Essential Medicines, 16th list (updated). Geneva, Switzerland, World Health Organization, March 2010. Available at: http://www.who.int/medicines/publications/essentialmedicines/en/index.html. Accessed October 23, 2010.

9

Personality Issues

Srinivasan S. Pillay, M.D.

Personality characteristics are normative. Societies have certain expectations about how people should behave, but they also recognize that considerable variation in behavior exists. When people experience the strain of disaster, their usual personality characteristics may become exaggerated. Notably, when these traits exceed the usual responses to threat and loss in the context of a disaster, they may significantly undermine treatment efforts and recovery. For example, emotionally expressive behavior that is inappropriate to the social context may disrupt the entire postdisaster caregiver setting. This behavior itself may be an expression of underlying personality issues that are centered around the need to disrupt the caregiver setting when the patient feels as though he or she is not getting sufficient attention. In this chapter, the term *personality issues* refers to personality traits that are unmasked by a disaster but not yet diagnosable as personality disorders (Tyrer 2010).

The prevalence of personality disorders in the United States is 9.1% (Lenzenweger et al. 2007). However, it is notable that functional impairment is significantly associated with Axis I comorbidity, and people with personality disorders are very likely to have major mental disorders (Lenzenweger et al. 2007). For example, in one study, 30.2% of individuals with borderline personality disorder (BPD) were also diagnosed with posttraumatic stress disorder (PTSD), whereas 24.2% of individuals with PTSD were also diagnosed with BPD (Pagura et al. 2010). When this comorbidity exists, individuals may have a poorer quality of life and increased odds of a lifetime suicide attempt.

In the DSM-IV-TR Axis II framework, personality disorders fall into one of three broad categories: odd/eccentric, dramatic/emotional, and anxious/fearful (American Psychiatric Association 2000). In the disaster setting, these different characteristics may become especially important when they are disruptive or maladaptive. For example, a person with excessive sensitivity to abandonment may end up utilizing caregiver resources to the detriment of other survivors, or a survivor who tends to be histrionic may manipulate the staff to serve his or her needs. When possible, once personality issues are suspected, efforts should be made to ensure that appropriate attention is given to them to optimize treatment outcome. To help mental health practitioners meet the needs of patients with personality issues after a disaster, I discuss the following topics in this chapter:

1. How to assess whether a personality disorder is present
2. When personality issues are especially relevant in the disaster situation
3. How to manage personality issues in the disaster environment

Assessment

As in any other diagnostic assessment, the clinician diagnoses personality characteristics and disorders by doing a thorough review of symptoms, starting with the question, "Have you always been the type of person who…?" The response may help the caregiver to distinguish acute symptomatology from chronic, ingrained, enduring personality traits due to stress reactions. Depending on the context for the assessment, the initial inquiry in the acute disaster setting may highlight the main problematic characteristics of each personality or personality disorder, with later assessments in the postacute situation focusing on the details to further elucidate the specific personality issue at hand. In fact, there is often no luxury of time for complete assessment of personality issues, and detecting maladaptive traits may be sufficient. In later follow-up, personality issues or disorders can be explored in greater detail. Table 9–1 lists the three general categories (clusters) of personality disorder, the specific personality disorders that make up each cluster, the hallmark Criterion A features of each disorder from DSM-IV-TR, and an example of how each disorder might affect the postdisaster caregiver setting. It is notable that these characteristics are not always detected by specific symptom inquiry or patient self-report; as is often the case in assessing personality issues, they may be better observed or reported by others. Because personality issues and disorders are usually ego-syntonic, people rarely complain about having them. However, a thorough history and mental status examination may reveal certain personality issues, such as impulsive behavior, odd thinking, or paranoia.

TABLE 9–1. Quick-reference table for diagnosis of personality disorders

Cluster	Personality disorder	Hallmark symptom	Example
A (odd or eccentric)	Paranoid	Pervasive distrust and suspicion of others	Consumes caregiver resources with excessive questions
	Schizoid	Pervasive detachment from social relationships; restricted range of emotional expression	Creates self-consciousness among the expressive survivors due to excessively restricted emotional range
	Schizotypal	Reduced capacity for close relationships, with cognitive or perceptual distortions and eccentric behavior	Increases distress by introducing "mysterious" possible causes of disaster
B (dramatic, emotional, or erratic)	Antisocial	Disregard for and violation of rights of others	Manipulates caregiver with superficial charm
	Borderline	Instability of interpersonal relationships, identity, and affects; impulsivity	Disrupts calmness with frequent temper tantrums
	Histrionic	Excessive emotionality and attention seeking	Seduces caregiver and dominates time of responders
	Narcissistic	Grandiosity; need for admiration; lack of empathy	May be critical or degrade other survivors
C (anxious or fearful)	Avoidant	Social inhibition; inadequacy; hypersensitivity to negative evaluation	May exclude self from group processes in acute recovery period
	Dependent	Excessive need for caretaking with submissive and clinging behavior	May become hysterical over threat of being alone
	Obsessive-compulsive	Preoccupation with orderliness, perfectionism, and mental and interpersonal control	May object to need for flexibility (e.g., relocating) in the service of sticking to rules

Personality styles may impact the quality of care or expectation of outcome as well. For example, David Shapiro (1999) described four basic neurotic styles: obsessive-compulsive, paranoid, hysterical, and impulsive. Keeping these styles in mind can be helpful to the clinician when assessing the needs of people in the disaster situation. At the most extreme, personality disorders may be resistant to treatment and require long-term intervention. Identifying subtypes of patients or neurotic styles may help the caregiver focus on treating needed and relevant symptoms without expecting to address the more deeply ingrained characteristics. In the disaster situation, personality issues may not always be identifiable as clear "disorders" despite being disruptive. As illustrated in the following two case vignettes, deliberate assessment of personality issues can be vital to looking beyond the Axis I diagnosis, instituting an appropriate (and, where possible, evidence-based) treatment for the personality disorder, and evaluating the prognosis.

A 35-year-old male survivor was seen after the terrorist attacks on the World Trade Center (WTC) on 9/11. In the initial assessment, he appeared to be genuinely shocked by the recent events, and in the context of the enormity of what had just happened, this reaction was understandable. He was visibly shaken and seemed to go in and out of "communicative" mode. When he stopped talking, the assessing doctor would leave him alone for a while, but because he was still in the physical proximity of the assessing doctor, she could clearly see that when she left him, he appeared to be responding to internal stimuli. When she returned to check on him, he would deny that anything unusual was happening, but as soon as the doctor left, this behavior would start again. It became progressively more difficult for the doctor to decide what to do. Should she attend to what appeared to be psychotic symptoms? Or should she chalk this up to an exaggerated personality trait of needing attention? These two situations would require very different care.

A young artist prone to mood elevation and depression was drawn to the drama of the rescue effort at the WTC site and was unable to leave the site for 2 weeks. She slept in an abandoned hotel and was almost sexually assaulted. She presented to a WTC mental health program with PTSD in addition to borderline traits. It was also unclear if she had become hypomanic at site. She had a renewed life narrative sparked by her sense of heroism at the WTC site, with both victim and rescuer fantasies activated. Her WTC involvement became the catalyst for seeking mental health treatment for lifelong issues, including self-cutting and eating disorders.

Personality Issues of Relevance in Disaster Situations

Sometimes in an acute disaster, an individual may respond with regressive reactions, which may be part of the acute traumatic response and progressively diminish over time (Eksi and Braun 2009). This response should be distinguished from the individual's more enduring personality issues. In the acute disaster situation, the clinician should give the patient the benefit of the doubt if the patient does not pose a danger to self or others.

On occasion, people who fall into certain categories of personality disorder (especially antisocial and borderline) may present as "hateful patients" (Strous et al. 2006). This problematic behavior may serve as a clue to examine personality issues. Hateful patients may fall into one of four categories: dependent clingers, entitled demanders, manipulative help-rejecters, and self-destructive deniers (Groves 1978). In the disaster situation, each of these personality types may pose a challenge to the caregiver. For example, meeting a manipulative help-rejecter may cause a caregiver who left his or her home country to care for a disaster-struck community to be angry, dissatisfied, and less motivated to continue working in that environment. However, if the worker identifies this personality issue as being probably resistant to treatment, and focuses instead on treating what can be treated, both the patient and the caregiver may benefit from this awareness.

Survivors with any of the personality disorders mentioned in Table 9–1 may have valid reasons to substantiate their reactions: survivors may be pervasively paranoid after a bombing, or excessively dependent after being separated from loved ones, or rigid and compulsive as part of their efforts to cope. Also, some victims may feel entitled to care because they are victims of a major disaster.

In the disaster situation, it may be unrealistic for clinicians to expect to be able to discern subtle maladaptive personality traits from initial exaggerated reactions to the disaster. For that reason, clinicians would benefit from focusing on whether the behavior is disruptive to the victim or the treatment goals in that setting acutely or in the postacute situation, and based on that determination, institute the appropriate interventions.

Management of Personality Issues in Disaster Environments

When personality issues arise in the disaster environment, the clinician should keep in mind several general principles of treatment: be realistic, diagnose when possible, triage to the appropriate caregivers, recognize that there may be things the clinician cannot do, and treat what is possible by being focused on alleviating acute distress and possible disruptions to team efforts in the crisis situation. Although the need for psychosocial support has been widely recognized (Rao 2006), a recent article highlighted how caregivers may inadvertently do harm by using psychotherapeutic techniques that negate the goals of the treatment (Wessells 2009). Some of the technical errors to avoid include insensitivity to the culture in which one is working, an excessive focus on victimization, and use of dependency-creating interventions. Through critical self-reflection, the clinician can avoid these pitfalls in order to deliver the most effective care possible. Principles of biological and psychological care are outlined below.

Biological Management

A clinician should not allow survivors' personality issues and disorders to distract him or her from looking for Axis I conditions that may benefit from early treatment with medication (see Chapter 15, "Psychopharmacology: Acute Phase"; Chapter 16, "Psychopharmacology: Postacute Phase"; and Chapter 17, "Child and Adolescent Psychiatry Interventions"). Because most Axis I disorders have a "duration" specifier, it is almost impossible to make a definitive diagnosis of new-onset symptoms during the acute phase, but it is possible in the postacute phase. Practically speaking, acute phase treatment, therefore, is often symptom based. Certain target symptoms of personality issues may respond well to medication. For example, panic attacks may respond well to alprazolam in patients with an anxiety-prone cognitive style (Uhlenhuth et al. 2008).

Psychological Management: Countertransference

As cited in Waska (2008), Sandler pointed out the important benefit of the clinician's examining his or her own countertransference to contain the acute anxieties of patients and to provide an environment that is as comfortable as possible for the patient. Although this effort may not be possible in the acute situation of a disaster, it forms the backbone of any good supportive therapy as well.

The hateful patient can generate a significant amount of countertransference. Problematic *positive countertransference* may occur when a caregiver relates to the helplessness of a histrionic survivor to the detriment of others. *Negative countertransference* may occur when a caregiver resents a survivor who just can't "get his or her act together."

Such feelings of resentment or anger in the clinician are not always problematic, however, and may be used therapeutically. They can be helpful clues in identifying people whose affects and behaviors invite therapeutic interventions, including limit setting. For instance, those who repeatedly use self-destructive gestures to gain attention benefit from a combination of understanding and clear limit setting about the effects of their actions on others and the potential adverse consequence for themselves. Manipulative behaviors may be accentuated, or even sparked anew, by the regressive tendencies common after disasters. Similarly, those whose personality issues include making others feel resentful or fearful from threats also may benefit from understanding of their personality issues and interventions, including arriving at manageable limits, to reduce such behaviors (Yudofsky 2005). Limit setting may be all the more necessary in the chaos of disaster, when survivors with personality issues must confront boundary problems not only from within but also from without.

Personality disorders may also mask underlying feelings in the patient. For example, the schizoid patient may have an inner, heightened sensitivity and longing for closeness despite being externally distant (Thylstrup and Hesse 2009). The psychiatrist should approach such a patient bearing in mind the tremendous shame and ambivalence the patient may feel about asking for help, even in the disaster situation.

Psychotherapeutic Interventions

Various types of psychotherapy may be useful in a disaster situation, as discussed in the following subsections.

Supportive Therapy

In the context of a disaster, supportive therapy, which requires reinforcing the patient's healthy and adaptive thoughts and behaviors, is very appropriate. The goal is to enhance the resilience of the disaster victim. Resilience enhancement shifts the focus of psychological investigation onto increasing the positive coping mechanisms rather than reducing the negative impact of the disaster (Connor and Zhang 2006). It is important to distinguish this from debriefing, which involves asking the disaster victim to describe what happened in detail and often is done in groups close to the time of the event. Debriefing has been found to be more harmful than helpful in the disaster setting (Stoddard et al. 2010). (Debriefing is discussed in more detail in Chapter 13, "Group and Family Interventions.") In the disaster situation, the protection of human dignity is vital (Petrini 2010).

Cognitive-Behavioral Interventions

Certain types of symptoms—for example, excessive reactions of a person with paranoid or borderline issues—may benefit from cognitive reframing. Instruments such as the Beliefs About Emotions Scale may help in developing a reframing intervention for a survivor with borderline personality disorder whose beliefs about the unacceptability of experiencing or expressing negative emotions may exacerbate his or her emotional instability (Rimes and Chalder 2010). Although this type of assessment may not be possible in the acute setting, such scales may be helpful in the postacute setting (weeks to months after the disaster) for identifying areas of resilience on which to focus in psychotherapy (see also Chapter 14, "Psychotherapies").

Early Dialectical Behavioral and Acceptance–Based Interventions

Although dialectical behavioral therapy is unlikely to be instituted in an emergency setting, certain principles such as mindfulness and acceptance may be helpful in the treatment of personality issues. These principles are especially useful in resiliency training and supportive therapy. Early interventions, even over a 5-day period, may have a long-lasting impact (Yen et al. 2009). Also, acceptance-based interventions may help emotional regulation (Gratz 2007).

Conclusion

Personality issues in the disaster situation may range from transient personality traits to more enduring manifestations of a personality disorder. In the acute situation, early identification of personality issues, followed by supportive interventions focusing on enhancing resilience rather than debriefing, may help contain patients in the disaster environment.

■ Teaching Points

- Personality issues may occur in both disaster victims and disaster responders.
- Awareness of the four types of "hateful patients"—dependent clingers, entitled demanders, manipulative help-rejecters, and self-destructive deniers—may be helpful.
- Appropriate use of psychopharmacology and brief therapy to treat personality disorders is essential.
- Caregivers should be sensitive to cultural differences and avoid use of dependency-creating interventions.
- Self-reflection on countertransference may help set the stage for supportive interventions.

Review Questions

9.1   Which of the following characteristics is *not* typical of personality disorders?

A.   Enduring.
B.   Maladaptive.

C. Ego-dystonic.

D. Ingrained.

E. Early age at onset.

9.2 Categories of "hateful patients" described by Groves (1978) include all of the following *except*

A. Homicidal maniacs.

B. Dependent clingers.

C. Entitled demanders.

D. Manipulative help-rejecters.

E. Self-destructive deniers.

9.3 When working with people with personality disorders in disasters

A. It is important to stress victimization a lot.

B. It is important to really reach out and allow them to become dependent on you.

C. It is important to use whatever therapeutic technique is possible even if it cannot be sustained.

D. It is important to employ critical self-reflection in examining one's own countertransference.

E. None of the above.

9.4 Which of the following is relatively contraindicated in a disaster situation?

A. Supportive therapy.

B. Psychological debriefing.

C. Examination of countertransference.

D. Resiliency-focused interventions.

E. None of the above.

9.5 When working with an entitled patient in a disaster situation, the best response to a demand for treatment is

A. "I'd like to give you everything you want, but you're not the only one who needs treatment here."

B. "I think you need to be less entitled."

C. "Of course, we can do whatever you'd like."

D. "I think you should know you are stressing the system."

E. "I agree that you deserve the best; this is what is possible."

References

American Psychiatric Association: Diagnostic and Statistical Manual of Mental Disorders, 4th Edition, Text Revision. Washington, DC, American Psychiatric Association, 2000

Connor KM, Zhang W: Recent advances in the understanding and treatment of anxiety disorders. Resilience: determinants, measurement, and treatment responsiveness. CNS Spectr 11:5–12, 2006

Eksi A, Braun KL: Over-time changes in PTSD and depression among children surviving the 1999 Istanbul earthquake. Eur Child Adolesc Psychiatry 18:384–391, 2009

Gratz KL: Targeting emotion dysregulation in the treatment of self-injury. J Clin Psychol 63:1091–1103, 2007

Groves JE: Taking care of the hateful patient. N Engl J Med 298:883–887, 1978

Lenzenweger MF, Lane MC, Loranger AW, et al: DSM-IV personality disorders in the National Comorbidity Survey Replication. Biol Psychiatry 62:553–564, 2007

Pagura J, Stein MB, Bolton JM, et al: Comorbidity of borderline personality disorder and posttraumatic stress disorder in the U.S. population. J Psychiatr Res 44:1190–1198, 2010

Petrini C: Triage in public health emergencies: ethical issues. Intern Emerg Med 5:137–144, 2010

Rao K: Psychosocial support in disaster-affected communities. Int Rev Psychiatry 18:501–505, 2006

Rimes KA, Chalder T: The Beliefs About Emotions Scale: validity, reliability and sensitivity to change. J Psychosom Res 68:285–292, 2010

Shapiro D: Neurotic Styles (The Austen Riggs Center Monograph Series, No 5). New York, Basic Books, 1999

Stoddard FJ Jr, Katz CL, Merlino JP: Hidden Impact: What You Need to Know for the Next Disaster. A Practical Mental Health Guide for Clinicians. Sudbury, MA, Jones & Bartlett, 2010

Strous RD, Ulman AM, Kotler M: The hateful patient revisited: relevance for 21st century medicine. Eur J Intern Med 17:387–393, 2006

Thylstrup B, Hesse M: "I am not complaining": ambivalence construct in schizoid personality disorder. Am J Psychother 63:147–167, 2009

Tyrer P: Personality structure as an organizing construct. J Pers Disord 24:14–24, 2010

Uhlenhuth EH, Starcevic V, Qualls C, et al: Cognitive style, alprazolam plasma levels, and treatment response in panic disorder. Depress Anxiety 25:E18–E26, 2008

Waska R: Using countertransference: analytic contact, projective identification, and transference phantasy states. Am J Psychother 62:333–351, 2008

Wessells MG: Do no harm: toward contextually appropriate psychosocial support in international emergencies. Am Psychol 64:842–854, 2009

Yen S, Johnson J, Costello E, et al: A 5-day dialectical behavior therapy partial hospital program for women with borderline personality disorder: predictors of outcome from a 3-month follow-up study. J Psychiatr Pract 15:173–182, 2009

Yudofsky S: Fatal Flaws: Navigating Destructive Relationships With People With Disorders of Personality and Character. Washington, DC, American Psychiatric Publishing, 2005

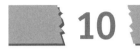

10

Injuries and Triage of Medical Complaints

Kristina Jones, M.D.

The mind-body connection has received increasing attention over the past few years in both the popular press and the psychiatric literature. In disaster psychiatry, this connection becomes a practical matter. For example, patients with no physical illness who fear that they have been exposed to a toxin during a disaster may develop psychogenic symptoms, including shortness of breath or palpitations. Also, patients with objective physical injury may be at increased risk for the development of posttraumatic stress disorder (PTSD).

In this chapter, I present two key areas in triage of patients presenting with both medical and psychiatric symptoms. During a disaster involving exposure to a nuclear, chemical, or biological weapon, and occasionally after a terrorist attack, patients may present with psychogenic presentations of illness. These are termed *medically unexplained physical symptoms* (MUPS). The first section of this chapter is concerned with acute psychiatric management of disaster survivors who present with MUPS, and includes discussion of typical symptoms, a cognitive model of such behavior, and guidelines for the disaster psychiatrist to help and to educate others on the disaster team about evaluating and managing this type of presentation.

The remainder of this chapter addresses psychiatric consultation for acutely injured patients, including those at disaster sites, in emergency settings, and in general hospitals. The psychiatrist's awareness of risk factors and early intervention may help prevent or mitigate psychiatric symptomatology in medically ill patients. The general psychiatrist may provide important psychiatric intervention, education, and management of patients, including high-risk patients, such as burn and trauma patients and those with uncontrolled pain.

Medically Unexplained Physical Symptoms Following Biological or Terrorist Events

After a bioterrorist event or accidental biological exposure, large numbers of people may present to the emergency department (ED) seeking evaluation and/or reassurance. For example, in March 1995, the Aum Shinrikyo cult released toxic sarin gas in the Tokyo subway system. The gas was odorless and colorless, and the symptoms were nonspecific. Twelve people died, and 5,510 people presented to the ED believing that they had been exposed. The ratio of those who died to those with nonsignificant symptoms was 1:500 (DiGiovanni 1999).

In 2001, the U.S. Postal Service was the vehicle used to disseminate letters containing weapons-grade *Bacillus anthracis* spores. Exposure to inhalational anthrax occurred in Florida, the District of Columbia, New Jersey, New York, Maryland, Pennsylvania, and Virginia. In the end, 22 people were infected, 11 with inhalational anthrax, 7 with cutaneous anthrax, and 4 with suspected cutaneous anthrax. Five of the patients infected with inhalational anthrax died. Although not effective at causing mass casualties, the anthrax incident created a general fear throughout the United States, causing significant expense and disruption. Media broadly reported that signs and symptoms of anthrax resembled the early signs of influenza or upper respiratory infection. Supplies of ciprofloxacin, reportedly the most effective treatment for anthrax, dwindled as health institutions and the public reportedly stockpiled supplies. An estimated 10,000 people received treatment for possible anthrax exposure. In this case, the ratio of deaths to persons seeking medical help was approximately 11:10,000 or 1:1,000 (Rodriguez et al. 2005).

After a disaster involving radioactive exposure or toxic exposure to a biological agent, mass panic may ensue. Although there are rare and isolated case reports of large numbers of patients presenting to EDs, usually after a false rumor of a gas leak or an unusual odor of some kind, mass panic is, fortunately, not a common or expected part of the public's reaction to an acute disaster event. The term *mass hysteria* now has a pejorative connotation, and is more usefully considered under DSM-IV-TR (American Psychiatric Association 2000) conceptual frameworks such as somatoform disorder or conversion disorder. *Mass panic* is generally defined as "the rapid spread of illness signs and symptoms affecting members of a cohesive group, originating from a nervous system disturbance involving excitation, loss or alteration of function, whereby physical complaints that are exhibited unconsciously have no corresponding organic etiology" (Bartholomew and Wessely 2002, p. 300). In general terms, natural and human-made disasters tend to mobilize communities, and impressive displays of cooperation and mutual aid often occur. The literature indicates that expressions of mutual aid are common and often predominate after disasters (Mawson 2008).

The term *surge capacity* describes the ability of emergency services to deal with a surge in mass casualties, which may include psychosomatic presentations. The disaster psychiatrist can contribute to the emergency response by offering information about the normal range of behavior after disaster, including brief anxiety and help-seeking behavior, and by being open to assisting in triage and evaluation of psychogenic complaints that may arrive in the ED under the guise of actual physical symptoms, such as shortness of breath, headache, palpitations, weakness, and emotional "shock."

The disaster psychiatrist working in a medical setting may need to serve as a point person and impromptu educator of both medical and nonmedical staff. Simplifying complex medical terminology and providing basic information at a level patients can comprehend is part of the mental health intervention. Providing information about normal reactions to disaster may be normalizing for patients and staff. The psychiatrist should be knowledgeable about the most current medical literature regarding the putative agent of exposure. Kman and Nelson (2008) provide an excellent illustrated review of all bioterrorism agents, including medical and psychiatric symptoms. As one example of a psychiatric manifestation, exposure to cyanide may result in mild symptoms of irritability, dizziness, headache, fatigue, and nausea, or a more moderate to severe symptom picture, involving dyspnea, altered mental status (including delirium), cardiac ischemia, syncope, coma, and seizure (Madsen 2005). The U.S. Department of Veterans Affairs National Center for PTSD maintains a Web site aimed at health professionals (www.ptsd.va.gov/PTSD/professional/) that contains training materials on how to counsel those at low risk, as well as children and families. It also offers such clinical pearls as typical presentations of major chemical exposures.

In discussing lessons learned from exposures involving severe acute respiratory syndrome (SARS), anthrax, and pneumonic plague, Rubin and Dickmann (2010) proposed strategies that can be employed to try to lower the number of low-risk patients arriving at the ED and potentially overwhelming the existing medical resources. These strategies include providing clear information about who should and should not go to hospitals; using the media and hospital telephone services to provide more detailed information and initial screening; employing rapid triage at hospital entrances, based, where possible, on exposure history and objective signs of illness; and following up by telephone those judged to be at low risk. These strategies were largely effective during the anthrax outbreak in that information to the public about the triad of high fever, cough, and significant respiratory problems was stressed, and fears about nonspecific symptoms, such as headache, dizziness, and fatigue, were minimized.

After a terrorist attack, or during and after a bioterrorism attack, there may be multiple presentations to EDs and clinics by patients seeking evaluation for symptoms they believe to be related to the attack. When relevant laboratory tests or imaging studies have been performed and objective findings are lacking, the ED, including the disaster psychiatrist, is confronted with the likelihood that the patient's presentation is that of MUPS, which is defined as physical symptoms that prompt the sufferer to seek health care but remain unexplained after an appropriate medical evaluation (Stoddard 2010).

Psychiatrists can understand MUPS as occurring within certain conceptual frameworks, such as undifferentiated somatoform disorder, conversion disorder, and somatic anxiety. In an excellent review of MUPS in medical practice, Richardson and Engel (2004) used the examples of fibromyalgia, chronic fatigue syndrome, and multiple chemical sensitivity (Gulf War syndrome) to formulate key features of MUPS and suggest strategies for psychiatric management of the doctor-patient encounter (Table 10–1).

Clinical strategies for physician communication in these challenging situations are helpful in managing patients with MUPS. The framework presented in Table 10–2 can guide the disaster psychiatrist to help a medical colleague communicate his or her findings to a patient in a nonpejorative, nonalienating way.

The disaster psychiatrist can help manage medical colleagues' considerable frustration and negative countertransference with patients with MUPS. For example, physicians must be counseled not to say to the patient "There is nothing wrong with you." Rather, the physician can educate the patient by correcting misunderstandings the patient may have regarding the body and its functions and can elicit the patient's reactions to being told that no serious disease or injury is present. A patient will accept that a rapid heart rate is due to adrenaline or fear, and not a heart attack, if the information is given in an empathic and professional manner (Disaster Psychiatry Outreach 2008).

It is essential that the psychiatrist and the primary care physician work collaboratively with each other and with the patient with MUPS to destigmatize the distress the patient is feeling and normalize the decision to seek

TABLE 10–1. Key features of medically unexplained physical symptoms (MUPS) in the doctor-patient relationship

Conflict in the doctor-patient dyad

Mismatch of patient's view that symptom is ominous and physician's view that it has no basis in disease

Patient minimizes the extent of psychological distress

Patient makes repeat emergency department visits or makes multiple physician visits at different locations

Patient questions physician's competence

Depression and anxiety are consistently associated with MUPS, although patient may be reluctant to admit such symptoms on history

Patient may experience vegetative symptoms such as fatigue, increased symptom sensitivity, changes in sleep, and altered autonomic nervous system functioning causing psychophysiological symptoms such as tremor or palpitations

MUPS serve as a mode of communicating distress

Patient's faulty explanatory beliefs set up a worsening cycle of anxiety, physiological arousal, and somatic symptoms

Source. Adapted from Richardson and Engel 2004.

TABLE 10–2. Physician communication techniques for patients with medically unexplained physical symptoms (MUPS)

Acknowledge uncertainty as to the causes of MUPS (e.g., "Doctors often see patients with symptoms like yours, and we do not know their exact cause").

Convey clinical experience (e.g., "I have seen many patients with unexplained symptoms similar to yours").

Offer hope (e.g., "Science has shown that there are things we can work on together that will help you feel and function better").

Promise action (e.g., "No matter what we decide to do, let's continue to meet on a scheduled basis until we agree that we've been effective").

Avoid potential adverse effects associated with indiscriminate medical therapies or invasive workups.

Source. Adapted from Richardson and Engel 2004.

mental health care. For example, as a segue into suggesting stress management techniques, relaxation training, or even a mental health referral for a patient, the primary care physician might state, "Terrorism or incidents of this type may cause a great deal of stress, which may have an impact on your heart rate, breathing, digestion, sleep, and other systems." Encouraging a patient to work with a single primary care physician rather than many is often helpful in containing the anxiety and behavioral help-seeking associated with MUPS. Although sedative-hypnotics or benzodiazepines may be useful, anxiolytics may actually impair coping in some individuals with MUPS by causing sedation or contributing to apathy or fatigue, which might decrease their seeking of social supports. It is important to discover the explanatory illness model that each patient has and to assess the patient's current psychosocial stressors (Richardson and Engel 2004); this involves, for example, exploring whether the patient has a fatalistic or pessimistic illness model and whether the patient can be encouraged to believe in his or her own ability to cope and have physical symptoms improve over time.

MUPS are psychiatrically complex. From research on Gulf War patients, many of whom presented with symptoms without objective findings, Hunt et al. (2002) conceptualized MUPS using a biopsychosocial model. They noted that predisposing, precipitating, and perpetuating factors may be present. Predisposing factors include heredity, biological diatheses, early life adversity, chronic illness, chronic distress, and mental illness. Immediate precipitating factors include biological stressors, such as exposure or presumed exposure; acute physical illness; psychosocial stressors; acute psychiatric disorders; and epidemic health concerns. Finally, perpetuating factors including harmful illness beliefs, labeling effects, misinformation, and workplace and compensation factors. Additional perpetuating factors include low social support factors, negative health habits, chronic illness, deconditioning, chronic illness, and poor integration into the treatment system (Hunt et al. 2002). The following case vignette illustrates the complexity presented by a patient with MUPS.

Ms. M, a 49-year-old Polish asbestos worker residing in New York City, had volunteered in the cleanup effort after 9/11, where she was exposed to World Trade Center (WTC) dust and found several body parts, including a severed finger and scalp. Two years later, she went to a free clinic complaining of shortness of breath, nausea, and a 25-pound weight loss. Ms. M was preoccupied with Polish newspaper stories about "heroes" of Polish origin who had helped clean the WTC site and then died of cancer. She believed that her weight loss meant that she had cancer and would die. In a passive suicidal gesture, Ms. M stopped taking her free asthma medicine, stopped eating, and stopped working. She met criteria for panic disorder and major depression. A medical workup revealed mild pulmonary disease but no evidence of malignancy. Upper endoscopy revealed significant reflux disease, for which she was unable to afford medication. The rash that Ms. M thought was WTC dust toxicity was discovered to be scabies, a result of her living accommodations. She reluctantly admitted to a history of postpartum depression, as well as depression following the death of her husband from cancer 2 years prior to 9/11. Ms. M's early life experience was one of extreme poverty. A precipitating stressor to her depression was the return of her son to Poland, leaving her alone in New York. She was poorly integrated into health care, uninsured, and undocumented, and she spoke poor English. Zoloft and Nexium were prescribed, and Ms. M gained 20 pounds over 3 months. She was connected to social services through her church and made a reasonable recovery.

The case highlights the point that MUPS may present long after a disaster. Similarly, in a study of 1,547 residents in the Netherlands surveyed 1 year before and 4 years after an explosion at a fireworks factory that killed 23 people, injured 900, and forced 1,200 from their homes, van den Berg et al. (2009) noted that 18 months postdisaster, 33% of survivors reported ≥10 symptoms, compared with 20.6% of control subjects who lived in the area but were neither injured nor forced from their homes by the explosion. The most frequently presented symptoms were back pain, cough, fatigue, neck problems, and shoulder symptoms. These represented, respectively, 10.3%, 5.0%, 5.0%, 4.6%, and 4.2% of all MUPS that presented to the general practitioner. The study found that predisposing factors were patient characteristics, including female gender, lower education level, unemployment, childhood medical illness, and maltreatment. Precipitating factors were events in the person's life, such as stressful life events and psychological problems, that resulted in the appearance of symptoms. Finally, perpetuating factors were those that maintained or exaggerated symptoms (e.g., financial problems and lack of social support).

One potential concern is the long-term effects on the mental health of patients who are exposed and affected by terrorist attacks. Follow-up mental health studies of individuals exposed to sarin gas or anthrax have yielded interesting results: Of 111 patients hospitalized at a Tokyo hospital after their exposure to sarin gas during the subway attack, one-third reported anxiety, fear, nightmares, insomnia, and irritability to their physicians. At 1 month after the incident, 32% of the patients treated at that hospital after the incident reported a fear of subways, 29% noted continuing sleep disturbances, and 16% reported flashbacks and depression. These symptoms persisted at 3- and 6-month follow-up visits to their physicians (Ohbu et al. 1997). Tucker et al. (2007) surveyed 60 survivors 7 years after the Oklahoma City bombing and found that although 66% felt they had fully recovered, 9% remained symptomatic and met full criteria for PTSD, compared with 1% of control subjects (age- and gender-matched Oklahoma City area community members).

Medical Illness: Triage and Evaluation of Medically Ill Survivors

After a major incident, the disaster psychiatrist in a hospital setting may be involved in the rapid triage and assessment of patients in the ED, as well as in medical or surgical wards. When mass casualties occur, some trauma patients will have psychiatric needs. The disaster psychiatrist may be called on to treat acute delirium and agitation, and to recognize early symptoms of mental trauma. In this section, I review the existing literature, highlight patients most at risk, offer techniques for evaluating critically ill patients, and briefly discuss common diagnoses, as well as a host of subclinical but important psychiatric dimensions of serious medical illness.

A review of the limited available literature, including that from military medicine and trauma journals, highlights that those patients with the most serious injuries are usually at higher risk for psychiatric disorders such as acute stress disorder (ASD). ASD includes symptoms such as insomnia, anxiety, irritability, hypervigilance, and, in extreme cases, dissociation. ASD by definition occurs only for 4 weeks, after which the diagnosis is PTSD. In a large population survey of 2,931 patients with physical trauma, patients were assessed with the PTSD Checklist after 12 months, and approximately 23% had symptoms consistent with PTSD. Greater levels of early postinjury anxiety and emotional distress, as well as physical pain, were positively associated with an increased risk of PTSD (Zatzick et al. 2007). Generally, the research literature supports the view that the more serious the injury, the more the risk, although this is not a perfectly consistent finding. Loss of a limb or loss of function is a significant risk, and burn patients are at particularly high risk for ASD and PTSD, with one study confirming PTSD in 15% of burn patients at 1-year follow-up (van Loey and Van Son 2003; van Loey et al. 2003). In a systematic review of PTSD in 1,104 survivors of burns, traumatic injuries, and intensive care unit (ICU) stays for other critical illnesses, Davydow et al. (2009) found a prevalence of PTSD in 19% of the patients, and reported that consistent predictors of post-ICU PTSD included prior psychopathology, greater ICU benzodiazepine administration, and post-ICU memories of ICU-related frightening and/or psychotic experiences. Female sex and younger age were less consistent predictors, and severity of illness was not a consistent predictor in this review. Patients with uncontrolled pain, burns, and facial disfigurement are also at high risk. Pain management and psychiatric medication interventions for adults and children are discussed in Chapters 15 and 16 on acute and postacute psychopharmacology and in Chapter 17, "Child and Adolescent Psychiatric Interventions."

Requests for psychiatric consultation for medical or surgical patients in disaster settings follow most of the principles for consultation requests from general medical and surgical setting practitioners, including those working in trauma. Common reasons for requesting a psychiatric consultation are listed in Table 10–3 (Stoddard et al. 2000).

TABLE 10–3. Reasons to request a psychiatric consultation for a medical or surgical patient

Patient has acute psychiatric symptoms (e.g., delirium, agitation, suicidal risk, anxiety, psychosis, depression); or capacity assessment ascertains patient's incapacity to refuse or consent to a surgical or medical procedure; or patient wishes to sign out against medical advice.

Family or nursing staff requests help in managing patient's psychological distress or patient's noncompliance with medical care.

Patient presents a diagnostic dilemma, regardless of whether a symptom is functional or organic. For example, patient is unwilling to participate in mobilization or physical therapy, or patient is overusing medication or requests what the team views as excessive or inappropriate pain control.

Source. Adapted from Stoddard et al. 2000.

In a few hospital settings, psychiatric consultation or screening of a medical or surgical patient occurs routinely. In the context of a disaster, it is unlikely that adequate resources will be available to allow for routine psychiatric screening. The psychiatrist can educate and show the medical staff how to perform triage to determine patients' needs for consultation where psychiatric staff are limited, and to focus the relevant questions. For example, delirious and agitated patients should take priority over the simply tearful or distressed patient, unless that patient is suicidal or presents a risk for elopement before being evaluated medically and psychiatrically. Curbside consults, often in the form of "schmoozing" or informal conversation, may allow some staff to "blow off steam" and process distressing emotions that result from the disaster or its impact (e.g., acute experiences from participating in amputations, major surgeries, and unsuccessful resuscitation efforts). Consultation can also be done via telepsychiatry, as discussed in Chapter 21, "Telepsychiatry in Disasters and Public Health Emergencies."

Types of Injury

The nature and severity of injuries vary depending on the event. Victims of natural disasters or of terrorist attacks may suffer blunt trauma, multiple wounds from broken glass or shrapnel, burns, or smoke inhalation. Bioterror agent exposure may result in symptoms of neuropsychiatric impairment, including confusion, dizziness, memory loss, and occasionally psychosis (Peer et al. 2007).

The surviving patient is subject to a broad range of stresses, including acute or chronic pain, exacerbated by effects of an injury, surgery, or other procedure; gastric stress ulcers; unavailability of analgesics; or the need for physical therapy to avoid bedsores or contractures. When a patient is in a state of relative sensory isolation, his or her fears may be magnified. Also, a patient may require isolation until the danger of infection has passed, or a necessary tracheostomy may interfere with communication (Wain et al. 2006). When a patient experiences acute vision loss, he or she is at high risk for delirium, psychosis, and dissociation (Wain et al. 2006).

Range of Mental Symptoms in Medically Ill Survivors

A key difference between disaster psychiatry and consultation psychiatry in general is that early after a disaster, the psychiatrist focuses on symptoms and may elect to treat these individually, before waiting for a diagnosable DSM-IV-TR disorder to be present. Medical illness, including that in the disaster setting, poses a number of psychological challenges for the patient, to which the psychiatrist must be alert. The hospital experience for the patient can evoke feelings of loss of control, loss of privacy, and dependence on others for the most basic tasks of feeding, toileting, ambulation, and so forth; this dependency is a challenge for the capable adult, and especially for the survivor of childhood neglect or abuse. The meaning of illness to the patient is important to ascertain, and will vary depending on personality type and character. The dependent patient may fear abandonment and need reassurance, whereas the obsessional patient may fear loss of control and require routine and choice about details of medical care where possible (Geringer and Stern 1986).

Important Symptoms

If time allows, a standard psychiatric evaluation screening for depression, anxiety, panic, psychosis, mania, and symptoms of ASD and PTSD should be performed. In the medical setting, the evaluation must include a brief cognitive screening for orientation and level of consciousness to assess for delirium, a common complication of narcotic analgesics used for pain management. Additional important symptoms to address are uncontrolled pain, insomnia, agitation, and suicidal ideation. Just because a patient does not present with a psychiatric history does not mean that he or she may not have a full-blown preexisting psychiatric disorder, such as untreated depression, or unreported alcohol or other substance abuse disorder.

Anxiety is common in the medical and surgical setting, and clinicians should observe patients for elevated pulse, respiratory rate, and other symptoms of acute stress, generalized anxiety, or panic. Medical illness may include palpitations and shortness of breath, both of which are symptoms of anxiety and warrant brief intervention with benzodiazepines, selective serotonin reuptake inhibitors (SSRIs), or even low-dose antipsychotics if comorbid with agitation or delirium. The fact that anxiety may be directly linked to a medical cause does not negate the need for psychiatric intervention if the patient is significantly distressed. ASD may also present with prominent numbing or detachment, and some patients, particularly male patients or patients in the uniformed services, may appear to be coping very well. In such a case, a systematic and detailed review of symptoms can reveal that the patient is suffering tremendous anxiety that may improve when treated with benzodiazepines or with sedative-hypnotics for sleep as needed. Male patients similarly have cultural expectations to express little emotion; the disaster psychiatrist can destigmatize appropriate expression of feelings and educate patients about the biological basis for immediate postdisaster hypervigilance, anxiety, and insomnia (Roberts et al. 2010). Patients can understand that their bodies are still on "high alert" and that the mind takes days or weeks to ramp down to a normal level.

ASD usually presents with significant anxiety, and the diagnostic screening should include a clinical review of symptoms, including assessment of dissociation. In the medical setting, psychological dissociation is easily confused with sedation or diminished neurological responsiveness. Rundell (2000), a prominent consultation-liaison psychiatrist, offers the following clinical technique for assessment of dissociative symptoms in the acute medical setting:

> Gently tap the patient on the shoulder and ask if there is anything they need and do they know where they are/what day it is. Watch for a muted but appropriate response in a dissociating person; this indicates his or her level of consciousness and orientation is grossly intact. Identifying otherwise uninjured disaster victims who are simply dissociating as having a grossly intact level of consciousness frees up scarce evaluation and treatment resources for other emergency patients. If dissociation becomes frequent, ongoing, and disabling the patient should be admitted for psychiatric observation and diagnostic clarification. Serial exams of the patient can help differentiate adaptive dissociation from dissociative disorder. Normally, initial dissociation should attenuate then disappear over several hours—after the threat is removed people should begin to call into play other coping mechanisms and psychological adjustment. (p. 250)

Insomnia in the ICU, medical, or surgical setting can foster pathological derealization and dissociation and prevent survivors from sustaining attention to recovery. Reviewing overnight nursing notes in the chart and asking the overnight nursing staff about a patient's sleep pattern can be helpful. Suicidal ideation in the acute care setting is not common but should not be overlooked. After terrorist events, clinicians must assess the occasional patients who harbor homicidal feelings, including those toward the perpetrators of terrorism or anyone from the nationality or religious group that perpetrated the terror.

Adjunctive Assessment Techniques for Medically Injured Survivors

In a chaotic disaster scene, a quiet private room in which to perform a focused mental status examination of a critically injured patient is unlikely to be available; therefore, the disaster psychiatrist must focus on high-yield observations and questions. First, the psychiatrist should note the patient's level of consciousness. Next, the psychiatrist should establish a method of communication. Patients who cannot communicate verbally can be asked to write answers on a piece of paper or a whiteboard, if possible. Writing may show spatial disorientation, misspellings, inappropriate repetition of letters (perseveration), and linguistic errors. If a patient is unable to speak or write, the psychiatrist may instruct him or her either to use an eyeblink method of communication (one blink for "yes," two blinks for "no") or to communicate by squeezing the clinician's finger with a hand (one squeeze for "yes," two squeezes for "no"). Questions can be phrased to allow for a yes or no response (e.g., "Are you feeling frightened?") (Rundell 2000). The need to recognize and treat dissociation is highlighted by the fact that dissociation in the peritraumatic periods has been documented by researchers to predict PTSD, including in a study of 715 police officers and other first responders (Marmar et al. 2006).

Pain Management and Posttraumatic Stress Disorder in Trauma Patients

In a recent controlled study, Holbrook et al. (2010) found that morphine use after combat injury may be effective for the secondary prevention of PTSD. In a survey of 696 patients from the Navy-Marine Corps Combat Trauma Registry Expeditionary Medical Encounter Database, the use of morphine during early resuscitation and trauma care was associated with a lower risk of PTSD after injury. In patients who did not develop PTSD, 76% had received morphine, whereas in patients who did develop PTSD, only 61% had received morphine, yielding an odds ratio of 0.47 ($P<0.001$). The authors of the study believe that pain control may decrease or impede memory consolidation and impede normalization of the associated conditioned response to fear after a person goes through a traumatic event. The issue of pain control is also of critical relevance in the treatment of children (Stoddard et al. 2002). In an important study of 70 children hospitalized for serious burns, morphine was found to decrease PTSD symptoms, especially those of arousal, in the months after major trauma (Stoddard et al. 2009).

Norman et al. (2008) found that self-reported pain levels within the first 48 hours of serious injury were significantly and strongly associated with subsequent risk of PTSD, with the risk increased by a factor of 5 at 4 months postinjury and by a factor of 7 at 8 months postinjury. In a larger study of 2,931 seriously injured patients admitted to acute care hospitals in the United States, Zatzick and Galea (2007) found that pain after injury was significantly related to an increased risk of PTSD 1 year after hospitalization.

Uncontrolled pain can be a stressor of catastrophic proportions that may lead to emotional trauma such as PTSD. Some patients associate pain with the severity of their injury, and this may also lead to anxiety, depression, loneliness, hostility, and sleep disturbances. Patients with significant pain often cannot respond to traditional psychotherapy interventions because sedation limits their ability to focus and attend, or because the pain is preoccupying and does not allow for concentration and reflection. Pain is often undertreated because both hospital staff and patients fear addiction; however, these fears are frequently exaggerated (Breitbart et al. 1999). This issue should be addressed assertively during the acute aftermath of a disaster to ensure that patients receive adequate pain control. The psychiatrist must educate both patients and staff about pain and fear of addiction. The disaster psychiatrist can offer adjunctive medications, such as SSRIs, serotonin-norepinephrine reuptake inhibitors (SNRIs), and judicious use of hypnotics, benzodiazepines, or anticonvulsants, to improve pain control. The recognition of pain as a key risk factor for PTSD and the psychiatrist's role in the management of adjunctive medication for pain may assist in preventing the development of PTSD from the initial injury or from the treatment of the injury in the hospital setting.

Special Considerations in Burn and Trauma Patients

Burns and other traumatic injuries incurred in disasters are important due to their impact on the patients, their families, and responders; the benefit of psychiatric consultation in the care of these individuals; and the likelihood of significant physical and psychiatric morbidity and mortality (Brennan et al. 2010; Stoddard and Saxe 2001; Stoddard et al. 2006). Patients with significant (not always severe) burns and trauma may be sent to specialized level 1 burn centers and trauma centers in major urban hospitals. As mentioned above, burn patients have consistently high rates of PTSD even at 1 year after the burn injury (van Loey and Van Son 2003; van Loey et al. 2003). Acute burn management is a complex procedure undertaken by a burn team. The disaster psychiatrist can treat delirium that often results from massive fluid shifts and may result from narcotics necessary to control burn pain. Delirium has been recognized as a source of psychological trauma. Patients may recall psychotic symptoms, commonly visual hallucinations, experienced during delirium, as well as the extreme pain experienced during debridement and dressing changes (DiMartini et al. 2007).

The psychiatrist can be helpful in advocating for the burn or trauma patient and by addressing concerns (usually unrealistic) that pain control will lead to addiction in an otherwise healthy patient (Powers and Santana 2005). Undertreatment of pain can lead to worsening delirium, anxiety, and other management problems. A common error is not waiting 10–15 minutes for adequate distribution of parenteral narcotics before beginning blunt debridement. Another common error is relying on benzodiazepines for pain control. If pain is managed adequately but the patient has anticipatory anxiety, oral or intravenous benzodiazepines can be very helpful (Powers and Santana 2005).

Visible scars from trauma or illness, particularly on the face and hands, may cause more psychological difficulty than those affecting other body areas, and may cause later social stigmatization. Patients should be given honest explanations and prognoses but should not be encouraged to view their injuries until ready; they may choose to wait several days or even weeks before looking in a mirror. Social skills interaction training, a variant of cognitive-behavioral therapy, is sometimes required to help severely injured patients adjust to permanent disfigurement and changes in body image (Lansdown et al. 1997). Facial burns and injuries highlight the overall high-risk nature of burn injuries and trauma in general for psychological sequelae: in one study, 35.3% of burn patients met criteria for PTSD at 2 months, 40% met the criteria at 6 months, and 45.2% met the criteria at 12 months postinjury (Perry et al. 1992).

Role of the Psychiatrist in the Hospital Setting

In a few hospitals where disaster survivors have been treated, psychiatric consultants 1) recommend that all patients be routinely triaged, without specific consultation requests, in order to set initial treatment goals; and 2) collaborate in providing early interventions where indicated. Initial interventions might include discussion of various topics, such as the concept of a therapeutic alliance; showing empathic understanding; identifying personality styles and defenses; and discussing how transference and countertransference issues may be relevant to care. Additional topics for staff include how to help normalize patients' expression of strong emotion and how to use specific psychological brief counseling approaches such as cognitive reframing, psychoeducation about managing anxiety, and relaxation and self-hypnosis techniques. Therapies meriting discussion include brief medical psychotherapy and cognitive therapy for insomnia and adjustment, which are very helpful to the medical patient who must endure long hospital stays or ICU boredom and isolation. Pharmacology is only one of the many things available in the psychiatric arsenal, a fact often forgotten in current psychiatric and general medical practice. The presence of the psychiatrist as part of the team, visiting all patients to check on mental health, depathologizes the consultation. Going on rounds with medical-surgical colleagues is an essential part of bringing psychiatric concepts to the team, and can help to decrease morbidity, prepare patients for discharge, and ensure their adjustment to posttrauma life. Additional benefits of the psychiatrist's involvement include decreased length of hospital stay and improved discharge planning following surgery.

Conclusion and Cautions

Essential psychiatric evaluation skills, judicious use of psychopharmacology, and liberal use of psychoeducation are extremely effective in the management of postdisaster medical injury and its psychological and psychiatric sequelae. For anxious patients affected by disaster who have no objective physical findings that correlate with their self-reported physical symptoms, the psychiatrist plays an important role by helping to diagnose new-onset or reactivated psychopathology, and by helping medical colleagues manage the psychological trauma that manifests as psychosomatic symptoms. By understanding that "medically unexplained" does not mean "biologically unexplained," the psychiatrist helps the patient and staff bridge the mind-body gap, and thereby intervenes in an effective way during the disaster response. For the hospitalized medically ill patient, the psychiatrist can offer psychopharmacological interventions for delirium, insomnia, anxiety, and other symptoms. The disaster psychiatrist can advocate for rational use of psychotropic medications by medical teams who often understand that intervention is necessary but lack the advanced assessment and psychiatric diagnostic skills needed to assist the patient. In these ways, the psychiatrist is able to play a role in the prevention of PTSD and other postdisaster psychiatric illness.

■ Teaching Points

- Patients may present to the ED with multiple somatic complaints without objective physical findings.
- MUPS can be understood as somatic expressions of anxiety.
- Management of MUPS includes psychiatric management of the patient's anxiety, as well as assisting medical colleagues to acknowledge the reality of the patient's distress and to communicate understanding to the patient with nonpejorative, low-conflict responses.

• Patients with serious medical injury following disaster are at risk for PTSD, depression, and other psychiatric complications. Most studies of ICU and trauma and burn patients show a 15%–20% rate of PTSD and high rates of comorbid depression.

• Benzodiazepines for anxiety disorders and antipsychotics for delirium are important interventions in the acute setting.

• In the acute setting, opiate treatment for pain from injuries may prevent the emergence of PTSD symptomatology.

• Psychoeducation regarding the psychiatric impact of disasters for patients and staff is an invaluable resource in the team's response to patients with MUPS and those with physical injuries.

Review Questions

10.1 "Mass hysteria" can most accurately be described as

    A. A likely consequence after a bioterrorism attack.
    B. Psychological symptoms in a physically ill person.
    C. Related to somatoform or conversion disorder.
    D. Common after a terrorist attack.
    E. An outdated term that inaccurately describes group response to a disaster event.

10.2 Strategies to help prevent "low-risk" patients from flooding the ED and hospitals after a bioterrorism attack include

    A. Giving clear information about who should and should not come to ED.
    B. Using media and telephone services to provide detailed information and initial screening.
    C. Employing rapid triage at hospital entrances based on objective signs of illness and likely exposure.
    D. Educating primary care staff on appropriate reassurance techniques.
    E. All of the above.

10.3 Effective strategies for doctor-patient communication for MUPS include all of the following *except*

    A. Acknowledging uncertainty.
    B. Telling patients they are overreacting.
    C. Offering hope.

    D. Avoiding additional invasive testing.

    E. Promising action.

10.4 What percentage of patients with facial burns and disfigurement are likely to have PTSD 12 months postinjury?

    A. 10%.

    B. 25%.

    C. 30%.

    D. 45%.

    E. 60%.

10.5 A symptom often missed in the acute phase assessment of postdisaster patients is

    A. Pain.

    B. Hypervigilance.

    C. Dissociation.

    D. Horror.

    E. Helplessness.

References

American Psychiatric Association: Diagnostic and Statistical Manual of Mental Disorders, 4th Edition, Text Revision. Washington, DC, American Psychiatric Association, 2000

Bartholomew RE, Wessely S: Protean nature of mass sociogenic illness. Br J Psychiatry 180:300–306, 2002

Breitbart W, Kaim M, Rosenfeld B: Clinician's perceptions of barriers to pain management in AIDS. J Pain Symptom Manage 18:203–212, 1999

Brennan MM, Ceranoglu TA, Fricchione GL, et al: Burn patients: psychopharmacological management of children and adolescents, in Massachusetts General Hospital Handbook of General Hospital Psychiatry, 6th Edition. Edited by Stern TA, Fricchione GL, Cassem NH, et al. Philadelphia, PA, Saunders Elsevier, 2010, pp 383–396

Davydow D, Katon W, Zatzick D: Psychiatric morbidity and functional impairments in survivors of burns, traumatic injuries, and ICU stays for other critical illnesses: a review of the literature. Int Rev Psychiatry 21:531–538, 2009

DiGiovanni C: Domestic terrorism with chemical or biological agents: psychiatric aspects. Am J Psychiatry 156:1500–1505, 1999

DiMartini A, Dew M, Kormos R, et al: Posttraumatic stress disorder caused by hallucinations and delusions experienced in delirium. Psychosomatics 48:436–439, 2007

Disaster Psychiatry Outreach: The Essentials of Disaster Psychiatry: A Training Course for Mental Health Professionals (Course Syllabus). New York, Disaster Psychiatry Outreach, 2008. Available as DPOCourseSyllabus_052108.pdf at: https://sites.google.com/a/disasterpsych.org/blog/File-Cabinet. Accessed December 21, 2009.

Geringer ES, Stern T: Coping with medical illness: the impact of personality types. Psychosomatics 27:251–261, 1986

Holbrook TL, Galarneau MR, Dye JL, et al: Morphine use after combat injury in Iraq and post-traumatic stress disorder. N Engl J Med 362:110–117, 2010

Hunt SC, Richardson R, Engel C: Clinical management of gulf war veterans with medically unexplained symptoms. Mil Med 167:414–420, 2002

Kman N, Nelson RN: Infectious agents of bioterrorism: a review for emergency physicians. Emerg Med Clin North Am 26:x–xi, 517–547, 2008

Lansdown R, Rumsey N, Bradbury E, et al: Visibly Different: Coping With Disfigurement. New York, Oxford, Butterworth-Heinemann, 1997

Madsen J: Terrorism and Disaster What Clinicians Need to Know: Sarin. Chicago, IL, Rush University Medical Center, 2005. Available at: http://www.centerforthestudyoftraumaticstress.org/csts_items/CSTS_CME_RUSH_USU_sarin_attack.pdf. Accessed March 30, 2010.

Marmar C, McCaslin S, Metzler T et al: Predictors of posttraumatic stress in police and other first responders. Ann NY Acad Sci 1071:1–18, 2006

Mawson AR: Understanding mass panic and other collective responses to threat and disaster. Psychiatry 68:95–113, 2008

Norman SB, Stein MB, Dimsdale JE, et al: Pain in the aftermath of trauma is a risk factor for post-traumatic stress disorder. Psychol Med 38:533–542, 2008

Ohbu S, Yamashina A, Takasu N, et al: Sarin poisoning on Tokyo subway. South Med J 90:587–593, 1997

Peer R, Hannan D, Amyot E, et al: A Physician's Education Program on Biological, Blast and Nuclear Preparedness 2007 Update. Albany, NY, Medical Society of the State of New York Bioterrorism and Emergency Preparedness Faculty, 2007. Available at: http://cme.mssny.org/index.jsp. Accessed March 30, 2010.

Perry SW, Difede J, Musngi G, et al: Predictors of posttraumatic stress disorder after burn injury. Am J Psychiatry 149:931–935, 1992

Powers P, Santana C: Surgery, in Textbook of Psychosomatic Medicine. Edited by Levenson J. Washington, DC, American Psychiatric Publishing, 2005

Richardson RD, Engel CC: Evaluation and management of medically unexplained physical symptoms. Neurologist 10:18–30, 2004

Roberts NP, Kitchiner NJ, Kenardy J, et al: Early psychological interventions to treat acute traumatic stress symptoms. Cochrane Database of Systematic Reviews 2010, Issue 3. Art. No.: CD007944. DOI: 10.1002/14651858.CD007944.pub2.

Rodriguez R, Reeves J, Houston S, et al: The effect of anthrax bioterrorism on emergency department presentation. Cal J Emerg Med 2:28–32, 2005

Rubin GJ, Dickmann P: How to reduce the impact of "low-risk patients" following a bioterrorist incident: lessons from SARS, anthrax, and pneumonic plague. Biosecur Bioterror 8:37–43, 2010

Rundell JR: Psychiatric issues in medical-surgical disaster casualties: a consultation-liaison approach Psychiatr Q 71:245–258, 2000

Stoddard F: Medically unexplained physical symptoms, in Hidden Impact: What You Need to Know for the Next Disaster: A Practical Mental Health Guide for Clinicians. Edited by Stoddard FJ, Katz CL, Merlino JP. Sudbury, MA, Jones & Bartlett, 2010, pp 79–86

Stoddard F, Saxe G: Ten-year research review of physical injuries. J Am Acad Child Adolesc Psychiatry 40:1128–1145, 2001

Stoddard F, Sheridan R, Selter L, et al: General surgery: basic principles, in Psychiatric Care of the Medical Patient, 2nd Edition. Edited by Stoudemire A. New York, Oxford University Press, 2000, pp 969–987

Stoddard F, Sheridan R, Saxe G: Treatment of pain in acutely burned children. J Burn Care Rehabil 23:135–156, 2002

Stoddard F, Levine JB, Lund K: Burn injuries, in Psychosomatic Medicine. Edited by Blumenfield M, Strain J. Philadelphia, PA, Lippincott Williams & Wilkins, 2006, pp 309–336

Stoddard F, Sorrentino EA, Ceranoglu TA, et al: Preliminary evidence for the effects of morphine on posttraumatic stress disorder symptoms in one- to four-year-olds with burns. J Burn Care Res 30:836–843, 2009

Tucker P, Pfefferbaum B, North C, et al: Physiologic reactivity despite emotional resilience several years after direct exposure to terrorism. Am J Psychiatry. 164:230–235, 2007

van den Berg B, Yzermans CJ, van der Velden PG, et al: Risk factors for unexplained symptoms after a disaster: a five-year longitudinal study in general practice. Psychosomatics 50:69–77, 2009

van Loey N, Van Son M: Psychopathology and psychological problems in patients with burn scars: epidemiology and management. Am J Clin Dermatol 4:245–272, 2003

van Loey N, Maas C, Faber A, et al: Predictors of chronic posttraumatic stress symptoms following burn injury: results of a longitudinal study. J Trauma Stress 16:361–369, 2003

Wain H, Grammer G, Stasinos J, et al: Psychiatric intervention for medical and surgical patients following traumatic injuries, in Interventions Following Mass Violence and Disasters: Strategies for Mental Health Practice. Edited by Ritchie EC, Watson PJ, Friedman MJ. New York, Guilford, 2006, pp 278–299

Zatzick DF, Galea S: An epidemiologic approach to the development of early trauma focused intervention. J Trauma Stress 20:401–412, 2007

Zatzick DF, Rivara FP, Nathens AB, et al: A nationwide US study of post-traumatic stress after hospitalization for physical injury. Psychol Med 37:1469–1480, 2007

11

Grief and Resilience

Chad M. Lemaire, M.D., R.N., B.S.N.

A patient presented with depressive symptoms and a chief complaint that "they found half my brother" in the rubble after the attacks of September 11. When he was asked which half, the patient tearfully related that the bottom half of his brother had been found. He was then asked what part was most important, and responded "the heart, of course." From the patient's perspective, the symbolic value of the heart meant that his brother was still buried, and not recovered. This impeded his grieving, leaving him unable to work. In a complex family dynamic, he was the designated mourner. As everyone else returned to functioning, this patient remained incapacitated by grief long after his loss. (Jones et al. 2004)

One of the biggest challenges in the postdisaster setting is responding to pervasive grief among survivors. Everyone will experience potentially traumatic events or suffer losses at various points in their lives, but trauma and loss are ubiquitous in times of disaster. Grief is a common and understandable response to disaster. Despite this, research has shown that resilience is more common than once thought and often underestimated after trauma or loss (Bonanno 2004). Grief and resilience are, in fact, not mutually exclusive experiences, and one can shape the other. However divergent they are, grief and resilience are universal elements of all disaster survivors' experience, and it is for this reason that they are considered together in this chapter. When working with disaster survivors, it may be helpful for the mental health provider to assess, and even promote, factors that make someone more resilient to the effects of grief. This chapter will cover the usual course of and assessment of grief. Topics include distinguishing bereavement from depression; the concept of complicated or prolonged grief; guidance in working with the bereaved, including existential, countertransferential, and cultural issues; and biopsychosocial factors associated with resilience.

Loss and Grief

After a disaster, variable amounts and types of losses are experienced. These can include the death of family or friends, significant personal injuries, loss of property and possessions, loss of personal identity, loss of social order, and loss of one's sense of safety. For example, since Hurricane Katrina in 2005, in addition to the loss of homes and the deaths of loved ones, survivors have continued to mourn the loss of their city's pre-Katrina sociocultural identity. The landscape of New Orleans, a city in which many generations of a survivor's family may have lived, was forever changed, and many residents have permanently relocated to other cities or struggled to rebuild. The loss of personal identity can include loss of a familial role (i.e., as parent, sibling, spouse, etc.). For example, the Monongah, West Virginia, mining disaster in 1907 killed several hundred men and boys, leaving behind hundreds of widows and over 1,000 children (McAteer 2007). More recent disasters, such as the Asian tsunami in 2004 and the earthquake in Haiti in 2010, left multitudes dead or severely injured, with many family members (including scores of orphans) left to go on with life after immense losses.

Bereavement is usually defined as the loss or death of a significant other. *Grief* involves the psychological, emotional, and cognitive reactions to a significant loss, although this is not limited to death of a loved one. *Trauma* can involve physical and psychological injury, and usually refers to a stressful or life-threatening situation that overwhelms someone's ability to manage. Although grief and trauma are different phenomena, their outcome trajectories show similar patterns (Bonanno 2004). *Traumatic grief* was a term used previously to describe the intense grief reactions to a sudden, unexpected, or traumatic death. However, after the 9/11 attacks in 2001, the groups that studied traumatic grief reverted to the term *complicated grief* to help distinguish grief reactions from other disorders such as posttraumatic stress disorder (PTSD) (Zhang et al. 2006). *Complicated grief* refers to unresolved, prolonged, and intense grief that is associated with substantial functional impairment (Zisook and Shear 2009).

Regardless of the term used to describe these grief responses, loss associated with disaster can generate intense reactions, including shock, despair, anger, guilt, denial, depression, and hopelessness. Also, grief reactions after a disaster can be different from usual grief reactions (e.g., those following prolonged illness), because the former is usually not preceded by a period of anticipatory bereavement. It is important to note that although most people will experience grief after losses, only a minority (anywhere from 5% to 20%) will exhibit long-standing complications (Love 2007; Zhang et al. 2006; Zisook and Shear 2009). Predicting which survivors will develop these complications remains difficult, however.

Although it is challenging to distinguish "normal" from "abnormal" grief, especially initially, there are general principles that guide when—and, perhaps as important, when *not*—to intervene. As discussed later in "Cultural Issues in Assessing and Responding to Grief," this determination is especially difficult when working with cultures outside of one's own, because of sociocultural factors that influence what is considered a "normal" response to loss. Most people find ways to incorporate a significant loss into their life narrative and move forward in a meaningful way. Many of the bereaved will experience transient distress and manage to function at a reasonable level (Bonanno 2004, 2006).

The initial waves of often intense, distressing symptoms can be frightening, especially to individuals who have not experienced them before. Initial shock, disbelief, denial, and immense dysphoria can give way to yearning, longing, and searching behaviors (Raphael et al. 2006). Also difficult to deal with are associated angry, ambivalent, and guilty reactions, including survivor guilt and rumination about what one could have or should have done differently. There may also be a preoccupation with images of the deceased, including, at times, hallucinations. Grief may move forward in fits and starts; fluctuations between being preoccupied with or consumed by grief and reengaging in life in a functional way are common (Walsh 2007; Zisook and Shear 2009). The usual course of grief, though variable from person to person, involves pangs of yearning and dysphoria that decrease in frequency and intensity over time (Shear et al. 2006). These waves are often associated with reminders of the loss, including significant anniversaries (Zisook and Shear 2009). Despite past suggestions to the contrary, it is also important to not label a lack of observable grief as pathological, because there is a paucity of evidence that validates this lack as being a risk factor for delayed grief or further complications. In fact, there is significant evidence to the contrary (Bonanno 2006; Zisook and Shear 2009).

Bereavement and Related Depression

Signs and symptoms of grief have much overlap with various other psychiatric disorders, and it is important to determine when these experiences are within the normal range and when further intervention may be necessary. DSM-IV-TR (American Psychiatric Association 2000) includes bereavement as a V code under the heading "additional conditions that may be a focus of clinical attention." It also states that "the duration and expression of 'normal' bereavement vary considerably among various cultural groups" (pp. 740–741). Consideration is given to the overlap with major depressive episode symptoms. DSM-IV-TR lists symptoms that may help differentiate bereavement from a major depressive episode. Table 11–1 presents the full DSM-IV-TR description for bereavement.

Under the criteria for a major depressive episode, DSM-IV-TR guides practitioners not to diagnose major depressive disorder (MDD) in the context of bereavement until 2 months have passed after the loss, or unless the symptoms are "characterized by marked functional impairment, morbid preoccupation with worthlessness, suicidal ideation, psychotic symptoms, or psychomotor retardation" (American Psychiatric Association 2000, p. 356). Zisook and Shear (2009) suggest that positive emotions alongside negative ones, with waves of symptoms coming in the manner previously described, often around reminders or anniversaries, is more indicative of grief, whereas pervasive sad mood with an inability to feel any positive emotion is more indicative of major depression. They also note that while only a minority of people who are bereaved meet full DSM-IV-TR criteria for a major depressive episode, studies have found bereavement-related major depression to be similar to non-bereavement-related major depression, including its response to treatment. At least six studies have shown efficacy of various antidepressants in treating bereavement-related major depression, and, interestingly, depressive symptom improvement was more robust than any improvement in grief. Although no studies have shown efficacy of psychotherapy in bereavement-related depression, there is no indication that psychotherapy would be any less efficacious than in non-bereavement-related depression (Zisook and Shear 2009). In the months following disaster, consideration needs to be given to the possibility that MDD has developed, because when it is present, treatment of depression is often required to facilitate the grieving process (Love 2007).

Complicated or Prolonged Grief

Although the grief process is usually never fully completed, even after many years, there are some signs that indicate a more pathological grief reaction. In the past, there have been numerous attempts to describe these types of grief reactions. Terms such as *pathological, abnormal, atypical,* and *traumatic bereavement or grief* have been used, often with much overlap. In recent years, the concepts of *complicated grief disorder* (CGD) or *prolonged grief disorder* (PGD) have received significant attention. Several groups have previously proposed criteria for CGD, but more recently, criteria for PGD were psychometrically validated and are being reviewed for possible inclusion in DSM-5 (Prigerson et al. 2009); Table 11–2 provides the proposed criteria. Although the PGD criteria have much overlap with previous criteria for CGD, the name was changed to "prolonged" to emphasize the chronicity of symptoms and to distinguish this newest set of validated cri-

TABLE 11–1. DSM-IV-TR description of bereavement (V62.82)

This category can be used when the focus of clinical attention is a reaction to the death of a loved one. As part of their reaction to the loss, some grieving individuals present with symptoms characteristic of a major depressive episode (e.g., feelings of sadness and associated symptoms such as insomnia, poor appetite, and weight loss). The bereaved individual typically regards the depressed mood as "normal," although the person may seek professional help for relief of associated symptoms such as insomnia or anorexia. The duration and expression of "normal" bereavement vary considerably among different cultural groups. The diagnosis of major depressive disorder is generally not given unless the symptoms are still present 2 months after the loss. However, the presence of certain symptoms that are not characteristic of a "normal" grief reaction may be helpful in differentiating bereavement from a major depressive episode. These include 1) guilt about things other than actions taken or not taken by the survivor at the time of the death; 2) thoughts of death other than the survivor feeling that he or she would be better off dead or should have died with the deceased person; 3) morbid preoccupation with worthlessness; 4) marked psychomotor retardation; 5) prolonged and marked functional impairment; and 6) hallucinatory experiences other than thinking that he or she hears the voice of, or transiently sees the image of, the deceased person.

Source. Reprinted from the *Diagnostic and Statistical Manual of Mental Disorders,* 4th Edition, Text Revision. Washington, DC, American Psychiatric Association, 2000, pp. 740–741. Copyright © 2000 American Psychiatric Association. Used with permission.

teria (H.G. Prigerson, personal communication, January 2010). Because it is unclear which name will be used if the diagnosis is included in DSM-5, the terms are used interchangeably in this chapter, depending on how they were used in the literature cited.

Whatever term is used, the severity or prolonged nature of grief symptoms suggests the need for clinical attention. The symptoms of PGD have been shown to be associated with increased suicidal ideation and attempts, various medical conditions (cancer, immunological dysfunction, hypertension and cardiac events), functional impairments, and reduced quality of life, even after controlling for depression and anxiety (Prigerson et al. 2009). Although CGD is fairly frequently comorbid with MDD and/or PTSD, studies have shown symptom clusters in CGD distinct from bereavement-related depression and anxiety (Zhang et al. 2006). In CGD, sadness and anhedonia are focused on missing the deceased, whereas in MDD, these symptoms are pervasive (Shear et al. 2006). The precipitating event in CGD is the loss of a positive relationship rather than the threat to someone's safety, as is common in PTSD. Also, sadness is prominent in CGD, but fear is common in PTSD (Shear et al. 2006). With CGD, there is often an increased focus on reminders of the deceased rather than the avoidance seen with PTSD (Zhang et al. 2006), although avoidance of reminders can also occur in CGD in a complex and variable manner (Shear et al. 2006). Finally, with numerous traumatic

---

TABLE 11–2.   Criteria for prolonged grief disorder proposed for DSM-5 and ICD-11

A. Event: Bereavement (loss of a significant other)

B. Separation distress: The bereaved person experiences yearning (e.g., craving, pining, or longing for the deceased; physical or emotional suffering as a result of the desired, but unfulfilled, reunion with the deceased) daily or to a disabling degree.

C. Cognitive, emotional, and behavioral symptoms: The bereaved person must have five (or more) of the following symptoms experienced daily or to a disabling degree:

    1. Confusion about one's role in life or diminished sense of self (i.e., feeling that a part of oneself has died)

    2. Difficulty accepting the loss

    3. Avoidance of reminders of the reality of the loss

    4. Inability to trust others since the loss

    5. Bitterness or anger related to the loss

    6. Difficulty moving on with life (e.g., making new friends, pursuing interests)

    7. Numbness (absence of emotion) since the loss

    8. Feeling that life is unfulfilling, empty, or meaningless since the loss

    9. Feeling stunned, dazed or shocked by the loss

D. Timing: Diagnosis should not be made until at least 6 months have elapsed since the death.

E. Impairment: The disturbance causes clinically significant impairment in social, occupational, or other important areas of functioning (e.g., domestic responsibilities).

F. Relation to other mental disorders: The disturbance is not better accounted for by major depressive disorder, generalized anxiety disorder, or posttraumatic stress disorder.

Source.   Reprinted from Prigerson HG, Horowitz MJ, Jacobs SC, et al: "Prolonged Grief Disorder: Psychometric Validation of Criteria Proposed for DSM-V and ICD-11." *Public Library of Science Medicine* 6:e1000121, 2009, Table 3. Used with permission from Holly Prigerson.

---

aspects of disaster (including traumatic death), CGD and PTSD may be comorbid (Zhang et al. 2006).

Although CGD or PGD is not currently a formal DSM diagnosis, the psychiatrist should intervene when the condition is suspected in the months after a disaster. The distinction between CGD or PGD and other disorders, such as bereavement-related major depression, is pertinent because the responses to treatment may be different. For example, in one randomized placebo-controlled clinical trial, nortriptyline and nortriptyline plus interpersonal psychotherapy significantly improved bereavement-related major depression but not CGD symptoms (Zhang et al. 2006). Although there have been no randomized controlled pharmacotherapy trials showing reduction in grief symptomatology, there have been some open trials of antidepressants that have shown some promise in reducing symptoms of CGD (Zhang et al. 2006). Shear and colleagues have validated a specific complicated grief treatment (CGT) that integrates interpersonal psychotherapy, cognitive-behavioral therapy, motivational interviewing, and exposure techniques. CGT was shown to be superior to interpersonal psychotherapy in a randomized controlled trial that measured CGD response rates and time to response (Shear et al. 2006; Zhang et al. 2006; Zisook and Shear 2009). In a naturalistic study of pharmacotherapy use in the CGT trial, compared with patients not taking an antidepressant, those patients taking antidepressant medication were more likely to complete CGT (91% vs. 58%) and achieved additional benefit from the CGT (Simon et al. 2008; Zisook and Shear 2009). Piper's interpretive and supportive therapy and Horowitz's integrated cognitive-dynamic approach show promise for CGD, but conclusive data from randomized controlled trials are needed (Zhang et al. 2006).

Talking and Listening to the Bereaved

There is much that a disaster psychiatrist can do to help the bereaved. The impulse to help should be grounded in awareness of the paucity of data about the efficacy of early intervention for grief, especially after disaster. Interventions are therefore informal and grounded in clinical experience. Some evidence even suggests that formal grief counseling, especially early on, may do more harm than good for some bereaved (Bonanno 2004). A recent meta-analysis showed that specific bereavement interventions had a small posttreatment effect that was not long lasting. However, the researchers noted that those individuals with marked difficulty adapting to loss had more favorable outcomes, and that some of the lack of separation from control subjects in the long term may be due to the tendency of the bereaved to improve over time regardless of intervention (Currier et al. 2008). Other meta-analyses have shown that grief-specific therapies are either inefficacious or, on average, less effective than other forms of therapy (Bonanno 2004). However, despite small overall effect sizes of most bereavement interventions noted in meta-analyses, benefits are often most noted for the at-risk bereaved, such as those with CGD (Zhang et al. 2006).

Despite this equivocal evidence for formal grief interventions, disaster psychiatrists would benefit from some guidance on talking and listening to the bereaved after disaster. Often, there is a pull to want to *do* something for the bereaved after a disaster. Many times, however, the most useful intervention is empathic listening. The value of the disaster psychiatrist's "bearing witness" to survivors' losses or emotions after disaster cannot be overestimated. After assessing physical (i.e., medical, food, shelter) and safety needs, and alongside the provision of Psychological First Aid (covered in Chapter 12), effective communication with the bereaved is essential. It is important to avoid forcing someone to talk about the details of their loss or the emotions that follow unless they are ready to do so. Being sensitive to the bereaved individual's readiness for sharing is of paramount importance, because disaster victims may have varying levels of readiness to deal with what has occurred (Raphael et al. 2006). Facilitating the sharing of the emotional and cognitive components of grief can be beneficial for many survivors who actually want to talk about their grief. Reviewing the symptoms and normal course of grief with survivors may be helpful for both normalizing the experience and decreasing anxiety for the bereaved. In addition, discussing differences between grief after traumatic loss and nontraumatic bereavement may be helpful. Acknowledging the bereaved individual's loss and emotional response, while not trying to provide explanations that may be patronizing (e.g., "It is God's will," "It will all be better soon," "I know how you feel"), can be a meaningful step in opening the lines of communication and validating the person's feelings. Maintaining a nonjudgmental stance and not prematurely cutting off the flow of emotion due to the disaster psychiatrist's own discomfort are vital. Directly expressing sympathy while acknowledging that the practitioner does not know what the bereaved is going through, using the deceased person's name, and asking about how the bereaved individual is coping are reasonable suggestions (Shear 2008). It is often unhelpful and invalidating to set an arbitrary time limit on grieving or give a message that one needs to move on (Love 2007). The disaster psychiatrist can help the bereaved identify how they may have successfully coped with loss or trauma in the past and how to mobilize or utilize support systems.

Furthermore, seemingly simple things a psychiatrist can do, such as sitting down and making direct eye contact, turning a cell phone off, and not looking at a watch, can help people feel more listened to and cared about. The use of touch (e.g., a gentle touch on the shoulder) may be more acceptable in brief grief counseling in the field than it is in many other clinical psychiatry settings. It is also prudent to consider that the informal grief interventions provided by the psychiatrist after a disaster are often brief, and thus there must be consideration early on about referral to a local resource that can provide ongoing care, if needed. Caution should be taken because the disaster-based professional relationship typically "terminates" sooner than do other psychotherapeutic relationships, possibly adding to the burden of individuals' grief.

Managing Hopelessness, Existential Issues, Meaning Making, and Countertransference

In the aftermath of disaster, managing overwhelming feelings of hopelessness in the face of death and destruction can be difficult. After a disaster, existential questions arise about the meaning of life. Survivors may face significant death anxiety as they come to terms with fear of their own mortality. A survivor's worldview may be shattered, especially if he or she tended to see the world as a safe and good place. The same can be said about religious or spiritual views: survivors may have significant cognitive dissonance about how a higher power that they felt was benevolent could let a widespread tragedy like a disaster occur. For example, one Sri Lankan survivor of the 2004 tsunami said this to a team of disaster psychiatrists: "I lost my daughter, my wife, my boat. I even actually lost the shirt off of my back. Where is the meaning? What's to be done?…What can you do for me?" (C. L. Katz, personal communication, 2010). There may also be additional fears of continued threat that contribute to hopelessness (Raphael et al. 2006). For example, victims of a terrorist attack may fear ongoing attacks, and the victims of the 2010 earthquake in Haiti had to live with the ongoing fear of aftershocks in the days after the initial earthquake. Also, modern technology brings survivors closer to the actual death and suffering (e.g., via cell messages from the deceased prior to their death on 9/11, constant media coverage, instant access to information via the Internet), which may intensify their emotional reactions (Lindy and Lindy 2004). Helping survivors deal with all of these feelings, including existential despair, is a difficult part of disaster relief work. Although it may be impossible to answer some existential questions, a disaster psychiatrist can help survivors navigate these painful straits, including feelings of self-blame, survivor guilt, and shame (Walsh 2007). Helping survivors communicate feelings of sadness, anger (e.g., at the government after Hurricane Katrina, at a perpetrator of a human-made disaster), despair, or confusion may be beneficial (Raphael et al. 2006). It is also often helpful to normalize a survivor's sense of hopelessness and despair as an understandable and common reaction to tragedy (Walsh 2007).

One technique widely studied and written about is that of "meaning making." Studies of grief work suggest that a central process in healing from trauma or loss is reconstructing meaning (Armour 2006; Walsh 2007). Meaning making can occur solely in a survivor's mind; however, it can also include finding meaning through one's actions, such as joining a cause that has some connection to the tragedy the survivor faced. Although for most, efforts to fathom some meaning occur after the acute stages of bereavement, for others there are attempts to do this early on after loss. Making meaning of a tragedy may help a person to regain some sense of coherence during a time when he or she is experiencing inner turmoil regarding the meaning and purpose of life (Armour 2006). Even after all of the devastation of the Asian tsunami in 2004, many survivors reconstructed meaning by noting a positive change in their worldview. Specifically, many noted viewing the world as a better place, because a large number of people were willing to help from all around the world (Rajkumar et al. 2008). As Viktor Frankl noted, although it is difficult to make meaning for others, it is possible to foster others' efforts to do this for themselves (Walsh 2007). Making sense of a loss has been shown to be a robust predictor of adjustment to bereavement, whereas being unable to do so is associated with complicated grief (Holland et al. 2006). Thus, assisting survivors in meaning making can be a helpful task in helping to restore order and purpose to their lives.

Countertransference issues are relevant when working with disaster survivors. It is often difficult for the disaster psychiatrist to maintain a healthy distance from the suffering following an event, especially when the psychiatrist is part of that community or is being constantly barraged with images of loss and trauma. For example, after 9/11, keeping an optimal empathic distance was almost impossible for mental health professionals; the sense of "we're in this together" made it seem almost cruel to maintain a neutral stance (Lindy and Lindy 2004). Glen Gabbard (2002), in writing about an interaction with a therapy patient on 9/11, reflected on how mutual self-disclosure about responses to the tragic events of that day affected the patient, and concluded that authenticity, genuineness, and being human were probably what was called for in that situation. Common dynamic themes that may arise in the countertransference of disaster workers include force and destruction, confrontation with death, helplessness, anger, loss, attachments, elation, guilt, and voyeurism (Raphael and Wilson 1994). The disaster psychiatrist faces dealing with his or her own countertransference, the vicarious traumatization he or she may experience, and the potential direct traumatization from the nature of working at a disaster site (Katz and Nathaniel 2002). The disaster psychiatrist may feel overwhelmed by a sense of helplessness while trying to help others in dire situations and, if so, may benefit from seeking counsel. More information is provided in Chapter 3, "Rescuing Ourselves."

Psychiatrists may also have countertransference reactions of either avoidance or overidentification (Lindy and Lindy 2004). Avoidance can include distancing to protect oneself from being overwhelmed, which can be exacerbated by a survivor's own unwillingness to discuss what he or she is experiencing. However, avoidance can also lead to a level of detachment and numbness that may not be optimal for a disaster psychiatrist (Disaster Psychiatry Outreach 2008). Overidentification is sometimes manifested in becoming an overinvolved, hero-type, idealized other who may try to be an omnipotent, comforting resource to a survivor. Some relief workers may even feel guilty about having any positive feelings of fulfillment in the midst of so much suffering (Lindy and Lindy 2004). Other potentially problematic responses of disaster relief workers include anger, paternalism, numbness, overdedication, and burnout (Disaster Psychiatry Outreach 2008). Being aware of these potential countertransference reactions can help the disaster psychiatrist navigate his or her reactions to the immense suffering of disaster survivors.

Cultural Issues in Assessing and Responding to Grief

Whether in the United States or abroad, psychiatrists responding to a disaster will encounter individuals from various cultures. When psychiatrists extend themselves to communities and even countries outside of their own after a disaster, they may be seen as strangers, and it is often necessary to involve the local community as much as possible to facilitate the grieving process. Important cultural implications must be considered when assessing grief. In Western cultures, there is often a focus on the individual experience of grief, whereas in many Eastern cultures, there are collectivist views that shape an individual's response to loss (Bonanno 2006). This difference was described in a report on a small Indian community after the December 26, 2004, tsunami: "Individuals of this hardy community had a fatalistic attitude and a tendency to collectivize their personal sorrow. They tended to view themselves as integral units of a larger traumatized society and not as lonely sufferers. They cherished their survivorhood as a gift from their God and desired not to view themselves as victims requiring external solace" (Rajkumar et al. 2008, p. 848).

Varying degrees of and ways of mourning are observed across different cultures (as well as perhaps between genders). In some cultures, demonstrative weeping, including wailing and falling to the ground, may be normal or even expected. In others, being very silent may be the norm. The psychiatrist may find it beneficial to be aware of some responses to the stress of loss that are common, such as *ataque de nervios* in Hispanic cultures, as well as the common occurrence of hallucinations of the deceased in many cultures (Ng 2005). Additionally, people from some East Asian and Latin American cultures may exhibit somatic symptoms in the face of grief (Bonanno 2006). Rituals of mourning are also very different across various cultures. In some cultures, people may experience added distress if a burial or cremation is not possible due to the inability to find or identify remains of the deceased (Ng 2005). Individuals from some cultures may accept and even seek out someone to speak to about their grief, whereas people from other cultures may consider a stranger asking about grief as an invasion of privacy or an insult. It may be prudent for the psychiatrist to collaborate with and involve local spiritual or other community advisers who may be more aware of local cultural implications. More information regarding cultural aspects of disaster response, including some culture-bound syndromes, is provided in Chapter 6, "Special Populations."

Resilience

Resilience has received much attention in recent years. Among the numerous definitions of resilience, many of which refer to the absence of pathology or specific diagnoses (e.g., depression or PTSD), some are pertinent to the disaster situation. These include the "absence of an expected bad outcome" (Shalev and Errera 2008, p. 149); the ability "to maintain relatively stable, healthy levels of psychological and physical functioning" in the face of significant adversity (Bonanno 2004, p. 20); and "the ability to successfully adapt to stressors, maintaining psychological well-being in the face of adversity" (Haglund et al. 2007, p. 889). There is much argument that the complex concept of resilience cannot be easily understood in terms of absence of a specific disorder, symptoms, or variables. Some authors feel that resilience is the default condition because there is evidence that most people who are exposed to loss or potentially traumatic events are resilient (Bonanno 2004).

Although most people exposed to a traumatic event experience some level of psychological distress, usually only a minority go on to develop chronic psychiatric disorders (Friedman et al. 2006). In fact, some even exhibit what has been termed *posttraumatic growth* (Kilmer and Gil-Rivas 2010). Although the disaster psychiatrist should avoid pathologizing common reactions, determining who may be more vulnerable or resilient can inform the approach taken. Some interventions, such as psychological debriefing, have been shown to worsen outcomes in the most vulnerable survivors, and the most resilient may benefit from not having any formal intervention while being allowed to recover spontaneously (Friedman et al. 2006). However, it is difficult to accurately predict who will be more resilient after a traumatic event such as a disaster in the face of a lack of consistent clinically applicable predictors of resilience to guide the disaster psychiatrist (Friedman et al. 2006). Although many risk and resilience factors have been studied in various settings, the interactions among the multiple factors are complex, and it remains difficult to ascertain how influential these factors are versus other unexplained variance in outcome (Shalev and Errera 2008).

Biopsychosocial Factors Implicated in Resilience

In recent years, there has been a movement toward studying biopsychosocial aspects of vulnerability and resilience in those exposed to loss and trauma, including during disasters. Despite the varying definitions of resilience across studies, many authors conclude that an array of biopsychosocial factors either confer resilience or make survivors more vulnerable to negative outcomes. Among the biological factors, numerous hormones and neurotransmitters have been implicated. These include cortisol, corticotropin-releasing hormone (CRH), dehydroepiandrosterone (DHEA), dopamine, norepinephrine, serotonin, neuropeptide Y, galanin, testosterone, and estrogen (Charney 2004). Detailed reviews of these biological factors are available (Charney 2004; Haglund et al. 2007). Also linked to resilience is the stress inoculation theory, which posits that prior exposure to manageable stress helps to create a neurobiological profile that confers resilience (Haglund et al. 2007). Even if the prior stressors are unrelated to the current one, these experiences seem to confer a level of protection. However, if the prior stressors were not adequately managed, they may lead to additional vulnerability during future stressors. It is difficult, though, to determine how much of the stress inoculation theory is due to biological versus psychological mechanisms, both of which are probably at play.

When studying resilience, there is often a chicken or egg argument, as researchers struggle to determine whether resilience is innate and confers lower risk for adverse outcomes after trauma or loss, or whether resilience is a process/outcome itself. A host of psychosocial factors have been associated with resilience. Although a thorough review of them is beyond the scope of this chapter, a brief mention of some of the commonly studied ones is necessary. Noted resilience factors across studies include social support, cognitive flexibility, having a moral compass, active coping, positive outlook, and physical exercise (Disaster Psychiatry Outreach 2008). A study of resilience (focusing on lack of PTSD and low levels of depressive symptoms and substance use) after the 9/11 attacks showed that the most robust predictor of resilience was the absence of additional life stressors. In the same study, increased social support, less income loss, fewer chronic diseases, less direct impact from the attacks, and fewer past and additional subsequent traumatic events all predicted resilience (Bonanno et al. 2007).

Bonanno (2004) had previously reviewed various factors linked to resilience, including hardiness, self-enhancement, repressive coping, and positive emotion. Hardiness involves "being committed to finding meaningful purpose in life, the belief that one can influence one's surroundings and the outcome of events, and the belief that one can learn and grow from both positive and negative life experiences" (p. 25). Self-enhancement, a trait associated with high self-esteem but also with narcissism, can be protective after disaster. Repressive coping involves some level of emotional dissociation or detachment, which in many normal settings may be maladaptive; however, in the extreme stress of trauma and loss, repressive coping has been shown to be protective and adaptive. Finally, Bonanno pointed out that whereas positive emotion and laughter in the face of adversity were formerly thought to be forms of unhealthy denial, more recent studies on trauma and loss are showing that these actions reduce negative emotions and increase social support and contact.

Recent reviews of psychobiological mechanisms of resilience agree that optimism and a sense of humor are related to resilience (Haglund et al. 2007; Southwick et al. 2005). Other notable features of resilience include active coping (i.e., problem solving rather than passive coping mechanisms such as resignation or avoidance); cognitive flexibility (ability to reappraise and explain adverse events in a positive light and possibly even find meaning or value in them; accepting things that cannot change but switching back to an active coping style if there is a possibility of change); living with a moral compass (guiding one's life by meaningful principles, including but not limited to religion, spirituality, and altruism); physical exercise; and social support, including having positive role models and mentors (Haglund et al. 2007; Southwick et al. 2005).

Social support is a widely studied and fairly consistent predictor of improved outcomes across a variety of adverse events such as trauma and loss associated with disaster (Southwick et al. 2005). Although one's social network is often fragmented after disaster, the disaster psychiatrist can help both to promote what social supports still exist and to create new ones within the existing society or culture. As illustrated in the following case vignette, psychiatrists sometimes have to do this in unexpected ways.

Two days after 9/11, volunteer psychiatrists began staffing the family assistance center set up to assist survivors, families of victims, and community members. Psychiatrists were prepared to evaluate and treat acute symptoms of grief and trauma, including with short-term medications. However, it quickly became apparent that traditional psychiatric practice was not nearly as relevant as was addressing peoples' desire to find their family members. Psychiatrists therefore began staffing tables to help families review lists of admitted patients from local area hospitals. Not only did this service speak to peoples' fundamental needs at that time, but it also created an opportunity to offer grief counseling and support to the overwhelming majority of people who did not locate loved ones.

Awareness of vulnerability and resilience factors has practical clinical implications in times of disaster. A discussion of vulnerability and risk factors is included in Chapter 5, "Psychiatric Evaluation." Vulnerability factors should be mitigated, if possible, and if they are static factors, they should be considered in the overall assessment. Although past research indicates that preparation and reducing risk exposure are vital (Watson et al. 2006), many disaster psychiatrists work with survivors *after* a disaster. Despite the lack of empirical data currently available about fostering resilience after a disaster, some general recommendations can be made. The psychiatrist can actively promote factors that are associated with resilience, taking into account the individual's innate coping style, as well as what has worked and not worked for him or her after previous stressors. Also, by educating survivors about resilience factors suggested by past evidence, the disaster psychiatrist can help to promote the development or acquisition of some of these factors (Disaster Psychiatry Outreach 2008). Focusing not on negatives or pathology, but rather on what one *can* do or *can* change, such as developing new goals or achieving some short-term successes, may lead to life satisfaction even if life may look different than it did before the disaster (Shalev and Errera 2008). By assisting disaster survivors in setting achievable goals, the psychiatrist can help them to experience repeated successes and reestablish some sense of control over their outcome (Watson et al. 2006). These are all suggestions that may help the disaster survivor get through an extremely difficult time.

The Web sites of the American Psychiatric Association (www.psych.org/Resources/DisasterPsychiatry.aspx) and the American Psychological Association (www.apa.org/helpcenter/road-resilience.aspx) have multiple resources available on disaster psychiatry. The American Psychological Association also has some online brochures specifically covering resilience (e.g., after hurricane, during war) as well as a module focusing on building resilience.

Conclusion

Disaster relief work by a psychiatrist is likely to involve helping survivors process intense emotional reactions, including grief. *Bereavement* is usually defined as the loss or death of a significant other. *Grief* involves the psychological, emotional, and cognitive reactions to a significant loss, although this is not limited to death of a loved one. After a disaster, many types of losses are experienced, including the death of family or friends, significant personal injuries, loss of property and possessions, loss of personal identity, loss of social order, and loss of one's sense of safety. The sudden and traumatic nature of disasters leads to responses among survivors that require perspective and flexibility from the disaster psychiatrist as well as a working knowledge of the many manifestations of grief and related interventions.

Signs and symptoms of grief have much overlap with various psychiatric disorders. It is important to differentiate symptoms that are within the normal range from those for which further intervention may be necessary. There is overlap with symptoms of major depression, which should not be diagnosed in the context of bereavement until 2 months have passed after the loss, or unless the symptoms are very severe. *Complicated grief* refers to unresolved, prolonged, or intense grief that is associated with substantial functional impairment. Varying degrees of and ways of mourning are observed across different cultures and between genders. In some cultures, demonstrative weeping, including wailing and falling to the ground, may be normal or even expected. In others, being very silent may be the norm. The duration and expression of "normal" bereavement varies considerably across cultural groups.

At the same time, recent research has shown that resilience is common and often underestimated. It may be helpful to assess and promote biopsychosocial factors associated with resilience, including social support, cognitive flexibility, active coping, positive outlook, humor, and physical exercise. Other factors are hardiness, self-enhancement, repressive coping, living with a moral compass (including but not limited to religion, spirituality, and altruism), and having positive role models and mentors.

There is much that a disaster psychiatrist can do to help the bereaved. The impulse to help should be grounded in awareness of the paucity of data about the efficacy of early intervention. Facilitating the sharing of the emotional and cognitive components of grief can be beneficial for many survivors who actually want to talk about their grief. Reviewing the symptoms and normal course of grief with survivors may be helpful for both normalizing the experience and decreasing anxiety for the bereaved. Additionally, being aware of factors that are implicated in resilience can help the disaster psychiatrist to foster hope and healing. Formal grief counseling early on may do more harm than good for some bereaved persons, and the benefits of specific interventions may not be long lasting.

Many times the most useful intervention for bereaved disaster survivors is empathic listening. Studies suggest that a central process in healing from trauma or loss is reconstructing meaning, a process that the disaster psychiatrist may foster. Making meaning of a tragedy may help a person to regain some sense of coherence during a time when he or she is experiencing inner turmoil regarding the meaning and purpose of life.

For more information, the Web sites of the American Psychiatric Association (www.psych.org/Resources/DisasterPsychiatry.aspx) and the American Psychological Association (www.apa.org/helpcenter/road-resilience.aspx) have multiple resources available on disaster psychiatry. The American Psychological Association also has some online brochures specifically covering resilience (e.g., after hurricane, during war) as well as a module focusing on building resilience.

■Teaching Points

- Responding to pervasive grief among disaster survivors is one of the most challenging aspects of disaster work.
- Differentiating bereavement from depression, complicated or prolonged grief, and other disorders with overlap can have important implications in treatment.
- Listening and talking to the bereaved, managing hopelessness and existential issues (including by making meaning), and monitoring countertransference are vital skills in disaster work with the bereaved.
- Working with disaster survivors who are outside of one's own culture requires cultural competence, including the enlistment of help from local community or spiritual advisers as needed.
- Knowledge of resilience factors can help inform the interventions of psychiatrists after disaster.

Review Questions

11.1 According to DSM-IV-TR, all of the following may indicate a diagnosis of major depressive disorder after bereavement *except*

A. Guilt about things other than actions taken or not taken by the survivor at the time of the death.
B. Thoughts of death other than the survivor's feeling that he or she would be better off dead or should have died with the deceased person.
C. Morbid preoccupation with worthlessness.
D. One month has passed since the bereavement without resolution of symptoms.
E. Prolonged and marked functional impairment.

11.2 When talking to a bereaved person, which of the following is the most appropriate statement?

    A. "It is God's will."
    B. "It will all be better soon."
    C. "I know how you feel."
    D. "I am sorry for your loss."
    E. "Your loved one is in a better place."

11.3 Which of the following statements regarding bereavement-related major depression is *true*?

    A. Bereavement-related major depression seems to respond to treatments that are effective in non-bereavement-related major depression.
    B. In antidepressant studies in bereavement-related major depression, improvements in grief are more robust than improvements in depressive symptoms.
    C. Almost all bereaved individuals will meet criteria for a major depressive episode.
    D. Bereavement-related major depression does not need to be treated because it is an expected part of bereavement.
    E. Bereavement-related major depression does not need to be differentiated from complicated or prolonged grief disorder because the responses to treatment are the same.

11.4 Factors found to be associated with resilience across studies include all of the following *except*

    A. Adequate social support.
    B. Cognitive flexibility.
    C. A positive outlook.
    D. A preexisting psychiatric condition.
    E. Physical exercise.

11.5 Potential ways of fostering resilience in people after a disaster include all of the following *except*

    A. Promoting and reinforcing social supports that remain in the postdisaster setting.
    B. Helping to create new social supports within the existing society or culture.
    C. Assisting in developing attainable short-term goals.

    D. Employing a strengths-based approach that encourages the use of coping mechanisms that have been beneficial during previous stressors.

    E. Focusing on psychopathology in survivors.

References

American Psychiatric Association: Diagnostic and Statistical Manual of Mental Disorders, 4th Edition, Text Revision. Washington, DC, American Psychiatric Association, 2000

Armour MP: Meaning making for survivors of violent death, in Violent Death, Resilience and Intervention Beyond the Crisis. Edited by Rynearson EK. New York, Routledge, 2006, pp 101–121

Bonanno GA: Loss, trauma, and human resilience: have we underestimated the human capacity to thrive after extremely aversive events? Am Psychol 59:20–28, 2004

Bonanno GA: Grief, trauma, and resilience, in Violent Death, Resilience and Intervention Beyond the Crisis. Edited by Rynearson EK. New York, Routledge, 2006, pp 31–46

Bonanno GA, Galea S, Bucciarelli A, et al: What predicts psychological resilience after disaster? The role of demographics, resources, and life stress. J Consult Clin Psychol 75:671–682, 2007

Charney DS: Psychobiological mechanisms of resilience and vulnerability: implications for successful adaptation to extreme stress (review). Am J Psychiatry 161:195–216, 2004

Currier JM, Neimeyer RA, Berman JS: The effectiveness of psychotherapeutic interventions for bereaved persons: a comprehensive quantitative review. Psychol Bull 134:648–661, 2008

Disaster Psychiatry Outreach: The Essentials of Disaster Psychiatry: A Training Course for Mental Health Professionals (Course Syllabus). New York, Disaster Psychiatry Outreach, 2008. Available as DPOCourseSyllabus_052108.pdf at: https://sites.google.com/a/disasterpsych.org/blog/File-Cabinet. Accessed December 28, 2009.

Friedman MJ, Ritchie EC, Watson PJ: Overview, in Interventions Following Mass Violence and Disasters: Strategies for Mental Health Practice. Edited by Ritchie EC, Watson PJ, Friedman MJ. New York, Guilford, 2006, pp 3–15

Gabbard GO: Gibraltar shattered. Am J Psychiatry 159:1480–1481, 2002

Haglund ME, Nestadt PS, Cooper NS, et al: Psychobiological mechanisms of resilience: relevance to prevention and treatment of stress-related psychopathology. Dev Psychopathol 19:889–920, 2007

Holland JM, Currier JM, Neimeyer RA: Meaning reconstruction in the first two years of bereavement: the role of sense-making and benefit-finding. Journal of Death and Dying 53: 175–191, 2006

Jones K, Kelly K, Cammarata C: Bodies and minds: PTSD in the FDNY. Presented at the American Psychiatric Association Annual Conference, New York City, May 5, 2004

Katz CL, Nathaniel R: Disasters, psychiatry, and psychodynamics. J Am Acad Psychoanal 30:519–529, 2002

Kilmer RP, Gil-Rivas V: Exploring posttraumatic growth in children impacted by Hurricane Katrina: correlates of the phenomenon and developmental considerations. Child Dev 81:1211–1227, 2010

Lindy JD, Lindy DC: Countertransference and disaster psychiatry: from Buffalo Creek to 9/11. Psychiatr Clin North Am 27:571–587, 2004

Love AW: Progress in understanding grief, complicated grief, and caring for the bereaved. Contemp Nurse 27:73–83, 2007

McAteer D: Monongah: The Tragic Story of the 1907 Monongah Mine Disaster, The Worst Industrial Accident in US History. Morgantown, West Virginia University Press, 2007

Ng AT: Cultural diversity in the integration of disaster mental health and public health: a case study in response to bioterrorism. Int J Emerg Ment Health 7:23–31, 2005

Prigerson HG, Horowitz MJ, Jacobs SC, et al: Prolonged grief disorder: Psychometric validation of criteria proposed for DSM-V and ICD-11. PLoS Med 6:e1000121, 2009

Rajkumar AP, Premkumar TS, Tharyan P: Coping with the Asian tsunami: perspectives from Tamil Nadu, India on the determinants of resilience in the face of adversity. Soc Sci Med 67:844–853, 2008

Raphael B, Wilson JP: When disaster strikes: managing emotional reactions in rescue workers, in Countertransference in the Treatment of PTSD. Edited by Wilson JP, Lindy JD. New York, Guilford, 1994, pp 333–350

Raphael B, Stevens G, Dunsmore J: Clinical theories of loss and grief, in Violent Death, Resilience and Intervention Beyond the Crisis. Edited by Rynearson EK. New York, Routledge, 2006, pp 3–29

Shalev AY, Errera YLE: Resilience is the default: how not to miss it, in Intervention and Resilience After Mass Trauma. Edited by Blumenfield M, Ursano RJ. New York, Cambridge University Press, 2008, pp 149–172

Shear K: Fact Sheet: Managing Grief After Disaster. Washington, DC, National Center for PTSD, 2008. Available at: http://www.ncptsd.va.gov/ncmain/ncdocs/fact_shts/fs_grief_disaster.html. Accessed January 17, 2010.

Shear K, Gorscak B, Simon N: Treatment of complicated grief following violent death, in Violent Death, Resilience and Intervention Beyond the Crisis. Edited by Rynearson EK. New York, Routledge, 2006, pp 157–174

Simon NM, Shear MK, Fagiolini A, et al: Impact of concurrent naturalistic pharmacotherapy on psychotherapy of complicated grief. Psychiatry Res 159:31–36, 2008

Southwick SM, Vythilingam M, Charney DS: The psychobiology of depression and resilience to stress: implications for prevention and treatment. Annu Rev Clin Psychol 1:255–291, 2005

Walsh F: Traumatic loss and major disasters: strengthening family and community resilience. Fam Process 46:207–227, 2007

Watson PJ, Ritchie EC, Demer J, et al: Improving resilience trajectories following mass violence and disaster, in Interventions Following Mass Violence and Disasters: Strategies for Mental Health Practice. Edited by Ritchie EC, Watson PJ, Friedman MJ. New York, Guilford, 2006, pp 37–53

Zhang B, El-Jawahri A, Prigerson HG: Update on bereavement research: evidence-based guidelines for the diagnosis and treatment of complicated bereavement. J Palliat Med 9:1188–1203, 2006

Zisook S, Shear K: Grief and bereavement: what psychiatrists need to know. World Psychiatry 67–74, 2009

PART III

INTERVENTION

Frederick J. Stoddard Jr., M.D.,
Section Editor

12

Psychological First Aid

Edward M. Kantor, M.D.
David R. Beckert, M.D.

Dr. Hardy, a private practice psychiatrist in Charleston, South Carolina, heard about the Haiti earthquake on the news one evening in January 2010. A volunteer paramedic prior to medical school, he reflected on his past emergency experience and decided he might be of some use in the relief effort. During his initial Internet search, he came across a journal article on the mental health needs after major disasters such as earthquakes and hurricanes. He wasn't sure where to start, and was concerned that he didn't speak Creole or know much about the Haitian culture, but he was healthy and willing, so he decided to figure out how best to get involved. After an extensive Web search, he realized he lacked any specific training or experience in disaster mental health interventions, such as Psychological First Aid, as suggested by most of the U.S. and international response agencies.

Major response agencies and training groups recommend Psychological First Aid (PFA) for use in early response to the emotional needs of those affected by disaster and major traumatic events (Hobfoll et al. 2009; National Institute of Mental Health 2002; Ng and Kantor 2010). The core elements of PFA are contact and engagement, safety and comfort, stabilization, information gathering, practical assistance, connection with social supports, information on coping, and linkage with collaborative services. PFA has great merit and promises to reduce variations in the approach to early intervention as it evolves into the standard tool for mental health professionals and first responders alike.

In this chapter we outline the history and evolution of PFA, describe the goals and basic elements that inform its implementation, and review key components and resources for intervention with specific populations.

History and Evolution

After 9/11, early mental health interventions for disaster survivors received increased attention. Federal support for disaster response planning required that states address mental health issues to receive funding. Although sources vary in reporting its origin, PFA, as a basic concept, is not new in the psychological literature. In the military and civilian response communities, various forms of Critical Incident Stress Debriefing (CISD) formerly prevailed as the primary intervention for police, fire, and emergency medical services workers, even as late as 2005 (McEvoy 2005). Otherwise, a great variety of approaches were used by unaffiliated mental health responders, who applied their individual or group early treatment of choice to victims of disaster. As a result of several expert consensus conferences and literature reviews (National Institute of Mental Health 2002), it became clear that components of psychological debriefing, such as CISD, could worsen stress symptoms in some people and did not appear to prevent the posttraumatic psychological effects of disasters. (*Psychological* debriefing is distinct from *operational* debriefing, which is used to evaluate organizational effectiveness and learn about what worked and what might be improved.)

Although the evidence is still evolving, it appears that early interventions that reconnect victims with family, social supports, and known resources may prove to be the most effective in facilitating recovery (Hobfoll et al. 2009; Orner et al. 2006). At its essence, PFA is an attempt to attune to the specific human needs and emotional style of the individual and his or her expressed needs at the moment of intervention. It emphasizes empathic listening coupled with nonjudgmental responses, as well as an attempt to support individual coping styles and connect the individual to helpful social supports.

The roots of PFA can be found in the evolving literature of crisis intervention and traumatic stress. As far back as the 1950s, a special article in the *Journal of the American Medical Association* titled "Psychological First Aid in Community Disasters" (Drayer et al. 1954), written by the American Psychiatric Association Committee on Civil Defense (forerunner of the association's Committee on Psychiatric Dimensions of Disaster), outlined many of the basic premises used in more formal PFA training. Twenty years later, Beverly Raphael (1977) used the term and added some basic approaches to bereavement intervention. Much of the recent disaster literature continues to support interventions and objectives, as outlined in Table 12–1, that promote safety, help to return a sense of control, and link individuals to relevant supports in the community or to people or institutions of particular significance to the survivor (Orner et al. 2006).

TABLE 12–1. Basic objectives of Psychological First Aid

Establish human connection in nonintrusive, compassionate manner.

Enhance immediate and ongoing safety and provide physical and emotional support.

Calm and orient emotionally overwhelmed and distraught survivors.

Help articulate immediate needs and concerns; gather information as appropriate.

Offer practical assistance and information to address needs.

Connect survivors with relevant support networks, family, friends, and helping resources.

Support positive coping and empower survivors to take an active role in recovery.

Provide information to help cope with psychological impact of disasters.

Facilitate continuity and ensure linking to other sources of support when leaving.

Source.   Adapted from Brymer et al. 2006.

The Developing Standard

In the United States, "Psychological First Aid" often refers to a very specific, organized approach for mental health workers to use in responding to disaster survivors, developed through the National Child Traumatic Stress Network (NCTSN) and the National Center for PTSD (NCPTSD). From what was previously a generic term for these basic interventions, a semistructured field guide has evolved for use by mental health providers who are well trained in their basic practice but not in crisis and disaster work. PFA guidelines emerged as evidence accumulated against the use of psychological debriefing due to its potential for worsening symptoms and increasing the risk of developing posttraumatic stress disorder (PTSD) (see Chapter 13, "Group and Family Interventions, and Chapter 14, "Psychotherapies"). Those findings and the lack of alternate safe practices have cemented PFA concepts into general use. NCCTS and NCPTSD released the first edition of the PFA Field Operations Guide immediately after Hurricane Katrina (Brymer et al. 2005). This was revised to accommodate new materials and information, and a second edition was released in 2006 (Brymer et al. 2006). A later version of the field guide—PFA for Medical Reserve Corps—resulted from collaboration of NCTSN with the Civilian Volunteer Medical Reserve Corps (MRC) National Mental Health Work Group (Brymer et al. 2008). The widespread dissemination of the PFA Field Operations Guide, including its eventual adoption by the American Red Cross for an updated mental health training course, further supported its acceptance by public health agencies, the military, and state and local governments (National Child Traumatic Stress Network 2009).

The PFA Field Operations Guide attempts to utilize the available literature in order to do no harm. In its introduction, the document claims that PFA is an "evidence-informed" rather than evidence-based strategy, because much of the material is drawn from the crisis, trauma, and bereavement literature and all recommendations have not yet been scientifically validated in disaster (Brymer et al. 2006; Ruzek et al. 2007). The rapidity of response, the inherent chaos and danger, and the limited resources have so far made it challenging to conduct studies of the effectiveness of various interventions during the immediate disaster response. Taking this into account, authors of the PFA Field Operations Guide considered the concerns and warnings in the literature, and there is a growing consensus of support for PFA among mental health experts.

Basics of Psychological First Aid

Detailed knowledge of the elements and goals of PFA will inform its accurate implementation. The basic elements are described in Table 12–2.

Among the key resources in the PFA Field Operations Guide are a series of specific techniques and sample scripts meant to serve as examples for responders working with survivors. Recommendations for learning PFA include an initial didactic understanding through readings and classroom or online material, as well as supervised practical exercises.

Special Populations

The PFA Field Operations Guide includes specific resources for working with children, elderly individuals, bereaved persons, and other special populations. Several adaptations and translations of the guide have evolved from the original. In particular, adaptations of the PFA Field Operations Guide were created for community-based religious professionals and school-based responders (adaptations and variations of the guide are available from the NCTSN Web site [www.nctsn.org/trauma-types/natural-disasters/psychological-first-aid]). It has since been translated into Spanish, Japanese, German, Swedish, and Italian. After the May 2008 earthquake in China, the guide was translated into Mandarin and simplified Chinese.

Cultural Implications

The needs and responses of individuals from different cultures and backgrounds play a part in early disaster response initiatives, including PFA. More information is coming to light, but very little is known for certain about how generic mental health assumptions and interventions should be

TABLE 12–2. Elements and goals of Psychological First Aid

1. **Contact and engagement:** To respond to contacts initiated by survivors, or to initiate contacts in a nonintrusive, compassionate, and helpful manner

2. **Safety and comfort:** To enhance immediate and ongoing safety, and to provide physical and emotional comfort

3. **Stabilization:** To calm and orient emotionally overwhelmed or disoriented survivors

4. **Information gathering—current needs and concerns:** To identify immediate needs and concerns, gather additional information, and tailor Psychological First Aid interventions

5. **Practical assistance:** To offer practical help to survivors in addressing immediate needs and concerns

6. **Connection with social supports:** To help establish brief or ongoing contacts with primary support persons and other sources of support, including family members, friends, and community helping resources

7. **Information on coping:** To provide information about stress reactions and coping to reduce distress and promote adaptive functioning

8. **Linkage with collaborative services:** To link survivors with available services needed at the time or in the future

Source. Adapted from Brymer et al. 2006.

defined or modified for a specific group of people. The World Health Organization (WHO) has issued a directive asking response organizations to discourage mental health professionals from responding to disaster areas where they are not familiar with the language or the culture (Inter-Agency Standing Committee 2007). The PFA Field Operations Guide has been translated into a number of languages, but the relevance and effectiveness studies are yet to be completed. By NCTSN statistics, over 10,000 copies of these translated guides were downloaded from the NCTSN Web site. The simplified Chinese version was published in China, and more than 10,000 copies were distributed to the earthquake region (National Child Traumatic Stress Network 2009). This distribution effort has not been without controversy. International providers have implied that simply translating and exporting the PFA Field Operations Guide may create a "Westernization" of the crisis and grief response, and may not have relevance in other cultures (Watters 2010). An emerging strategy for effective intervention may be to pair up international responders with local mental health professionals who know the culture and social system, or to pair them with native social supports, such as religious, community service, or educational professionals. Even so, there have been questions about the relevance and usefulness of materials developed in the United States for those in non-Western cultures. In an effort to address these concerns, the

PFA Field Operations Guide includes nonspecific "culture alerts" interspersed throughout to alert providers to sensitive areas of understanding and intervention as they relate to other cultures.

These culture alerts are useful for clues on how to initially approach and interact with survivors, but they do not speak in depth to specific cultural norms. As pointed out by the WHO's Inter-Agency Standing Committee (2007) in its guidance for mental health professionals thinking of responding to other countries, there is no substitute for having a solid understanding of the regional culture and language, prior disaster experience, and knowledge of the legal environment at the disaster scene. One example is the update issued by the American Psychological Association, based on the Inter-Agency Standing Committee guideline mentioned above, for mental health professionals considering participation in the 2010 Haiti earthquake relief effort. The association recommended that unaffiliated volunteers be discouraged from traveling to affected regions without meeting specific culture-based criteria or sponsorship by established relief organizations (Inter-Agency Standing Committee 2010). Cultural issues surrounding disaster response are discussed further in Chapter 6, "Special Populations."

Children and Adolescents

The PFA Field Operations Guide integrates strategies throughout that are designed to facilitate working with children and their parents (see Chapter 17, "Child and Adolescent Psychiatry Interventions"). It also offers child-specific tip sheets for parents and other caregivers on how to work with their own kids. Variations focus on how parents can help their own children and how school personnel can use the techniques at times of disaster or school crises.

Conclusion

Although this chapter is not intended to convey the totality of PFA, the goals and basic elements are presented. Some components are knowledge based and can be obtained through readings or a short online training course. More significant is the need to develop the skills and attitudes that translate these concepts and interventions into practice. This is best accomplished through live scenarios and through practical skill sessions mentored by seasoned instructors. Many agencies and courses utilize the PFA concepts, including the American Red Cross, the MRC, the American Psychiatric Association, and other disaster response organizations. Efforts are under way to further evaluate PFA. Despite the difficulty of conducting disaster outcomes research in a timely and ethical way, the widespread adoption of PFA is likely to lead to more specific data regarding its effectiveness as an intervention tool and to further inform its use as an early intervention. As physicians, psychiatrists must approach disaster settings aware of their own skills as well as the full range of potential medical and psychiatric issues that may move beyond the basic elements of PFA. Although PFA involves initially attending to basic needs, such as food, shelter, safety, and referral, the use of PFA by psychiatrists in acute disaster settings may eventually lead to more specific assessment, diagnosis, and therapeutic interventions as the disaster phases unfold and psychiatric illness emerges.

■ Teaching Points

- Disaster mental health professionals should make an effort to do the following:
  - Understand the origin and evolution of Psychological First Aid (PFA) in disaster response.
  - Be aware of the strengths and limitations of PFA as an evidence-informed approach.
  - Become familiar with the basic goals and principles of PFA.
  - Recognize that any mental health intervention, including PFA, may have cultural implications.
  - Obtain information about the major PFA training resources.

Review Questions

12.1 Which of the following organizations in the United States has adopted PFA as a major component of its disaster mental health curriculum?

   A. National Child Traumatic Stress Network (NCTSN).
   B. Civilian Volunteer Medical Reserve Corps (MRC).
   C. American Red Cross.
   D. All of the above.
   E. None of the above.

12.2 In its Introduction, the PFA Field Operations Guide self-discloses as utilizing which of the following strategies?

   A. Evidence-based.
   B. Evidence-informed.
   C. Case-controlled
   D. Expert-informed.
   E. Expert-controlled.

12.3 Basic objectives of PFA include all of the following *except*

    A. Establish a human connection in a nonintrusive and compassionate manner.

    B. Support positive coping skills and empower survivors to take an active role in their recovery.

    C. Enhance the immediate and ongoing safety of the individual by providing physical and emotional support.

    D. Offer practical assistance and connect survivors with relevant support networks.

    E. Facilitate emotional processing through psychological debriefing of survivors using Critical Incident Stress Management techniques.

12.4 True or False: The PFA Field Operations Guide integrates strategies for working with children and their parents and also offers child-specific tip sheets, for parents and other caregivers, on how to work with children.

12.5 Which of the following statements regarding the cross-cultural relevance of PFA is *false*?

    A. The PFA Field Operations Guide has been translated into a number of languages.

    B. An emerging strategy for effective intervention may be to pair up foreign mental health responders with either local mental health professionals or other native service providers, such as religious, community service, or educational professionals, who are already familiar with the culture and social norms.

    C. PFA can be applied universally to all cultures, and the relevance and usefulness of materials developed in the United States outside of Western culture has been well established.

    D. Nonspecific "culture alerts" are interspersed throughout the PFA Field Operations Guide to alert providers to sensitive areas of understanding and intervention as they relate to other cultures.

    E. There is no substitute for having a solid understanding of the regional culture and language, prior experience, and knowledge of the legal environment at the disaster scene.

References

Brymer M, Layne C, Pynoos R, et al. (National Child Traumatic Stress Network/ National Center for PTSD): Psychological First Aid: Field Operations Guide. September 2005. Available at: http://www.vdh.state.va.us/EPR/pdf/PFA9-6-05Final.pdf. Accessed February 8, 2011.

Brymer M, Jacobs A, Layne C, et al. (National Child Traumatic Stress Network/ National Center for PTSD): Psychological First Aid: Field Operations Guide, 2nd Edition. July 2006. Available at: http://www.naccho.org/topics/ HPDP/infectious/upload/PsyFirstAid-2.pdf. Accessed February 8, 2011.

Brymer M, Jacobs A, Layne C, et al. (National Child Traumatic Stress Network/ National Center for PTSD/MRC National Mental Health Work Group): Psychological First Aid for Medical Reserve Corps Field Operations Guide. March 2008. Available at: http://www.nctsn.org/sites/default/files/assets/pdfs/ MRC_PFA_04_02_08.pdf. Accessed February 8, 2011.

Drayer CS, Cameron DC, Woodward WD, et al: Psychological first aid in community disasters. Prepared by the American Psychiatric Association Committee on Civil Defense. JAMA 156:36–41, 1954

Hobfoll SE, Watson P, Bell CC, et al: Five essential elements of immediate and mid-term mass trauma intervention: empirical evidence. Focus 7:221–242, 2009

Inter-Agency Standing Committee: IASC Guidelines on Mental Health and Psychosocial Support in Emergency Settings. Geneva, Switzerland, Inter-Agency Standing Committee, 2007. Available at: http://www.who.int/mental_health/ emergencies/guidelines_iasc_mental_health_psychosocial_june_2007.pdf. Accessed July 13, 2010.

Inter-Agency Standing Committee: International Resources: Guidance Note for Mental Health and Psychosocial Support Haiti Earthquake Emergency Response, January 2010. Washington, DC, American Psychological Association, 2010. Available at: http://www.apa.org/international/resources/haiti-guidelines.pdf. Accessed July 13, 2010.

McEvoy M: Psychological first aid: replacement for critical incident stress debriefing? Fire Engineering 12:63–66, 2005 Available at: http://www.fireengineering. com/index/articles/display/243037/articles/fire-engineering/volume-158/ issue-12/features/psychological-first-aid-replacement-for-critical-incident-stress-debriefing.html. Accessed July 13, 2010.

National Child Traumatic Stress Network/: PFA Information Brief, November 2009. Los Angeles, CA, National Child Traumatic Stress Network, 2009. Available at: http://www.nctsn.org/nccts/nav.do?pid=abt_nccts. Accessed July 13, 2010.

National Institute of Mental Health: Mental Health and Mass Violence: Evidence-Based Early Psychological Intervention for Victims/Survivors of Mass Violence. A Workshop to Reach Consensus on Best Practices (NIH Publ No 02-5138). Washington, DC, U.S. Government Printing Office, 2002

Ng AT, Kantor EM: Psychological first aid, in Hidden Impact: What You Need to Know for the Next Disaster: A Practical Mental Health Guide for Clinicians. Edited by Stoddard FJ, Katz CL, Merlino JP. Sudbury, MA, Jones & Bartlett, 2010, pp 115–122

Orner R, Kent A, Pfefferbaum BJ, et al: The context of providing immediate post event intervention, in Interventions Following Mass Violence and Disasters: Strategies for Mental Health Practice. Edited by Ritchie EC, Watson PJ, Friedman MJ. New York, Guilford, 2006, pp 121–133

Raphael B: Preventive intervention with the recently bereaved. Arch Gen Psychiatry 34:1450–1454, 1977

Ruzek JI, Brymer MJ, Jacobs AK, et al: Psychological first aid. J Ment Health Couns 29:17–49, 2007

Watters E: The Americanization of mental illness. The New York Times Magazine, January 10, 2010, p MM40. Available at: http://www.nytimes.com/2010/01/10/magazine/10psyche-t.html. Accessed July 13, 2010.

Additional Online Resources

Center for Disaster Medicine and Emergency Preparedness: Psychological First Aid: Helping People Cope During Disasters and Public Health Emergencies (program with a self-text). 2006. Rochester, NY, University of Rochester. Available at: www.centerfordisastermedicine.org/disaster_mental_health.html

Disaster Psychiatry Outreach: The Essentials of Disaster Psychiatry: A Training Course for Mental Health Professionals (Course Syllabus). New York, Disaster Psychiatry Outreach, 2008. Available as DPOCourseSyllabus_052108.pdf at: https://sites.google.com/a/disasterpsych.org/blog/File-Cabinet

National Child Traumatic Stress Network: Psychological First Aid for Youth Experiencing Homelessness. 2009. Available at: www.hhyp.org/downloads/HHYP_PFA_Youth.pdf

National Child Traumatic Stress Network: Psychological First Aid Online (includes a 6-hour interactive course that puts the participant in the role of a provider in a post-disaster scene). Available at: http://learn.nctsn.org

Nebraska Disaster Behavioral Health: Nebraska Psychological First Aid Curriculum. Lincoln, University of Nebraska Public Policy Center, 2005. Available at: http://www.disastermh.nebraska.edu/psychfirstaid.html

Ready.gov: Psychological First Aid for Students and Teachers. 2006. Available at: http://www.ready.gov/kids/_downloads/PFA_SchoolCrisis.pdf

University of Rochester: Psychological First Aid for Employers and Supervisors. Available at: http://www.omh.state.ny.us/omhweb/disaster_resources/pfa/Employers.pdf

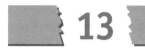

Group and Family Interventions

Anand Pandya, M.D.

After Hurricane Katrina, large numbers of New Orleans residents moved to Houston and Baton Rouge, and smaller numbers were dispersed throughout the United States. These individuals were physically separated from their neighbors, church congregations, and coworkers. Despite this wide scattering, cities as far away as New York had large enough numbers of evacuees from Katrina to develop specialized services for them. Regardless of location, psychiatrists working with evacuees likely heard a common statement: "You cannot understand because you were not there." An experienced disaster psychiatrist would know that many individuals who experience trauma express this concern, as do many war veterans when treated by civilians. At the same time, however, this assertion seemed to be a convenient way to dismiss mental health treatment, which often carries significant societal stigma.

For psychiatrists treating these evacuees, group psychotherapy could solve a variety of problems. Survivors' knowledge that other evacuees are attending groups has the potential to reduce the stigma by normalizing the need for help. In the post-Katrina group, survivors could feel more certain that they were understood when they referred to local places and things that they missed or when they talked about their mix of feelings about New Orleans. More important, group members who felt that "you had to be there to understand" could open up about their specific experiences of the disaster trauma knowing that the other group members experienced the flooding and evacuation, even if the group leader did not. A few months after the hurricane, many evacuees had left emergency shelters and were dispersed into communities that were no longer focused on Katrina. In this context, a group could provide evacuees a surrogate community and reduce their sense of isolation. Furthermore, groups can be a cost-effective intervention, because no disaster mental health response system has sufficient resources to provide individual psychotherapy to every individual expressing distress from his or her experience of a disaster.

An important consideration is what type of group intervention would help. In the first part of this chapter, I provide recommendations for postdisaster group interventions. I then look at family interventions that can serve as a complementary perspective on the "social" end of the biopsychosocial spectrum.

Group Interventions

Peer-led support groups and professional-led therapeutic groups are among the most popular interventions in postdisaster settings. For the purposes of this chapter, group interventions are divided into two broad categories: 1) single-session interventions intended to address acute distress and/or to reduce the risk of developing full psychiatric disorders and 2) multiple-session interventions intended to prevent posttraumatic stress disorder (PTSD), treat PTSD, and/or address grief.

Single-Session Acute Group Interventions: Debriefings

Few topics in disaster psychiatry have created as much controversy as single-session acute group interventions. Such interventions are generally referred to as "debriefings," although this term has been used to describe a variety of processes, including interventions intended primarily for information gathering rather than for therapeutic effects. The term *debriefings* has been used to describe group interventions and individual interventions, as well as interventions conducted in varying time frames. In this chapter, I use the term to refer to one-time group interventions that have a therapeutic intent and are conducted in the first few days after a traumatic event.

Although various types of psychological debriefing may differ in their formal structure, many debriefing models include both an experiential part, in which individuals who were exposed to the trauma are given an opportunity to describe their experience, and an informational part, in which the group leader educates the group members about normal responses to stress and coping strategies. In some debriefing models, each individual in the group is given an opportunity to share the facts of the event and a separate opportunity to discuss his or her responses to the experience. Debriefings do not presume that the intervention is provided by a mental health professional, although there are well-developed training and educational materials for the two most popular models for debriefings: Critical Incident Stress Debriefing (CISD) and the Community Crisis Response Team (CCRT).

CISD, the best-studied model for debriefings (Flannery and Everly 2004), is part of a more comprehensive intervention called Critical Incident Stress Management (CISM), which includes defusing, a less formal intervention conducted on the day of the event, and the availability of follow-up after the debriefing. Therefore, the data supporting the use of CISD cannot be generalized to interventions lacking the other elements of CISM.

CCRT, a second debriefing model in common use, is disseminated by the National Association of Victims Assistance.

A Cochrane review of 15 randomized controlled trials of debriefing (conducted after traumas that included nondisaster traumas) did not find a reduction in subjective distress and found no short-term (3- to 5-month) decrease in the risk of PTSD (Rose et al. 2002). Of more concern, however, one of the trials reported an *increase* in PTSD at 1 year posttrauma. Although the Cochrane review is the most definitive analysis of debriefing to date, it had some limitations. It defined *debriefing* as including single-time interventions up to 1 month after the event, which is a relatively long time frame. Some CISD supporters have argued that CISD may be effective for the subpopulation of emergency service personnel even if it is not effective for "primary victims" who directly experienced the trauma (Jacobs et al. 2004). Despite the fact that CISM has had an impact on the culture of some groups of first responders—and, indeed, the strongest evidence for the effectiveness of debriefing has come from situations in which it was given to groups that work as a team (Raphael and Wooding 2004)—the available data do not support debriefing as a recommended intervention. This is the consensus of multiple groups of experts (Disaster Psychiatry Outreach 2008; Medical Reserve Corps et al. 2006; National Center for PTSD 2010), even if it is possible that future research may identify specific situations in which debriefing is helpful.

Evidence base aside, psychological debriefing is still frequently requested after a disaster, so psychiatrists may not be in a position to eliminate the practice. They may find that some groups are not willing to accept any alternative form of psychological intervention. In these cases, the psychiatrist should at least try to ensure that such debriefing is not mandatory for all participants and to flexibly frame the intervention as an opportunity for affected people to potentially be heard, supported, and psychoeducated. Also, although therapeutic debriefing is not supported, "operational" debriefing, or informational debriefing to review facts and figures, *is* supported and appears useful to the work of responders who are organizing their teams and coordinating information flows through the stages after a disaster.

Multiple-Session Group Interventions

Many researchers have examined multiple-session group interventions used for survivors of disasters in the postacute phase. Such interventions can have diverse goals, including addressing bereavement and grief, reducing the risk of PTSD, and, at times, treatment of PTSD. Posttrauma groups described in the peer-reviewed literature include psychodynamic groups, cognitive-behavioral therapy (CBT) groups, and supportive psychotherapy groups.

Posttraumatic Stress Disorder Groups

The most studied group model to treat PTSD in individuals who already meet criteria for this disorder is trauma-focused CBT (TF-CBT). TF-CBT can include exposure therapy, the addressing of cognitive distortions, and the teaching of stress management and relaxation techniques. In a Cochrane review of four studies of group TF-CBT, this treatment was found to be more effective than a wait-list control (Bisson and Andrew 2007). Notably, the Cochrane review focused on all individuals with PTSD and not merely those with PTSD after a disaster, and it includes studies on veterans, who may differ considerably from disaster survivors both in the nature of trauma experienced and in the demographic characteristics of the exposed population. The trials did not prevent the individuals from receiving individual therapy and pharmacological management at the same time as TF-CBT. Nonetheless, this evidence supporting TF-CBT suggests a beneficial role in the postdisaster setting.

The trauma focus in TF-CBT differentiates it from present-centered CBT, in which references to the trauma are excluded. A variety of coping strategies and symptom reduction strategies can be incorporated into present-centered therapy. Results from one study of different types of present-centered CBT suggest that a focus on anger management can be effective in reducing aggression and that a focus on stress management can decrease reports of depression and can improve reports of overall life satisfaction (Bolton et al. 2004). Of note, in a randomized comparison of present-centered CBT versus TF-CBT in Vietnam War veterans, no significant difference was found (Schnurr et al. 2003), although the chronicity of the PTSD in this population and the lack of a non–active treatment control group limit the generalizability of this study. Therefore, the available studies suggest a stronger evidence base for TF-CBT than for present-centered

CBT but do not provide enough information to conclude whether TF-CBT is a better treatment.

Other forms of group psychotherapy that have been described in the postdisaster setting include psychodynamic groups, interpersonal therapy groups, process-oriented groups, and supportive groups (Shea et al. 2009). These therapies all focus on the trauma to varying degrees. A review of this broad array of groups noted a range from 6 to 52 sessions, with a mean of 12 sessions and with sessions that tended to be in the 1.5- to 2-hour range (Shea et al. 2009). Despite the heterogeneity of theoretical models, Shea et al. note that most successful groups are closed to new members at some point, allowing maturation of the group process. In addition to using a closed-group format, other recommendations from a separate review of the literature include using two co-leaders, ensuring that groups include individuals who have survived the same disaster, and selecting group members based on relative homogeneity in the severity of trauma exposure and stage of life (Foy 2008).

Although early postdisaster groups may have other goals aside from treating PTSD, it is important to note that a Cochrane review of multiple-session psychological interventions after traumas did not find sufficient evidence that any therapy, either group or individual, is effective at reducing the risk of PTSD (Roberts et al. 2009).

Bereavement and Grief Groups

Individual treatment for bereavement and grief is covered separately (see Chapter 11, "Grief and Resilience"). In addition to such individual treatment, groups for grief are common. Using a manualized intervention model, Rynearson et al. (2002) describe a form of group psychotherapy for family members of homicide victims that is divided into two 10-week blocks. The first block focuses on how to cope with the criminal process after such deaths, whereas the second block uses more typical bereavement techniques, focusing on commemoration and shifting the narrative toward a more balanced memory of the deceased that is not dominated by the traumatic death. Preliminary data suggest that this group format is well tolerated and that people improve over the course of the treatment, although no control subjects were used to compare this intervention to the rate of spontaneous recovery. This group format was used in New York City after 9/11, although the data about its effectiveness in that population have not been published. In addition to this manualized model, less structured support groups are common for bereavement, both in disaster settings and for non-disaster-related deaths. Support groups differ from traditional group psychotherapy in that support groups are not necessarily led by a mental health professional. Although this is a popular format for group interventions, it is difficult to determine how effective such groups are compared with professional-led groups.

Child and Adolescent Groups

In addition to groups for adults, a variety of groups have been used after disasters for children and adolescents. There are relatively few controlled studies for group interventions. However, preliminary evidence suggests that groups may be effective in reducing PTSD symptoms for survivors of disasters (Chemtob et al. 2002; Salloum and Overstreet 2008; Tol et al. 2008) and for individuals exposed to non-disaster-related traumas (Stein et al. 2003). These group interventions ranged from 4 to 15 sessions, and the published studies provide preliminary support for the use of group interventions with children ages 6–15. Two studies that compared individual therapy with group therapy for children and adolescents did not find a significant difference in outcome between these two forms of therapy (Chemtob et al. 2002; Salloum and Overstreet 2008), although one of these studies noted that the children in group therapy dropped out of treatment less than the children in individual therapy (Chemtob et al. 2002). Aside from a focus on PTSD symptoms, group interventions have been used to address grief in children (Cohen et al. 2004; Layne et al. 2001; Tompsett 2004). In addition, Cohen et al. (2007) found TF-CBT to be effective for traumatized children in a study comparing it with sertraline alone and in combination.

As in adult group psychotherapy after trauma, CBT elements are common in the group treatments that have the greatest evidence of success with children (Chemtob et al. 2002; Stein et al. 2003; Tol et al. 2008). However, unlike adult groups, many trauma groups for children use creativity and play as alternative modes of expression (Chemtob et al. 2002; Tol et al. 2008; Tompsett 2004).

Couples and Family Interventions

Mrs. S moved to Los Angeles, where her new husband had a job as a bouncer in a nightclub. She had two children within a couple of years of this move. Between the pregnancies and child rearing, she did not have time to develop friends in the area. Six years after the move, a shooting occurred at the nightclub where Mr. S worked. The news of this shooting was broadcast on television, and Mrs. S immediately began worrying that her husband had been shot. Mrs. S attempted to call Mr. S at work but did not get an answer. Mrs. S stayed awake for hours wanting to go to the club but unwilling to leave her young children alone or to wake them and take them with her to a crime scene. Later that night, a news program reported that one of the many fatalities was a club employee. Mrs. S felt so sure that Mr. S was dead that she began to rehearse how she would inform relatives. She realized that without Mr. S, she could not support herself and she could not get a job because she could not afford child care. Shortly before dawn, Mr. S returned home, having spent most of the night at a hospital with coworkers and the wife of the deceased coworker. It had not occurred to him that his wife would know about the shooting and would be worried.

Over the next months, the couple began to resent each other. Mrs. S could not shake the thoughts that she had the night of the mass shooting. She felt that she should go home to visit her family, realizing that they would be the people she would depend on if anything happened to Mr. S. She wanted Mr. S to go with her, but his attention was diverted to planning a benefit for the families of those who died in the shooting. He poured tremendous energy and many hours into this event. He noticed how stoic and dignified his coworker's widow appeared in contrast to his own wife, whom he felt was being overly anxious and demanding. He could not understand Mrs. S's histrionic reactions; she was never in harm's way and she did not know any of the dead. Mrs. S became increasingly resentful of the time that her husband spent away. She complained that he should call her more often to let her know that he was OK. Mr. S felt that his wife did not appreciate the demands of his job.

At this time, their older child began to have problems in school. In contrast to Mr. S, who continued to function despite the trauma, his son was performing so poorly that his teacher recommended a psychiatric evaluation. The parents understood that their son's problems were probably linked to the disaster. Somehow, he had been traumatized enough by the event to require some type of psychotherapy. But what type of treatment is appropriate for someone one step removed from the trauma?

This case vignette exemplifies the many ways that a trauma can "bounce around" among family members, creating significant dysfunction and distress among individuals who neither personally experienced a life-threatening event nor experienced the loss of a loved one. One of the most richly studied examples of this phenomenon comes from the study of children of Holocaust survivors. Literally hundreds of reports examine what has been termed the "transgenerational transmission of trauma" (Kellermann 2001) and how the effects of genocide may be transmitted across generations, including a possibly greater vulnerability to PTSD, but not PTSD itself. This greater vulnerability to PTSD and the term *transgenerational transmission of trauma* should not be misunderstood to mean that the diagnosis of PTSD can be directly transmitted to offspring. As conceived in DSM-IV-TR (American Psychiatric Association 2000), one cannot develop PTSD to a trauma that one did not experience.

In addition to the risk of psychopathology in children, other problems have been reported in families of survivors of mass trauma events, such as increased anger identified in survivors of the Cambodian genocide (Hinton et al. 2009) and higher rates of domestic violence in survivors of hurricanes and in veterans (Norris and Uhl 1993; Norris et al. 1999; Price and Stevens 2010). Some of the most dramatic evidence of the effect of trauma on families comes from research on war veterans. Veterans who develop PTSD have higher rates of parenting problems, marital problems, family violence, and sexual problems. Vietnam veterans, with or without PTSD, had high rates of divorce; 38% of marriages failed within 6 months of veterans' returning from Southeast Asia (Price and Stevens 2010). Galovski and Lyons (2004) hypothesized, based on a review of the literature, that different PTSD symptoms may lead to different types of problems, with the numbing and avoiding (Criterion C) symptoms leading to problems with communication and attachment with loved ones. In this model, violence, aggression, and anger would correspond to the hyperarousal signs and symptoms (Criterion D). More concerning, at least one study suggests that not only are veterans with PTSD more violent toward their spouses, but their spouses admit to being more violent toward others (Jordan et al. 1992).

Limited data exist on family interventions in postdisaster settings. Most of the literature describes interventions for couples rather than for larger family systems. Among the literature on couples, the dominant interventions described are forms of couples therapy, but there are also interventions that target spouses separately. Family and couples interventions may focus on improvement of symptoms in the traumatized individual (or individuals) or on functional outcomes such as a decrease in a destructive pattern of arguments or improvement in family relationships. The best practices for family interventions for survivors of civilian disasters must be extrapolated from the larger literature on interventions in families of veterans (Galovski and Lyons 2004; Glynn et al. 1999; Monson et al. 2004; Rabin and Nardi 1991) and survivors of trauma in general (Williams-Keeler and Johnson 1998).

In its practice guidelines for PTSD treatment, the International Society for Traumatic Stress Studies rates two therapies that incorporate CBT methodologies—behavioral family therapy (BFT) and behavioral marital therapy (BMT)—as the practices with strongest evidence (Riggs et al. 2009). Of note, the one randomized controlled study of BMT is not published in the peer-reviewed literature, and the only controlled trial of BFT in the treatment of a traumatized population in the peer-reviewed literature did not show additional benefits for exposure therapy plus family therapy (16 sessions over 6 months) compared with exposure therapy alone for the symptoms of PTSD (Glynn et al. 1999). Nonetheless, in that study, BFT may have helped veterans with problem-solving skills. BMT in eight 2-hour weekly sessions did show improvement in a variety of measures of relationship functioning and a reduction in PTSD symptoms.

Findings suggest the benefit of psychoeducational therapy models for veterans and their spouses (Devilly 2002; Rabin and Nardi 1991; Riggs et al. 2009). Devilly (2002) found small improvements in PTSD symptoms using a 1-week course, whereas Rabin and Nardi's (1991) study did not show improvements in PTSD symptoms but showed improvements in social relations at work, marital relations, parenthood, self-control, and problem-solving ability using group interventions for veterans, separate psychoeducational groups for spouses, and group sessions that included both spouses. However, these results do not differentiate the 33 veterans who participated with their spouses from the 7 other veterans whose spouses did not participate in the program. Furthermore, it is notable that many of the reports on couples interventions allowed the traumatized veteran to simultaneously receive individualized treatment for PTSD symptoms (Galovski and Lyons 2004), making it difficult to ascertain which benefits resulted from which treatment. Other adaptations of CBT for couples have been tried with some success, and some reports support the utility of emotionally focused marital therapy, which focuses on the pattern of emotional responses and is based in attachment theory (Williams-Keeler and Johnson 1998). Although emotionally focused marital therapy has empirical support for its use to address marital conflict in general, the case for its use in trauma is based largely on theory and clinician impressions. More systematic data in disaster-exposed populations are still needed.

On the basis of findings from the previously mentioned studies, psychiatrists in the postdisaster setting should consider developing family interventions, especially those that incorporate CBT techniques. The selection of a family intervention may be dictated by a variety of logistical factors, such as whether couples are willing or able to be seen together and whether there are sufficient spouses to initiate separate group interventions for spouses. In addition, in that different techniques have been shown to be effective for different goals, psychiatrists should be thoughtful about whether the goal of these interventions is to reduce PTSD symptoms or to improve family functioning. Because family interventions have not been as well studied as the group interventions described earlier in this chapter, no single family intervention can be considered a "gold standard" treatment at this point. Nonetheless, there is substantial evidence of psychological and interpersonal problems when a family member has experienced a trauma. Therefore, more than any specific intervention, the most fundamental recommendation is that psychiatrists must remain mindful of the impact of a disaster on the family as a whole.

Conclusion

Because disasters directly and indirectly effect a large number of people, family and group interventions address an obvious clinical problem. There is more evidence for the efficacy of group interventions for PTSD, especially groups using CBT, although it is important to note that the best evidence is for treatment of PTSD rather than for bereavement and grief or for the prevention of PTSD. Although fewer studies have looked at family interventions, there is ample evidence of family dysfunction in families of individuals who have been exposed to trauma. Such interventions may be aimed at reducing the trauma-related symptoms of the individual who was traumatized, at addressing family dysfunction, or at both. The best-studied family interventions have focused on couples; however, further research is needed to control for the effects of concurrent individual treatment.

■Teaching Points

- Single-session group interventions such as psychological debriefing do not appear to reduce distress or the risk of PTSD.
- Multiple-session group interventions may be effective for the treatment of PTSD, but there is insufficient evidence to suggest that they can prevent PTSD.
- Trauma-focused cognitive-behavioral therapy (TF-CBT) groups have the strongest evidence for the treatment of PTSD and include the use of exposure therapy, the addressing of cognitive distortions, and the teaching of stress management and relaxation techniques.
- Other CBT foci in groups may help to reduce specific signs or symptoms in individuals with PTSD (e.g., anger management reduces acts of aggression).
- Group CBT may be adapted for children by using art, play, and other creative modalities.
- PTSD is not transmitted directly from disaster survivors to their children, but children of sustained disasters such as the Holocaust may be more vulnerable to developing PTSD if they are exposed to trauma.
- According to data from veterans, PTSD increases the risk of domestic violence, parenting problems, sexual problems, and divorce.
- Preliminary evidence suggests that family interventions (e.g., couples therapy or psychoeducation for spouses) may reduce the symp-

toms of PTSD and may reduce marital distress. However, this therapy should be in addition to, not instead of, individual treatment.

Review Questions

13.1 Which of the following statements about debriefing is *true?*

    A. The consensus is that it reduces the risk of PTSD at 1 year.

    B. The consensus is that it reduces the risk of PTSD at 3–5 months.

    C. The consensus is that it decreases distress.

    D. It is used in both the Critical Incident Stress Management and the Community Crisis Response Team models.

    E. All of the above.

13.2 Which type of group therapy has the most evidence for the treatment of PTSD?

    A. Psychodynamic psychotherapy.

    B. Interpersonal psychotherapy.

    C. Trauma-focused cognitive-behavioral therapy.

    D. Process-oriented therapy.

    E. Present-centered cognitive-behavioral therapy.

13.3 Group psychotherapy models shown to be effective in the treatment of children after a disaster include which of the following?

    A. Play.

    B. Creative expression such as art.

    C. Cognitive-behavioral therapy.

    D. All of the above.

    E. None of the above.

13.4 Studies of postdisaster group interventions support which of the following approaches?

    A. Focusing on single-time interventions, given the fluidity of the postdisaster environment.

    B. Allowing rolling membership so that participants can experience the therapeutic forces of hope and altruism when they interact with other patients at different stages of recovery.

    C. Selecting members from different disasters or different levels of exposure to the same disaster so that group members can develop more perspective on their experience.

    D. Using two co-leaders and closing the group membership at some point.

    E. None of the above.

13.5 Which of the following statements about couples and families exposed to trauma is *false?*

    A. Vietnam veterans with PTSD have high rates of domestic violence.

    B. Vietnam veterans have high rates of divorce.

    C. Preliminary evidence suggests that couples therapy reduces the symptoms of PTSD.

    D. Preliminary evidence indicates that couples therapy reduces marital distress when a couple is affected by trauma.

    E. Studies suggest that couples therapy is an effective alternative to individual treatment for PTSD.

References

American Psychiatric Association: Diagnostic and Statistical Manual of Mental Disorders, 4th Edition, Text Revision. Washington, DC, American Psychiatric Association, 2000

Bisson J, Andrew M: Psychological treatment of post-traumatic stress disorder (PTSD). Cochrane Database of Systematic Reviews 2007, Issue 3. Art. No.: CD003388. DOI: 10.1002/14651858.CD003388.pub3.

Bolton EE, Lambert JF, Wolf EJ, et al: Evaluating a cognitive-behavioral group treatment program for veterans with posttraumatic stress disorder. Psychol Serv 1:140–146, 2004

Chemtob CM, Nakashima JP, Hamada RS: Psychosocial intervention for postdisaster trauma symptoms in elementary school children: a controlled community field study. Arch Pediatr Adolesc Med 156:211–216, 2002

Cohen JA, Mannarino AP, Knudsen K: Treating childhood traumatic grief: a pilot study. J Am Acad Child Adolesc Psychiatry 43:1225–1233, 2004

Cohen JA, Mannarino AP, Perel JM, et al: A pilot randomized controlled trial of combined trauma-focused CBT and sertraline for childhood PTSD symptoms. J Am Acad Child Adolesc Psychiatry 46:811–819, 2007

Devilly GJ: The psychological effects of a lifestyle management course on war veterans and their spouses. J Clin Psychol 58:1119–1134, 2002

Disaster Psychiatry Outreach: The Essentials of Disaster Psychiatry: A Training Course for Mental Health Professionals (Course Syllabus). New York, Disaster Psychiatry Outreach, 2008. Available as DPOCourseSyllabus 052108.pdf at https://sites.google.com/a/disasterpsych.org/blog/File-Cabinet. Accessed December 28, 2009.

Flannery RB, Everly GS: Critical Incident Stress Management (CISM): updated review of findings, 1998–2002. Aggress Violent Behav 9:319–329, 2004

Foy DW: On the development of practice guidelines for evidence-based group approaches following disaster. Int J Group Psychother 58:567–574, 2008

Galovski T, Lyons JA: Psychological sequelae of combat violence: a review of the impact of PTSD on the veteran's family and possible interventions. Aggress Violent Behav 9:477–501, 2004

Glynn S, Eth S, Randolph E, et al: A test of behavioral family therapy to augment exposure for combat-related posttraumatic stress disorder. J Consult Clin Psychol 67:243–251, 1999

Hinton DE, Rasmussen A, Noud L, et al: Anger, PTSD, and the nuclear family: a study of Cambodian refugees. Soc Sci Med 69:1387–1394, 2009

Jacobs J, Horne-Moyer H, Jones R: The effectiveness of critical incident stress debriefing with primary and secondary trauma victims. Int J Emerg Ment Health 6:5–14, 2004

Jordan B, Marmar C, Fairbank J, et al: Problems in families of male Vietnam veterans with posttraumatic stress disorder. J Consult Clin Psychol 60:916–926, 1992

Kellermann NP: Psychopathology in children of Holocaust survivors: a review of the research literature. Isr J Psychiatry Relat Sci 38:36–46, 2001

Layne CM, Pynoos RS, Saltzman WR, et al: Trauma/grief-focused group psychotherapy: school-based postwar intervention with traumatized Bosnian adolescents. Group Dyn 5:277–290, 2001

Medical Reserve Corps, National Child Traumatic Stress Network, National Center for PTSD: Position Statement and Guidance for MRC Units on Psychological Debriefing. Rockville, MD, Substance Abuse and Mental Health Services Administration, 2006. Available at: http://www.medicalreservecorps.gov/File/MRC_Resources/MRC_PFA.doc. Accessed July 7, 2010.

Monson CM, Schnurr PP, Stevens SP, et al: Cognitive-Behavioral Couple's Treatment for posttraumatic stress disorder: initial findings. J Trauma Stress 17:341–344, 2004

National Center for PTSD: Types of Debriefing Following Disasters. Washington, DC, National Center for PTSD, 2010. Available at: http://www.ptsd.va.gov/professional/pages/debriefing-after-disasters.asp. Accessed July 7, 2010.

Norris F, Uhl G: Chronic stress as a mediator of acute stress: the case of Hurricane Hugo. J Appl Soc Psychol 23:1263–1284, 1993

Norris FH, Perilla JL, Riad JK, et al: Stability and change in stress, resources, and psychological distress following natural disaster: findings from Hurricane Andrew. Anxiety Stress Coping 12:363–396, 1999

Price JL, Stevens SP: Partners of Veterans With PTSD: Research Findings. National Center for PTSD Fact Sheet. Washington, DC, National Center for PTSD, June 15, 2010. Available at: http://www.ptsd.va.gov/professional/pages/partners_of_vets_research_findings.asp. Accessed January 6, 2011.

Rabin C, Nardi C: Treating posttraumatic stress disorder couples: a psychoeducational program. Community Ment Health J 27:209–224, 1991

Raphael B, Wooding S: Debriefing: its evolution and current status. Psychiatr Clin North Am 27:407–424, 2004

Riggs DS, Monson CM, Glynn SM, et al: Couple and family therapy for adults, in Effective Treatments for PTSD: Practice Guidelines From the International Society for Traumatic Stress Studies, 2nd Edition. Edited by Foa EB, Keane TM, Friedman MJ, et al. New York, Guilford, 2009, pp 458–478

Roberts NP, Kitchiner NJ, Kenardy J, et al: Multiple session early psychological interventions for the prevention of post-traumatic stress disorder. Cochrane Database of Systematic Reviews 2009, Issue 3. Art. No.: CD006869. DOI: 10.1002/14651858.CD006869.pub2.

Rose SC, Bisson J, Churchill R, et al: Psychological debriefing for preventing post traumatic stress disorder (PTSD). Cochrane Database of Systematic Reviews 2002, Issue 2. Art. No.: CD000560. DOI: 10.1002/14651858.CD000560.

Rynearson EK, Favell J, Saindon C: Group intervention for bereavement after violent death. Psychiatr Serv 53:1340, 2002

Salloum A, Overstreet S: Evaluation of individual and group grief and trauma interventions for children post disaster. J Clin Child Adolesc Psychol 37:495–507, 2008

Schnurr PP, Friedman MJ, Foy DW, et al: Randomized trial of trauma-focused group therapy for posttraumatic stress disorder: results from a Department of Veterans Affairs cooperative study. Arch Gen Psychiatry 60:481–489, 2003

Shea MT, McDevitt-Murphy M, Ready DJ, et al: Group therapy, in Effective Treatments for PTSD: Practice Guidelines From the International Society for Traumatic Stress Studies, 2nd Edition. Edited by Foa EB, Keane TM, Friedman MJ, et al. New York, Guilford, 2009, pp 306–326

Stein BD, Jaycox LH, Kataoka SH, et al: A mental health intervention for school-children exposed to violence: a randomized controlled trial. JAMA 290:603–611, 2003

Tol WA, Komproe IH, Susanty D, et al: School-based mental health intervention for children affected by political violence in Indonesia: a cluster randomized trial. JAMA 300:655–662, 2008

Tompsett ME: Working with fatherless children after September 11, 2001, in Disaster Psychiatry: Intervening When Nightmares Come True. Edited by Pandya A, Katz CL. Hillsdale, NJ, Analytic Press, 2004, pp 211–218

Williams-Keeler L, Johnson SM: Creating healing relationships for couples dealing with trauma: the use of emotionally focused marital therapy. J Marital Fam Ther 24:25–40, 1998

14

Psychotherapies

Srinivasan S. Pillay, M.D.

The importance of psychotherapies in the disaster situation has been widely recognized (Rao 2006), and postdisaster mental health recovery programs that include sustained psychosocial support are thought to be helpful after major disasters (Kun et al. 2009). Although short-term interventions are generally favored for postdisaster treatment, a review of the evidence for the full range of therapies helps ground the interventions of psychiatrists and other mental health professionals in a thorough understanding of both the psychology of patients and responders and the range of psychotherapeutic choices. In general, while medication may offer rapid relief of symptoms after a disaster, the evidence suggests that psychotherapy is often more effective (Stoddard 2010). This chapter addresses psychotherapies that can be beneficial after disasters and outlines practical implications of these therapies.

Determining Who Needs Psychotherapy After a Disaster

Although the literature indicates that most disaster programs offer debriefing and support, it is unclear whether all survivors need psychotherapy after a disaster (see Chapter 13, "Group and Family Interventions"). For example, one study showed that the majority of children are likely to be resilient after a tsunami and that only children with preexisting vulnerability require specific and specialized interventions (Vijayakumar et al. 2006; for additional information on psychotherapy in children, see Chapter 6, "Special Populations," and Chapter 17, "Child and Adolescent Psychiatry Interventions"). Less information is known about adults than children, but they probably vary widely in resilience.

PRACTICAL IMPLICATIONS

1. Mental health professionals should not assume that all survivors need psychotherapy.
2. Although there is no well-researched instrument to assess who may or may not be a candidate for therapy, as a course of action, a determination of need should be the first clinical decision. As a guideline, the following factors may identify those in greater need of psychotherapy:
    a. Physical proximity—Those who are closer to the primary site of the disaster appear to be more affected by the disaster and may be more in need of psychotherapy (Sharot et al. 2007).
    b. Individual resilience—Those who have less resilience after the disaster, upon monitoring, may have more need for psychotherapy than those who have greater resilience.
    c. Family and community support—Those who have less family and community support may need psychotherapy more than those who do not have this support.
    d. Clinical indication—Psychotherapy may be justified for those survivors with anxiety disorders, stress disorders, somatoform disorders, or other indications of psychological risk.
    e. Individual preferences—A recommendation of therapy should take into account patients' receptivity to psychotherapy, because they are unlikely to benefit unless they choose to participate in therapy.
3. In addition to the survivors needing psychotherapy, psychiatrists and other mental health professionals may also benefit from psychotherapy to cope with secondary traumatization, to prevent burnout, and to support themselves while they are exposed to the impact of massive trauma on others (Knobler et al. 2007; also see Chapter 3, "Rescuing Ourselves").

Psychological First Aid

Crisis management is often the first line of psychosocial intervention after a disaster (Milligan and McGuinness 2009). After a crisis, the first mental health responders have to be available to intervene psychologically, because during this period new learning occurs and memories are consolidated. Thus, psychotherapy could interrupt the formation of traumatic memories (Peres et al. 2007).

The American Red Cross psychosocial support program consists of four specific components: participatory crisis assessment, dealing with survivors' disconnection from the familiar environment, community mobilization, and community development. The program presupposes that after a disaster, survivors lose their sense of "place" (Diaz 2008). Thus, it focuses on reestablishing a sense of connection between the survivor and the physical environment. Other people also are a critical part of the physical environment.

Psychological First Aid (PFA), a technique for providing initial support for large numbers of impacted survivors, is a widely accepted form of crisis intervention used by the military and the American Red Cross, among others. Mental health professionals may assist in training and organizing first responders to provide PFA, and provide elements of it themselves. PFA provides initial support and connection to survivors. After informational debriefing and identifying the trauma of displacement and disconnection, mental health professionals should participate in organizing to connect survivors as groups, and should mobilize communities through brief group meetings with a positive focus, if possible. These efforts create a sense of connection and orientation for each individual survivor. (See Chapter 12 for the basic elements of PFA, and Chapter 17, "Child and Adolescent Psychiatry Interventions," for use of PFA with children. Descriptions of PFA vary somewhat, including those within this volume.) Also see the discussion of psychological debriefing in Chapter 13, "Group and Family Interventions" supported by the current research.

In addition, the Linking Human Systems Approach (Landau et al. 2008) focuses on tapping into the inherent strengths of individuals and their families and emphasizes resilience rather than vulnerability. This approach reconnects the trauma survivor with his or her social support system. Examples of this approach are reminding the survivor of how his or her predecessors managed adversity, or recruiting and coaching an individual family member who then serves as a natural agent of change. This technique has been successfully used in facilitating recovery from major trauma or disaster (Landau et al. 2008). Early interventions have also been shown to be feasible when delivered via the Internet (Ruggiero et al. 2006). The

Internet can be used to provide chat rooms for early support, or to answer e-mailed questions. In addition, a Web site can be set up to address frequently asked questions about a relevant disaster.

PRACTICAL IMPLICATIONS

Psychological First Aid is recommended as the most basic general psychosocial supportive intervention after a disaster. When more specific intervention is feasible, part of crisis intervention involves resiliency training, which uses the principles of positive psychology by focusing on the strengths in creating a narrative rather than focusing on the weaknesses of the survivors. For example, survivors can be made to be more aware of their initial body "shock reactions" as defenses rather than signs of vulnerability. This reframing allows survivors to focus on recovery rather than retelling their stories.

In summary, mental health professionals should be encouraged to introduce a crisis intervention plan in stages: PFA, assessment, and community mobilization (i.e., reaching out to one member of the family support system). Effectively, the last step involves speaking to individuals as well as to the support system as a whole. Use of Internet resources is increasing and appears to be helpful in reaching large numbers of people. After these steps, it may be appropriate, when indicated and feasible, to introduce psychotherapeutic interventions.

Short-Term Psychotherapies

Most of the recommended postdisaster therapies are short-term therapies because most survivors recover from their initial shock. The form of short-term therapy that has the most evidence substantiating its use is cognitive-behavioral therapy (CBT).

In the context of a disaster, CBT is a type of psychotherapy that focuses on alleviating suffering by modifying maladaptive behaviors and thought processes. CBT techniques relevant to the disaster situation include coping skills training, problem solving, imaginal and real-world exposure to anxiety-provoking stimuli, cognitive restructuring (identifying and modifying beliefs or thoughts that intensify or prolong distress), goal setting, progressive muscle relaxation, behavioral activation, guided imagery, breathing control, and relapse prevention strategies (Ruzek et al. 2008). Part of CBT may involve using the principles of the relaxation response, which stands in contrast to the fight-or-flight response in emergency situations (Benson et al. 1975). Effectively, CBT involves new learning. For example, exposure therapies involve asking survivors to confront stimuli associated with their traumatic experiences so as to reexperience their resilience. This "exposure" can be done through the use of verbal descriptions, imagining the situation, or in vivo situations that resemble the traumatic event. The following case vignette demonstrates the use of exposure.

> After 9/11, Ms. P was afraid of visiting downtown Manhattan and avoided going there at all costs. A psychiatrist used exposure therapy in which Ms. P was asked to imagine the following in a series of stages: 1) tall buildings, 2) people walking around these buildings, 3) a plane flying over the building, and 4) eventually herself actually visiting the downtown area. For each stage of the exposure, Ms. P was given enough time to process the stimulus and "adjust" to the initial shock value. This is known as *habituation*.

CBT has been shown to be an effective model for postdisaster interventions in several different populations of children and adults. It has much in common with disaster mental health services generally, especially if matched to the contexts of the disaster and the needs of individuals. CBT was found to be effective with Asian survivors of the 2004 tsunami (Udomratn 2008). In children, control-focused behavioral treatment, involving mainly encouragement for self-exposure to feared situations, is highly effective in facilitating recovery from earthquake trauma (Salcioglu and Basoglu 2008). In addition, CBT was found to be highly effective in adolescents after the 2003 earthquake in Bam, Iran (Shooshtary et al. 2008). In fact, treatment gains from short-term CBT in children were still apparent 4 years after the 1999 Athens earthquake (Giannopoulou et al. 2006). A study that examined the use of CBT in disaster workers found that CBT was effective but that dropout rates were associated with lower income, less education, and higher alcohol consumption (Difede et al. 2007). Notably, virtual reality may also be an effective add-on to exposure therapy in the treatment of posttraumatic stress disorder (PTSD) (Difede et al. 2006). CBT has been shown anecdotally to also help in prolonged postdisaster distress (Hamblen et al. 2006).

PRACTICAL IMPLICATIONS

1. The mental health professional should use or teach a culturally sensitive CBT protocol and should adapt existing materials to be relevant to the situation.

2. Initially, exposure therapy and response prevention (i.e., prevention of anxiety through learning to tolerate the associations with the trauma) appear to be quite effective. Virtual reality tools, such as virtual simulations of the disaster situation and virtual exposure to associated elements (e.g., exposure to an airplane after 9/11), may enhance the exposure technique.

Phillips (2009) reported that in her post-9/11work, she used the stages of safety, remembering and mourning, and reconnection to create a structure for postdisaster therapy. This staging is a fundamental aspect of CBT. When a worldwide panel of experts on the study and treatment of those exposed to disaster and mass violence gathered to extrapolate from related fields of research and to gain consensus on "immediate and midterm" (in this book, termed *acute* and *postacute*) intervention principles postdisaster, their articulated priorities were promoting 1) a sense of safety, 2) calming, 3) a sense of self- and community efficacy, 4) connectedness, and 5) hope (Hobfoll et al. 2009).

PRACTICAL IMPLICATIONS

When planning a CBT protocol, the mental health professional should first promote safety for the patient; then proceed to accompanying the patient in remembering and tolerating memories of the trauma or disaster, with the possibility of exposure; and follow that by reconnecting the patient with life, hope, and community support.

Alternative and Culturally Specific Therapies

Having knowledge of culturally specific therapies offers the clinician a wider array of therapeutic possibilities for working with patients. A review of therapies in southern India showed that a greater availability of culturally congruous forms of therapy increases the likelihood that an individual will find a therapy to which he or she responds (Halliburton 2004). For example, if meditation and yoga are familiar to a culture, patients will be more likely to respond to them, whereas if they are not familiar to a culture, patients will be less open to them as a form of intervention.

Yoga Breathing

Yoga breathing (pranayama) has been shown to be effective in reducing stress and increasing resilience after mass disasters (Brown and Gerbarg 2009). Where this practice is culturally acceptable, it may be useful in helping people focus their attention on the moment and away from the trauma of the recent past. Also, yoga has been shown to decrease the symptoms of PTSD, such as frequency of intrusions and hyperarousal (van der Kolk 2006).

Meditation

Meditation has also proved to be beneficial. For example, after the 2004 tsunami in Sri Lanka, one study showed that meditation and relaxation led to recovery in 71% of children (Catani et al. 2009).

Narrative Exposure Therapy

In narrative exposure therapy (NET), survivors tell the story of the most disturbing parts of the trauma, with the goal being habituation to the distressing elements of the recollection. After the 2004 tsunami in Sri Lanka, one study showed that NET resulted in recovery in 81% of children (Catani et al. 2009). Notably, there were no differences between meditation and NET in terms of target symptoms.

PRACTICAL IMPLICATIONS

Alternative and culturally specific therapies, such as yoga breathing, meditation, and NET, should be used only with great cultural sensitivity. The mental health professional should be familiar with the data backing up these techniques.

Family Support

Family support can be of great benefit following a disaster. This topic is discussed in Chapter 13, "Group and Family Interventions."

Long-Term Psychotherapies

Long-term psychotherapies for disaster survivors have also been investigated, but they are not available in remote disaster settings. In some urban centers, including New York City, long-term psychotherapy is still widely practiced. The World Trade Center Disaster Outcomes Study, a prospective cohort study of 2,368 New York City adults funded by the National Institutes of Health after the 9/11 attacks, found that those who received more conventional postdisaster interventions, such as formal psychotherapy sessions and/or psychotropic medicines, seemed to have poorer outcomes; only brief worksite interventions seemed to be effective postdisaster treatment interventions (Boscarino and Adams 2008). In selected cases, however, long-term psychotherapy, including intensive treatments such as psychoanalysis, can be useful (Bohleber 2007; Lewis 2009).

Another form of therapy that may be useful in the posttraumatic context is eye movement desensitization and reprocessing (EMDR), which integrates multiple therapies—including psychodynamic, cognitive-behavioral, interpersonal, experiential, and body-focused—into structured protocols (Bisson and Andrew 2007). EMDR is an information processing therapy that uses an eight-phase approach to address the experiential contributors of a wide range of pathologies (Shapiro 1999). Various procedures are used, including dual stimulation, which uses bilateral eye movements, tones, or taps. In the reprocessing phases, the client attends to past memories, present triggers, or anticipated future experiences while focusing on a set of external stimuli. During that time, clients may experience the emergence of insight, changes in memories, or new associations. The clinician assists the client in focusing on specific material before initiation of each subsequent reprocessing set.

PRACTICAL IMPLICATIONS

It is unclear whether long-term therapies work in treating disaster survivors. However, when instituting long-term therapies in this context, mental health professionals should institute these with care, recognizing that the evidence favors short-term therapies.

Side Effects of Therapy

Wessells (2009) stated that many therapists at the time of disaster might inadvertently do more harm than intended by emphasizing victimization and by using unsustainable short-term approaches that breed dependency. Activating dependency needs rather than the capacity for resilience will not be helpful in the longer term.

PRACTICAL IMPLICATIONS

Although psychotherapy is helpful postdisaster, it can also potentially have negative side effects, such as reducing autonomy and increasing dependency and shame. Therefore, a well-balanced program is much more likely to be effective than one that focuses entirely on one aspect of psychotherapy. Specifically, focusing on both resilience and vulnerability is important.

Conclusion

Psychotherapies are an important part of the disaster intervention if they are used when indicated, as part of a crisis intervention and within cognitive-behavioral protocols with exposure prevention. Also, mental health professionals should be aware of longer-term therapies but should recommend or use these only after careful consideration. Psychotherapists in disaster situations should not encourage assumption of an identity as a victim and should monitor dependency, both of which delay progress and recovery (Wessells 2009). An intelligent use of individual and group interventions may be very helpful to postdisaster psychological recovery. Figure 14–1 illustrates the main considerations in regard to choice of psychotherapy.

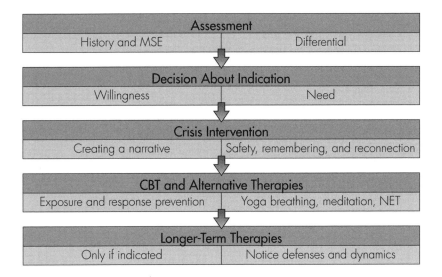

FIGURE 14–1.   Considerations in choice of psychotherapy.

CBT = cognitive-behavioral therapy; MSE = mental status examination; NET = narrative exposure therapy.

▮ Teaching Points

- Mental health professionals should not assume that all survivors need psychotherapy. A survivor who presents for care should first be assessed for indications for psychotherapy.

- Crisis management is the first-line psychosocial intervention after a disaster; Psychological First Aid is recommended as an efficient way of providing immediate basic psychosocial support to large numbers of survivors.

- Psychotherapeutic crisis intervention involves assessment, dealing with acute trauma and displacement, and community mobilization of social supports.

- An important focus of postdisaster psychotherapy is enhancing resilience.

- For short-term postdisaster therapy, the clinician should consider CBT.

- Exposure therapy and response prevention (habituating to strong emotions) may be very important during the acute phase.

- Virtual reality can be used to enhance exposure therapy and response prevention.

- Short-term therapy has three stages: establishing safety, remembering and tolerating memories of disaster, and reconnecting with life and community support.

- Yoga breathing, meditation and relaxation, and narrative exposure therapy can all be used as short-term therapies.

- Family support is critical in facilitating recovery from major trauma or disaster.

- Although long-term therapies are not to be considered a general treatment for disaster survivors, in selected instances they may be useful.

Review Questions

14.1 Which of the following statements about psychotherapy after a disaster is *true*?

A. Cognitive-behavioral therapy (CBT) should be immediately initiated for all survivors.

B. Long-term therapies are always preferred when possible.

C. A determination of need should precede any clinical action.

D. Therapy should primarily focus on survivors' vulnerabilities.

E. None of the above.

14.2 People who lived closer to the World Trade Center during 9/11

A. Were more traumatized than people who lived farther away.

B. Were less traumatized than people who lived farther away.

C. Experienced trauma equal to that of people who lived farther away.

D. Were not traumatized by 9/11.

E. None of the above.

14.3 Which of the following alternative therapies has *not* been found to be useful after a disaster?

A. Meditation.

B. Relaxation.

C. Yoga breathing.

D. Narrative therapy.

E. None of the above.

14.4 Which of the following statements regarding CBT as a postdisaster intervention is *false?*

A. CBT can be helpful if used early.

B. Exposure therapy is a valid behavioral approach after a disaster.

C. Virtual reality can enhance exposure therapy.

D. Dropout is associated with higher education.

E. Dropout is associated with alcohol consumption.

14.5 With regard to therapy in postdisaster situations, which of the following statements is *true?*

A. Psychological First Aid is the first-line psychosocial intervention after a disaster.

B. Psychodynamic therapy is an integral part of crisis management.

C. CBT addresses thoughts, not behaviors.

D. The efficacy of long-term therapy has been unequivocally demonstrated.

E. Family support appears to be less important in the postdisaster environment than in nondisaster settings.

References

Benson H, Greenwood MM, Klemchuk H: The relaxation response: psychophysiologic aspects and clinical applications. Int J Psychiatry Med 6:87–98, 1975

Bisson J, Andrew M: Psychological treatment of post-traumatic stress disorder (PTSD). Cochrane Database of Systematic Reviews 2007, Issue 3. Art. No.: CD003388. DOI: 10.1002/14651858.CD003388.pub3.

Bohleber W: Remembrance, trauma and collective memory: the battle for memory in psychoanalysis. Int J Psychoanal 88:329–352, 2007

Boscarino JA, Adams RE: Overview of findings from the World Trade Center Disaster Outcome Study: recommendations for future research after exposure to psychological trauma. Int J Emerg Ment Health 10:275–290, 2008

Brown RP, Gerbarg PL: Yoga breathing, meditation, and longevity. Ann NY Acad Sci 1172:54–62, 2009

Catani C, Kohiladevy M, Ruf M, et al: Treating children traumatized by war and tsunami: a comparison between exposure therapy and meditation-relaxation in North-East Sri Lanka. BMC Psychiatry 9:22, 2009

Diaz JO: Integrating psychosocial programs in multisector responses to international disasters. Am Psychol 63:820–827, 2008

Difede J, Cukor J, Patt I, et al: The application of virtual reality to the treatment of PTSD following the WTC attack. Ann NY Acad Sci 1071:500–501, 2006

Difede J, Malta LS, Best S, et al: A randomized controlled clinical treatment trial for World Trade Center attack-related PTSD in disaster workers. J Nerv Ment Dis 195:861–865, 2007

Giannopoulou I, Dikaiakou A, Yule W: Cognitive-behavioural group intervention for PTSD symptoms in children following the Athens 1999 earthquake: a pilot study. Clin Child Psychol Psychiatry 11:543–553, 2006

Halliburton M: Finding a fit: psychiatric pluralism in south India and its implications for WHO studies of mental disorder. Transcult Psychiatry 41:80–98, 2004

Hamblen JL, Gibson LE, Mueser KT, et al: Cognitive behavioral therapy for prolonged postdisaster distress. J Clin Psychol 62:1043–1052, 2006

Hobfoll SE, Watson P, Bell CC, et al: Five essential elements of immediate and mid-term mass trauma intervention: empirical evidence. Focus 7:221–242, 2009

Knobler HY, Nachshoni T, Jaffe E, et al: Psychological guidelines for a medical team debriefing after a stressful event. Mil Med 172:581–585, 2007

Kun P, Han S, Chen X, et al: Prevalence and risk factors for posttraumatic stress disorder: a cross-sectional study among survivors of the Wenchuan 2008 earthquake in China. Depress Anxiety 26:1134–1140, 2009

Landau J, Mittal M, Wieling E: Linking human systems: strengthening individuals, families, and communities in the wake of mass trauma. J Marital Fam Ther 34:193–209, 2008

Lewis JI: The crossroads of countertransference and attribution theory: reinventing clinical training within an evidence-based treatment world. Am J Psychoanal 69:106–120, 2009

Milligan G, McGuinness TM: Mental health needs in a post-disaster environment. J Psychosoc Nurs Ment Health Serv 47:23–30, 2009

Peres JF, Newberg AB, Mercante JP, et al: Cerebral blood flow changes during retrieval of traumatic memories before and after psychotherapy: a SPECT study. Psychol Med 37:1481–1491, 2007

Phillips SB: The synergy of group and individual treatment modalities in the aftermath of disaster and unfolding trauma. Int J Group Psychother 59:85–107, 2009

Rao K: Psychosocial support in disaster-affected communities. Int Rev Psychiatry 18:501–505, 2006

Ruggiero KJ, Resnick HS, Acierno R, et al: Internet-based intervention for mental health and substance use problems in disaster-affected populations: a pilot feasibility study. Behav Ther 37:190–205, 2006

Ruzek J, Walser RD, Naugle AE, et al: Cognitive-behavioral psychology: implications for disaster and terrorism response. Prehosp Disaster Med 23:397–410, 2008

Salcioglu E, Basoglu M: Psychological effects of earthquakes in children: prospects for brief behavioral treatment. World J Pediatr 4:165–172, 2008

Shapiro F: Eye Movement Desensitization and Reprocessing (EMDR) and the anxiety disorders: clinical and research implications of an integrated psychotherapy treatment. J Anxiety Disord 13:35–67, 1999

Sharot T, Martorella EA, Delgado MR, et al: How personal experience modulates the neural circuitry of memories of September 11. Proc Natl Acad Sci USA 104:389–394, 2007

Shooshtary MH, Panaghi L, Moghadam JA: Outcome of cognitive behavioral therapy in adolescents after natural disaster. J Adolesc Health 42:466–472, 2008

Stoddard FJ Jr: Psychological interventions, in Hidden Impact: What You Need to Know for the Next Disaster. A Practical Mental Health Guide for Clinicians. Edited by Stoddard FJ, Katz CL, Merlino JP. Sudbury, MA, Jones & Bartlett, 2010, pp 139–148

Udomratn P: Mental health and the psychosocial consequences of natural disasters in Asia. Int Rev Psychiatry 20:441–444, 2008

van der Kolk BA: Clinical implications of neuroscience research in PTSD. Ann N Y Acad Sci 1071:277–293, 2006

Vijayakumar L, Kannan GK, Ganesh Kumar B, et al: Do all children need intervention after exposure to tsunami? Int Rev Psychiatry 18:515–522, 2006

Wessells MG: Do no harm: toward contextually appropriate psychosocial support in international emergencies. Am Psychol 64:842–854, 2009

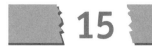

Psychopharmacology

Acute Phase

Kristina Jones, M.D.

> *All of a sudden there were people screaming. I saw people jumping out of the building. Their arms were flailing. I stopped taking pictures and started crying.*
>
> *Michael Walters,*
> *freelance photojournalist,*
> *Manhattan 2001*

Pharmacotherapeutics: Goals and Considerations in the Acute Disaster Setting

The psychiatrist in the acute disaster setting is challenged by a lack of evidence for many psychopharmacological interventions. In acute disaster care, treatment is directed at specific symptoms rather than specific syndromes or disorders. Insomnia and anxiety are the most common presentations, followed by panic, agitation and recurrence of depression, exacerbation of pre-existing psychiatric illness, and relapse of substance abuse and dependence.

Basis for Intervention

Key goals of acute phase intervention are to assure safety, reduce symptom burden, reduce anxiety and distress, and improve functioning. Because the evidence base for psychopharmacological interventions in the acute disaster setting is very limited, medications are usually prescribed on a short-term basis to reduce target symptoms, based on prior clinical experience in disasters and research with other acutely stressed populations. Despite the lack of medications approved by the U.S. Food and Drug Administration for acute stress disorder (ASD), standard clinical practice is to prescribe anxiolytic, sedative, or antipsychotic medications for "off-label" use to treat anxiety, insomnia, and agitation, similar to such practice in emergency psychiatry or primary care settings (Disaster Psychiatry Outreach 2008). According to Shalev (2009), evidence suggests that there is a window of opportunity, the so-called golden hour, to help those persons who are vulnerable to developing chronic posttraumatic stress disorder (PTSD) in the very early aftermath of trauma. Prescribing in an acute setting, especially one in which the clinician and victim may not have future contact, should be limited to a few days' supply of medication unless it is for purposes of continuing or resuming medication(s) lost amid the disaster. The clinician must document that a discussion with the patient regarding the risks and benefits of the psychopharmacological intervention occurred and was understood by the patient, and that follow-up plans were included in the intervention.

Types of Interventions

During the first few hours after a traumatic event, the primary clinical goal is to reduce a patient's terror and decrease neuronal imprinting. Theoretically, β-adrenergic blockers would be useful at this time (see subsection "Propranolol for Anxiety and Prevention of Posttraumatic Stress Disorder" later in this chapter). Moving the patient to safety may also reduce terrifying arousal or anxiety. In the next few days, β-adrenergic blockers and anxiolytic medications may help reduce conditioned fear and minimize consolidation of traumatic memory of the event (Shalev 2009). Psychopharmacology should not be applied indiscriminately or without other interventions. Marmar et al. (2002) advised that pharmacotherapy and cognitive therapy should be used in combination to optimize treatment efficacy. Psychopharmacology may be equally or even less effective for ASD than psychological treatments, such as exposure therapy, which shows promising results (Bryant et al. 2008).

Literature on disasters from 1980 to 2000 contains advice against use of psychotropic medication at the time of an acute trauma, due to concern that it might adversely affect a person's psychological processing of the event. This view has been replaced by a call for more research, including randomized controlled trials (RCTs). There is extremely limited support for the notion that psychopharmacology may actually be harmful (see "Benzodiazepines for Anxiety" later in this chapter). Because research that relies on RCTs is rarely feasible at disaster sites, it has been difficult to obtain the needed evidence for or against medication treatment. Much psychopharmacological intervention is guided by targeting putative disease mechanisms of ASD and PTSD, including dysregulation of the hypothalamic-pituitary-adrenal axis and of the norepinephrine, glutamate, and serotonin systems (Ravindran and Stein 2009).

A statistical review of studies that quantified psychopathology in the aftermath of disasters dating back to 1966 estimated that disasters are associated with a 17% mean increase in the best mean estimate prevalence of psychopathology in comparison with rates in predisaster or control groups (Katz et al. 2002). It is not clear what the expected rate of ASD is after natural or human-made disasters. The non-disaster-related lifetime prevalence of PTSD has been estimated at 6.8% in the general population, with a 12-month prevalence rate of 3.5% (Kessler et al. 2005). The fact that a disaster survivor does not meet full criteria for ASD (Table 15–1) does not mean that he or she is not at risk for PTSD. There is debate as to which symptoms are most predictive of PTSD, with some studies finding that anxiety and hyperarousal are predictive, and others finding that detachment, numbing, and dissociation predict future PTSD (Harvey and Bryant 2000). In some studies, ASD does not always lead to PTSD, and PTSD may occur acutely. For example, in a study of 596 admissions to trauma facilities in Australia, the majority of people who developed PTSD did not have ASD. Symptoms of PTSD at the time of acute assessment were more predictive of later development of PTSD than were symptoms of ASD (Bryant et al. 2008).

Psychiatrists need to be alert for acute changes in mental status of patients after a disaster. Therefore, they need to assess each patient's level of consciousness and orientation to day, date, month, and year; observe for dissociative symptoms by asking the patient where he or she is; and arrange for a focused medical history, including screening for any medical event specific to the type of disaster, a history of head injury and seizure, and a review of systems and medication allergies (Stevens et al. 2010).

Acute Psychopharmacological Interventions

An intentional exposure of workers to anthrax in a midtown Manhattan office building became known to public health officials after several patients presented to nearby emergency departments (EDs). Ms. A, a 37-year-old freelance writer, arrives at the ED asking for a ciprofloxacin prescription for anthrax, saying that she worked in the building. She reports no significant medical history and has stable vital signs. Although not in respiratory distress, Ms. A appears anxious. She reports that she has arrived back in New York City after vacation. Given her stable vital signs, Ms. A is asked to wait. An hour into her wait, Ms. A runs to the triage nurse complaining of short-

TABLE 15–1.   DSM-IV-TR diagnostic criteria for 308.3 acute stress disorder[a]

A. The person has been exposed to a traumatic event in which both of the following were present:

   (1) the person experienced, witnessed, or was confronted with an event or events that involved actual or threatened death or serious injury, or a threat to the physical integrity of self or others

   (2) the person's response involved intense fear, helplessness, or horror

B. Either while experiencing or after experiencing the distressing event, the individual has three (or more) of the following dissociative symptoms:

   (1) a subjective sense of numbing, detachment, or absence of emotional responsiveness

   (2) a reduction in awareness of his or her surroundings (e.g., "being in a daze")

   (3) derealization

   (4) depersonalization

   (5) dissociative amnesia (i.e., inability to recall an important aspect of the trauma)

C. The traumatic event is persistently reexperienced in at least one of the following ways: recurrent images, thoughts, dreams, illusions, flashback episodes, or a sense of reliving the experience; or distress on exposure to reminders of the traumatic event.

D. Marked avoidance of stimuli that arouse recollections of the trauma (e.g., thoughts, feelings, conversations, activities, places, people).

E. Marked symptoms of anxiety or increased arousal (e.g., difficulty sleeping, irritability, poor concentration, hypervigilance, exaggerated startle response, motor restlessness).

F. The disturbance causes clinically significant distress or impairment in social, occupational, or other important areas of functioning or impairs the individual's ability to pursue some necessary task, such as obtaining necessary assistance or mobilizing personal resources by telling family members about the traumatic experience.

G. The disturbance lasts for a minimum of 2 days and a maximum of 4 weeks and occurs within 4 weeks of the traumatic event.

H. The disturbance is not due to the direct physiological effects of a substance (e.g., a drug of abuse, a medication) or a general medical condition, is not better accounted for by brief psychotic disorder, and is not merely an exacerbation of a preexisting Axis I or Axis II disorder.

[a]See Appendix Table 15A–1 at the end of this chapter for DSM-5 proposed criteria for acute stress disorder.

Source.   Reprinted from the *Diagnostic and Statistical Manual of Mental Disorders,* 4th Edition, Text Revision. Washington, DC, American Psychiatric Association, 2000, pp. 471–472. Copyright © 2000 American Psychiatric Association. Used with permission.

ness of breath and chest pain. She looks very anxious, pale, and sweaty. Her respiratory rate is 20, and her vital signs are stable. She has pushed past the security guard and is yelling, "If I don't get help now, I will leave and spread this around the city." The nurse's attempts to reassure Ms. A agitate her further, and she is ushered into the subacute treatment area.

In the assessment, it becomes apparent that since her return from vacation, Ms. A has not been back to the building where the anthrax was discovered. She becomes more distressed and irritable when attempts are made to reassure her, and says she just wants to get the ciprofloxacin and leave. The history reveals that Ms. A has been having panic attacks for 2 months, ever since she and her husband separated. The person she was to interview for her writing assignment canceled his trip to New York due to the anthrax scare. Now Ms. A is alarmed that she will not finish her article, which makes her more worried about her finances now that she is raising her child on her own. ED staff ask Ms. A about social supports, past psychiatric history, and alcohol use, and give her lorazepam 0.5 mg. An electrocardiogram reassures both Ms. A and the ED staff that there is no cardiac disease and that she is not having a heart attack. Ms. A is referred to a crisis counseling line, is urged to reach out to friends for additional support, and is provided with phone referral to psychiatry services via the state's disaster resource helpline.

Benzodiazepines for Anxiety

Following a disaster, a person with panic symptomatology (such as Ms. A) may benefit from benzodiazepine treatment (see Table 15–2). Benzodiazepines enhance transmission of γ-aminobutyric acid and exert an inhibitory effect on the amygdala, which is involved in the processing of fear. Because PTSD shares many of its symptoms with other anxiety disorders for which benzodiazepines are effective, there is an evidence base for using this class of drugs to treat acute anxiety, agitation, and insomnia after a disaster, whether or not these symptoms develop into full-syndrome ASD or PTSD (Bandelow et al. 2008).

In a pilot study in the immediate aftermath of exposure to trauma, temazepam 30 mg was administered to four patients at bedtime for 5 days, followed by 15 mg for 2 days (Mellman et al. 1998). Evaluations 1 week after medication cessation showed improved sleep and reduced symptoms of posttraumatic stress. The authors speculated that the facilitation of a normal sleep pattern (thereby regulating hyperarousal) before the consolidation of PTSD may be important for preventing progression to illness.

Midazolam, a short-acting benzodiazepine with anxiolytic, amnestic, and sedative properties that is used in surgical procedures, has been posited to enhance memory of traumatic events by interfering with memory consolidation and processing of trauma. Researchers tested this hypothesis in a study of soldiers hospitalized for burns sustained in the Iraq war (McGhee et al. 2009). Rates of PTSD in the 142 soldiers given midazolam did not

---

TABLE 15–2.   Psychopharmacological interventions for anxiety

---

Benzodiazepines

Anxiety, including panic symptoms, can be effectively reduced with low-dose benzodiazepines.

Intervention for anxiety should include a prescription of 1 week's supply or less, to avoid tolerance and dependence.

Examples:

    Lorazepam 0.5 mg po qhs; can also be used bid or tid, to a maximum of 4 mg/ day for patients who are benzodiazepine naive

    Clonazepam 0.5 mg po qhs or bid for 7–14 days only; can also be used bid or tid to a maximum of 4 mg/day

Alternatives to benzodiazepines

    Diphenhydramine 25–50 mg qhs or bid

    Hydroxyzine 10–50 mg qhs or bid

Over-the-counter alternatives

    Acetaminophen with diphenhydramine acceptable for very mild anxiety

Risks, side effects, and drug interactions

Sedation and dizziness are most common side effects of benzodiazepines. In a few individuals, disinhibited behavior can occur. Caution must be used in elderly patients (who may experience slowed metabolism and increased CNS effects and drug interactions; see Chapter 18, "Geriatric Psychiatry Interventions"), in patients with substance abuse, and in patients with a history of dementia or delirium. Drug interactions of concern for benzodiazepines include any drug with CNS sedation as a risk, including narcotics, mood stabilizers, or antiseizure medications.

Benzodiazepine dependence

Evidence suggests that after 21 days, patient can become dependent, and that withdrawal may occur, with rebound insomnia and anxiety. Patient should use medication for first few nights, then taper if anxiety improves and use only on an as-needed basis.

Note.   CNS=central nervous system.

differ significantly from rates in the 69 soldiers who were not given midazolam, thus providing supportive evidence that intraoperative administration of midazolam does not amplify the intensity of traumatic memories or heighten the risk of developing PTSD.

Benzodiazepine administration can be considered safe, effective, and useful in the immediate postdisaster setting for acute symptoms of extreme arousal, insomnia, and uncontrollable anxiety, all of which may be considered greater risk factors for developing PTSD than the administration of a benzodiazepine per se (Simon and Gorman 2004). Potential drug interaction hazards for benzodiazepines include medications or substances that increase the risk of central nervous system (CNS) sedation, such as narcotics, mood stabilizers, anticonvulsants, and alcohol. The clinician needs to take a complete clinical history and screen for contraindications before prescribing benzodiazepines. These medications must be used only for a brief period postdisaster and must not be given to patients who are using or abusing alcohol or other drugs. Benzodiazepines are contraindicated in the setting of traumatic brain injury (TBI), where they have been associated with disinhibition and may increase delirium or enhance risk of seizure. Patients must be made aware of risks and benefits, informed of side effects, and cautioned strongly about tolerance, dependence, and potential for addiction.

Nonbenzodiazepine Agents for Sleep

Sleep imbalance may put the patient at risk for postdisaster trauma-related sequelae and for alcohol abuse. Agents that can be used safely for insomnia are listen in Table 15–3. Alcohol independently impedes encoding of traumatic memories. Compared with benzodiazepines, the nonbenzodiazepine compounds that bind to benzodiazepine receptors (e.g., zolpidem, zaleplon, eszopiclone) may have fewer side effects in terms of morning sedation or cognitive impairment (Lavie 2001). Evidence for the effectiveness of diphenhydramine and other sedating antihistamines is less convincing, except in children (Lavie 2001). The disaster psychiatrist should be alert for changes in the patient's heart rate and blood pressure, because some studies show elevated pulse (over a cutoff of 95) to be indicative of high responsiveness to stress and to be predictive of PTSD (Zatzick et al. 2005). The psychiatrist should be able to perform relevant elements of the physical exam if no medical personnel are available to do so. Pulse rate, blood pressure, and respiratory rate are essential, and a focused neurological exam is indicated where head injury or delirium is part of the psychiatric presentation.

Antidepressants for Anxiety and Acute Traumatic Stress

Although selective serotonin reuptake inhibitors (SSRIs) are recommended for use in treating PTSD, there is greater research support for use in chronic PTSD. The effect of SSRIs on ASD is poorly researched. No studies have established whether acute administration of SSRIs may prevent PTSD from developing. An RCT of escitalopram for acute PTSD found no positive effect of that drug over placebo or wait-list control; however, the small study sample (22 patients in each arm) calls for larger replication (Shalev et al. 2007; Ursano et al. 2004). There are few good studies of pharmacological interventions for patients with ASD. SSRIs and other antidepressants are reasonable clinical interventions that are supported by limited findings in

---

TABLE 15–3.   Psychopharmacological interventions for insomnia

No large trials have been reported of medication used for sleep disturbance in patients with acute stress disorder or posttraumatic stress disorder, although medications are widely used adjuncts for short-term treatment of insomnia (their FDA indication).

Prescriptions for 14 days may be appropriate, after which time patient should seek formal psychiatric consultation.

Interventions for insomnia

Zolpidem 10 mg po qhs

Zolpidem CR 6.25 or 12.5 mg po qhs

Eszopiclone 1, 2, or 3 mg po qhs

Ramelteon 8 mg po qhs

Trazodone 50 mg po qhs

Risks, side effects, and drug interactions

Sedation and dizziness are the most common side effects of medications for insomnia. In very few individuals, disinhibited behavior can occur. Caution must be used in patients who are elderly, who abuse substances, and who have a history of dementia or delirium. Drug interactions of concern for insomnia medication include any drug with CNS sedation as a risk, including benzodiazepines, narcotics, mood stabilizers, or antiseizure medications.

Note.   CNS=central nervous system; FDA=U.S. Food and Drug Administration.

---

patients with ASD, as well as by findings of therapeutic benefit in patients with PTSD. SSRIs may be helpful in treating specific symptom clusters in individual patients (Ursano et al. 2004; see also Chapter 16, "Psychopharmacology: Postacute Phase").

SSRIs in the acute phase have been shown in small open-label trials to be effective and safe. In one study, 15 adult acute burn victims were given citalopram daily for 6 months. All had improved wound healing, and none developed PTSD, whereas 50% of untreated control subjects developed PTSD (Bláha et al. 1999). In a study in children with acute burns, researchers compared the tricyclic antidepressant imipramine and the SSRI fluoxetine and found that 55% responded positively to placebo, 60% to imipramine, and 72% to fluoxetine. Within the parameters of the study, placebo was statistically as effective as either drug in treating symptoms of ASD (Robert et al. 2008). In a study performed 4 months after the 1999 earthquake in Turkey that killed more than 15,000 people, 103 patients were randomly assigned to fluoxetine, the monoamine oxidase inhibitor moclobemide, or the atypical antidepressant tianeptine; all of the patients completing the study had a greater than 50% decrease in PTSD symptoms assessed using validated standardized scales. The authors concluded that all three medications were equally effective (Onder et al. 2006).

Although no large RCTs have been performed with the atypical antidepressant mirtazapine, its mechanism of action would suggest a possible role in PTSD. Mirtazapine enhances both serotonergic and noradrenergic transmission via a dual mechanism of action: blockade of both presynaptic α_2 autoreceptors and α_2 heteroreceptors, as well as antagonism of postsynaptic 5-hydroxytryptamine (serotonin) type 2 and type 3 (5-HT_2 and 5-HT_3) receptors. An RCT of 29 patients with PTSD found rates of response of 64.7% for mirtazapine and 20% for placebo (Davidson et al. 2003).

In conclusion, in the acute setting it is usually not appropriate to start a medication intended for longer-term use (e.g., antidepressants), although disaster psychiatrists continue to consider this option. Case reports suggest that antidepressants may prevent the development of PTSD (Stein et al. 2007). The disaster psychiatrist could consider SSRIs for certain high-risk patients, such as those with prior history of PTSD or with a preexisting anxiety disorder (e.g., panic disorder) or those at high risk for recurrence of major depression (Ursano et al. 2004). It is critical that adequate follow-up be provided and that patients be monitored for switches into mania, as well as for the rare complication of developing suicidal ideation after starting an SSRI.

Prazosin for Posttraumatic Stress Disorder–Related Nightmares

Because PTSD results in part from hyperarousal associated with elevated α-adrenergic activation, α-adrenergic blockade should reduce arousal, including nightmares. This is the case, particularly for the agent prazosin, which has been studied in adults. Several studies, including a placebo-controlled study in 13 patients in a crossover design, indicate that prazosin is effective both in reducing nightmares and in increasing sleep time (Fraleigh et al. 2009; Taylor et al. 2008). Use of prazosin has steadily increased in the region (Tacoma, Washington) in which the original studies were conducted (Harpaz-Rotem and Rosenheck 2009).

Antipsychotics for Agitation and Extreme Anxiety

The off-label prescription of atypical antipsychotics for agitation and anxiety has increased, albeit without a strong evidence base. Atypical antipsychotics act on dopaminergic systems, and some also act on serotonergic systems; both systems have been implicated in the development of PTSD. Some of these antipsychotics also show affinity for α-adrenergic receptors, which have been demonstrated to be dysregulated in PTSD. In addition, through their antihistaminic effects, antipsychotics may help alleviate sleep-related symptoms of ASD or PTSD (Berger et al. 2009).

In a retrospective chart review of 10 adult burn patients, risperidone given 5 days after the injury appeared to reduce sleep disturbances, nightmares, and hyperarousal; this finding must be interpreted with caution, however, given the lack of randomized studies (Stanovic et al. 2001). Among six RCTs of risperidone, all in the chronic PTSD population, only one demonstrated its superiority over placebo as monotherapy; the others examined risperidone as adjunctive therapy with an SSRI. Similar small controlled studies exist for olanzapine, quetiapine, and clozapine (Berger et al. 2009).

In the acute disaster setting, antipsychotics should be reserved for individuals with extreme agitation, psychotic illness, or hypomania, or for those in whom a benzodiazepine might be contraindicated (see Table 15–4). Because significant side effects, such as acute dystonias and extrapyramidal reactions, can occur, antipsychotics should only be given in a setting in which the patient can be monitored. Restarting the patient on an antipsychotic for prophylaxis of mania or to prevent recurrence or exacerbation of chronic schizophrenia is a reasonable strategy for individuals with severe and persistent mental illness presenting in the acute disaster setting.

TABLE 15–4.   Psychopharmacological interventions for acute agitation

---

Although rare, agitation can be seen in the acute phase of disaster. Agitated patients warrant a psychiatric referral for evaluation; they often have an underlying mental illness, substance abuse, or other disorder.

Medical workup

For any patient presenting with agitation, a history must be obtained regarding recent alcohol or substance abuse, and appropriate urine or blood drug screens should be performed. A CT scan or MRI is indicated in any patient with a history of head injury or trauma or with complex underlying medical problems, such as cancer.

Interventions for agitation

Agitation is managed in the same way as any acute ED presentation if the survivor is dangerous, extremely agitated, or psychotic. In the ED, use:

   Haloperidol 0.5–2.0 mg po or intramuscular with an antiparkinsonian agent

   Lorazepam 1–2 mg po or intramuscular

   Diphenhydramine 50 mg po or intramuscular can be given if there is concern for dystonic reactions

Dose ranges per 24 hours in the ED:

   Haloperidol: 0.5–2.0 mg po or intramuscular q 4 hours

   Lorazepam: 1–2 mg po or intramuscular q 4 hours

   Diphenhydramine: 50 mg po or intramuscular q 4 hours

TABLE 15–4. Psychopharmacological interventions for acute agitation *(continued)*

Risks, side effects, and drug interactions

Sedation and dizziness are the most common side effects of medications for agitation. Haloperidol can cause dystonic reactions in vulnerable patients. Young African American males, patients with mood disorder histories, and elderly patients require close monitoring for a dystonic reaction. Giving 50 mg diphenhydramine in combination with haloperidol and lorazepam is a precautionary measure against dystonic reactions. For a longer duration of antiparkinsonian action, 2 mg benztropine mesylate may be prescribed instead.

Caution must be used in the elderly, in whom doses can be used at the lowest range and given less frequently. Benzodiazepines must be given with great caution in elderly patients due to risk of falls and hip fractures, or hypotension. Close monitoring and observation by a nurse is important (see Chapter 18, "Geriatric Psychiatry Interventions").

Drug interactions of concern include any drug with CNS sedation as a risk, including benzodiazepines, narcotics, mood stabilizers, or antiseizure medications, or other antipsychotics.

Mild agitation with extreme anxiety

In patients for whom a benzodiazepine is contraindicated, very-low-dose atypical antipsychotics (e.g., low-dose risperidone 0.5–1.0 mg po hs or bid, or low-dose quetiapine 25–50 mg po hs or bid) can be used to control agitation or extreme anxiety. All antipsychotic medications include a black box warning not to use them with patients who have dementia, due to risk of CVA. In at-risk patients, an ECG is advised if possible. Antipsychotic and other medications may cause QTc prolongation and cardiac complications. Additionally, documentation should be provided clarifying why conventional approaches to agitation (including benzodiazepines or diphenhydramine) are not indicated, or have been tried but found ineffective.

In a pilot study, 10 burn victims taking risperidone reported better sleep, reduced nightmares, and decreased flashbacks and hyperarousal (Eidelman et al. 2000). A case report of 4 burn patients found that risperidone led to improvement in acute stress disorder symptoms (Stanovic et al. 2001).

Quetiapine may be an appropriate agent to consider for off-label use, instead of a benzodiazepine, when patient is anxious or agitated or has insomnia, and when a benzodiazepine has been ineffective or is not appropriate. For example, quetiapine is useful in patients with substance abuse, during cocaine or amphetamine intoxication; or in patients who are taking methadone, where a benzodiazepine risks respiratory depression; or in patients with prior brain injury.

Note. CNS=central nervous system; CT=computed tomography; CVA=cerebrovascular accident; ECG=electrocardiogram; ED=emergency department; MRI=magnetic resonance imaging.

Source. Data from Gibson L: *Pharmacological Treatment of Acute Stress Reactions and PTSD.* Washington, DC, National Center for PTSD, February 2010. Available at: http://www.ptsd.va.gov/professional/pages/handouts-pdf/Pharmacological_Tx.pdf. Accessed January 1, 2011.

Propranolol for Anxiety and Prevention of Posttraumatic Stress Disorder

Animal data suggest that treatment with a β-adrenergic–blocking agent following an acute psychologically traumatic event could reduce subsequent PTSD symptoms. Theory suggests that blocking the adrenergic responses to a traumatic event might prevent its long-term encoding of the fear response into memory. In an open-label study, Vaiva et al. (2003) gave the β-blocker propranolol to 11 patients presenting in the ED after motor vehicle accidents or physical assault. At 2 months postincident, PTSD occurred in 1 of the 11 patients given propranolol and in 3 of the 11 patients who refused medication. In a randomized, double-blind controlled study, Pitman et al. (2002) administered propranolol to 32 trauma survivors who had an elevated initial heart rate within 6 hours of a traumatic event. The treatment failed to decrease the intensity of PTSD symptoms 3 months later. Although propranolol treatment did not change Clinician-Administered PTSD Scale scores at 1 month, it decreased the physiological response to script-driven traumatic imagery 3 months after the trauma. Stein et al. (2007) found that neither propranolol nor gabapentin reduced PTSD symptoms when administered within 48 hours of a traumatic injury. Further research is needed. It may be that for those patients with contraindications for benzodiazepines, propranolol may relieve panic symptoms acutely, even if it does not prevent PTSD (Benedek et al. 2009).

Posttraumatic Symptoms From Medications for Serious Medical Trauma

Important lessons from military psychiatry can be used by the disaster psychiatrist. It is important to be familiar with medications used in the acute medical setting and their psychiatric effects. Rundell (2000) noted that agents such as intravenous fluids, epinephrine, lidocaine, atropine, sedatives, nitroglycerin, and morphine are commonly used and have significant psychiatric or autonomic effects. These effects can mimic primary psychiatric disorders. For example, atropine causes significant anxiety and anticholinergic effects. Lidocaine in some patients can cause vivid visual hallucinations. Epinephrine causes blood pressure and heart rate elevations, as well as anxiety or panic. Morphine causes sedation and impairs orientation and responsiveness (Rundell 2000). In treating hospitalized patients, the psychiatrist should consult with consultation-liaison psychiatry colleagues. Excellent resources are available for management of delirium, agitation, anxiety, and their psychiatric conditions in the medical setting (Caplan et al. 2010; Wise and Rundell 2004).

Delirium in the Acute Disaster Setting

Delirium is a common presentation in acute medical trauma patients, including burn patients, postoperative patients, those who are seriously injured, and those exposed to chemical or biological toxins. A useful consultation intervention is to educate medical colleagues that giving benzodiazepines for agitation and confusion may make the patient even more delirious (Breitbart et al. 1996). Antipsychotics including haloperidol may be indicated in the management of delirium and agitation. Haloperidol or another antipsychotic should be prescribed at dosages sufficient to achieve therapeutic effect (i.e., remission of symptoms). Initially, haloperidol may be helpful to prevent patients from pulling out intravenous lines, drains, and nasogastric tubes, as well as to restore a normal sleep-wake cycle and prevent anxiety (Fricchione et al. 2008; Trzepacz and Meagher 2005). Intravenous haloperidol appears to have a lower incidence of extrapyramidal symptoms than the oral medication.

Conclusion and Cautions

Research data regarding psychopharmacological intervention in acute disaster settings are extremely limited. Nevertheless, existing emergency psychiatry principles and practice provide guidance for intervening effectively and safely in the acute disaster setting to relieve anxiety, panic, insomnia, traumatic bereavement, and symptoms of ASD. Psychopharmacological treatment should focus both on preexisting psychiatric disorders and substance abuse and on disaster-related stress, both of which may influence the patient's biological response to medication. The goals are to develop treatment relationships, manage symptoms, and assure that disaster survivors can access follow-up care in the postacute disaster phase. Important considerations during a disaster are relapse or new onset of major mental illness or substance abuse, which requires assessment, careful management, and referral when available. The clinician should be alert for elderly, impoverished, or severely medically or mentally ill patients who have discontinued their prescribed medications and relapsed. Because patient safety is paramount, disaster psychiatrists need to use common sense, intervene with the lowest effective dosages, and seek to ensure patient access to follow-up care in the community. All patients must consent to medications and be informed of potential adverse effects.

■ Teaching Points

- The goal of psychopharmacological treatment in the acute phase is to reduce symptoms—typically anxiety, shock, insomnia, depression, or agitation—that may interfere with postdisaster coping. Making a diagnosis of PTSD it *not* a goal at this early stage.

- The disaster psychiatrist should be aware of groups at high risk in the acute setting, including individuals with preexisting psychiatric disorders, current or past substance abuse disorders, or a family history of mood disorders.

- Special attention should be paid to individuals with physical injuries, such as burn patients and trauma patients, who are at high risk for postdisaster trauma-related sequelae and for whom adequate pain management and control of delirium may possibly prevent PTSD.

- Medication strategies for anxiety include short-term administration of low-dose benzodiazepines.

- Medication strategies for insomnia include the use of nonbenzodiazepine hypnotics; sedating antihistamines such as diphenhydramine; and, in certain populations, sedating antidepressants such as trazodone.

- Although SSRIs are effective in chronic PTSD, there is as yet no evidence base for their use in the acute disaster setting. Without adequate follow-up, SSRIs may provoke mania or even suicidal ideation and therefore are best used only in the postacute stage.

- Medication strategies for extreme agitation or psychotic illness include benzodiazepines; sedating antihistamines such as diphenhydramine; and, in supervised settings, low-dose antipsychotics.

- Biological factors affecting the absorption, metabolism, distribution, and excretion of medication should be considered. History of medication allergy, adverse reactions, and potential drug interactions must be evaluated.

- If the patient appears suicidal, he or she should be evaluated for immediate danger to self. Patients should be hospitalized if the threat of self-harm is acute or if they are intoxicated.

- Common diagnoses in the acute phase following a disaster include acute and posttraumatic stress disorders, major depression, and alcohol withdrawal; mania and drug-induced psychoses are less common.

Review Questions

15.1 Among acute disaster survivors, which of the following groups are likely to be at high risk for developing PTSD?

    A. Those with dissociation.
    B. Those with insomnia and hypervigilance.
    C. Those with physical injury.
    D. Those with loss of property and ongoing secondary stressors.
    E. All of the above.

15.2 In the acute care medical setting, which of the following medications may mimic symptoms of anxiety?

    A. Atropine.
    B. Lorazepam.
    C. Epinephrine.
    D. Morphine.
    E. A and C.

15.3 In the acute care medical setting, which of the following would likely be most effective for a patient with agitation and delirium?

    A. More morphine.
    B. Lorazepam.
    C. Physical restraint.
    D. A low-dose antipsychotic such as haloperidol.
    E. Propofol.

15.4 Which of the following medication classes is contraindicated in patients with traumatic brain injury?

    A. Antihistamines.
    B. Anticonvulsants.
    C. Benzodiazepines.
    D. SSRIs.
    E. Antipsychotics.

15.5 One of the most important reasons to avoid prescribing SSRIs in the acute disaster setting is the potential for

    A. Gastrointestinal side effects.
    B. Medication noncompliance.
    C. Development of extrapyramidal symptoms.

D. Triggering of mania in a patient with unknown bipolar disorder.
E. Anticholinergic side effects.

References

Bandelow B, Zohar J, Hollander E, et al: World Federation of Societies of Biological Psychiatry (WFSBP) guidelines for the pharmacological treatment of anxiety, obsessive-compulsive and post-traumatic stress disorders—first revision. World J Biol Psychiatry 9:248–312, 2008

Benedek DM, Friedman MJ, Zatzick D, et al: Guideline watch (March 2009): Practice Guideline for the Treatment of Patients With Acute Stress Disorder and Posttraumatic Stress Disorder. Washington, DC, American Psychiatric Publishing, 2009. Available at: http://www.psychiatryonline.com/content.aspx?aid=156498. Accessed January 1, 2011.

Berger W, Mendlowicz MV, Marques-Portella C, et al: Pharmacologic alternatives to antidepressants in posttraumatic stress disorder: a systematic review. Prog Neuropsychopharmacol Biol Psychiatry 33:169–180, 2009

Bláha J, Svobodová K, Kapounková Z: Therapeutic aspects of using citalopram in burns. Acta Chir Plast 41:25–32, 1999

Breitbart W, Marotta R, Platt MM, et al: A double-blind trial of haloperidol, chlorpromazine, and lorazepam in the treatment of delirium in hospitalized AIDS patients. Am J Psychiatry. 153:231–237, 1996

Bryant RA, Mastrodomenico J, Felmingham KL, et al: Treatment of acute stress disorder: a randomized controlled trial. Arch Gen Psychiatry 65:659–667, 2008

Caplan JP, Cassem NH, Murray GB, et al: Delirious patients, in Massachusetts General Hospital Handbook of General Hospital Psychiatry, 6th Edition. Edited by Stern TA, Fricchione GL, Cassem NH, et al. Philadelphia, PA, Saunders Elsevier, 2010, pp 93–104

Davidson JR, Weisler RH, Butterfield MI, et al: Mirtazapine vs. placebo in posttraumatic stress disorder: a pilot trial. Biol Psychiatry 53:188–191, 2003

Disaster Psychiatry Outreach: The Essentials of Disaster Psychiatry: A Training Course for Mental Health Professionals (Course Syllabus). New York, Disaster Psychiatry Outreach, 2008. Available as DPOCourseSyllabus_052108.pdf at: https://sites.google.com/a/disasterpsych.org/blog/File-Cabinet. Accessed December 28, 2009.

Eidelman I, Seedat S, Stein DJ: Risperidone in the treatment of acute stress disorder in physically traumatized in-patients. Depress Anxiety 11:187–188, 2000

Fraleigh LA, Hendratta VD, Ford JD, et al: Prazosin for the treatment of posttraumatic stress disorder-related nightmares in an adolescent male (letter to the editor). J Child Adolesc Psychopharmacol 19:475–476, 2009

Fricchione GL, Nejad SH, Esses JA, et al: Postoperative delirium. Am J Psychiatry 165:803–812, 2008

Harpaz-Rotem I, Rosenheck RA: Tracing the flow of knowledge: geographic variability in the diffusion of prazosin use for the treatment of posttraumatic stress disorder nationally in the Department of Veterans Affairs. Arch Gen Psychiatry 66:417–421, 2009

Harvey AG, Bryant RA: Two-year prospective evaluation of the relationship between acute stress disorder and posttraumatic stress disorder following mild traumatic brain injury. Am J Psychiatry 157:626–628, 2000

Katz CL, Pellegrino L, Pandya A, et al: Research on psychiatric outcomes and interventions subsequent to disasters: a review of the literature. Psychiatry Res 110:201–217, 2002

Kessler RC, Chiu WT, Demler O, et al: Prevalence, severity, and comorbidity of 12-month DSM-IV disorders in the National Comorbidity Survey Replication. Arch Gen Psychiatry 62:617–627, 2005

Lavie P: Sleep disturbances in the wake of traumatic events. N Engl J Med 345:1825–1832, 2001

Marmar CR, Neylan TC, Schoenfeld FB: New directions in the pharmacotherapy of posttraumatic stress disorder. Psychiatr Q 73:259–270, 2002

McGhee L, Maani C, Garza T, et al: The relationship of intravenous midazolam and posttraumatic stress disorder development in burned soldiers. J Trauma 66:S186–S190, 2009

Mellman TA, Byers PM, Augenstein JS: Pilot evaluation of hypnotic medication during acute traumatic stress response. J Trauma Stress 11:563–569, 1998

Onder E, Tural U, Aker T: A comparative study of fluoxetine, moclobemide, and tianeptine in the treatment of posttraumatic stress disorder following an earthquake. Eur Psychiatry 21:174–179, 2006

Pitman RK, Sanders KM, Zusman RM, et al: Pilot study of secondary prevention of posttraumatic stress disorder with propranolol. Biol Psychiatry 51:189–192, 2002

Ravindran LN, Stein MB: Pharmacotherapy of PTSD: premises, principles, and priorities. Brain Res 1293:24–39, 2009

Robert R, Tcheung WJ, Rosenberg L, et al: Treating thermally injured children suffering symptoms of acute stress with imipramine and fluoxetine: a randomized, double-blind study. Burns 34:919–928, 2008

Rundell JR: Psychiatric issues in medical-surgical disaster casualties: a consultation-liaison approach. Psychiatr Q 71:245–258, 2000

Shalev A: Posttraumatic stress disorder and stress-related disorders. Psychiatr Clin North Am 32:687–704, 2009

Shalev AY, Peleg T, Ankri Y, et al: Prevention of PTSD by early treatment: a randomized controlled study. Preliminary results from the Jerusalem Trauma Outreach and Prevention Study (J-TOPS) (poster), in American College of Neuropsychopharmacology 46th Annual Meeting General Program, Boca Raton, FL, December 9–13, 2007. Nashville, TN, American College of Neuropsychopharmacology, 2007, p 63

Simon A, Gorman J: Psychopharmacological possibilities in the acute disaster setting. Psychiatr Clin North Am 27:425–458, 2004

Stanovic JK, James KA, Vandevere CA: The effectiveness of risperidone on acute stress symptoms in adult burn patients: a preliminary retrospective pilot study. J Burn Care Rehabil 22:210–213, 2001

Stein MB, Kerrifge C, Dimsdale JE, et al: Pharmacotherapy to prevent PTSD: results from a randomized controlled proof of concept trial in physically injured patients. J Trauma Stress 20:923–932, 2007

Stevens JR, Fava M, Rosenbaum JF, et al: Psychopharmacology in the medical setting, in Massachusetts General Hospital Handbook of General Hospital Psychiatry, 6th Edition. Edited by Stern TA, Fricchione GL, Cassem NH, et al. Philadelphia, PA, Saunders Elsevier, 2010, pp 441–466

Taylor FB, Martin P, Thompson C, et al: Prazosin effects on objective sleep measures and clinical symptoms in civilian trauma posttraumatic stress disorder: a placebo-controlled study. Biol Psychiatry 63:629–632, 2008

Trzepacz P, Meagher D: Delirium, in Textbook of Psychosomatic Medicine. Edited by Levenson J. Washington, DC, American Psychiatric Publishing, 2005, pp 91–130

Ursano J, Bell C, Eth S, et al: Practice Guidelines for the Treatment of Patients With Acute Stress Disorder and Posttraumatic Stress Disorder. Work Group on ASD and PSTD. Washington, DC, American Psychiatric Association, 2004

Vaiva G, Ducrocq F, Jezequel K, et al: Immediate treatment with propranolol decreases posttraumatic stress disorder two months after trauma. Biol Psychiatry 54:947–949, 2003

Wise M, Rundell J: Clinical Manual of Psychosomatic Medicine: A Guide to Consultation-Liaison Psychiatry. Washington, DC, American Psychiatric Publishing, 2004

Zatzick DF, Russo J, Pitman RK, et al: Re-evaluating the association between emergency department heart rate and the development of post-traumatic stress disorder: a public health approach. Biol Psychiatry 57:91–95, 2005

Appendix 15A

DSM-5 Supplement to Table 15–1

APPENDIX 15A.   DSM-5 proposed criteria for DSM-IV-TR 308.3 acute stress disorder

A.   The person was exposed to one or more of the following event(s): death or threatened death, actual or threatened serious injury, or actual or threatened sexual violation, in one or more of the following ways:

1.   Experiencing the event(s) him/herself

2.   Witnessing, in person, the event(s) as they occurred to others

3.   Learning that the event(s) occurred to a close relative or close friend; in such cases, the actual or threatened death must have been violent or accidental

4.   Experiencing repeated or extreme exposure to aversive details of the event(s) (e.g., first responders collecting body parts; police officers repeatedly exposed to details of child abuse); this does not apply to exposure through electronic media, television, movies, or pictures, unless this exposure is work related

B.   Eight (or more) of the following symptoms are present that were not present prior to the traumatic event or have worsened since the event:*

Intrusion symptoms

1.   Spontaneous or cued recurrent, involuntary, and intrusive distressing memories of the traumatic event

2.   Recurrent distressing dreams in which the content and/or affect of the dream is related to the traumatic event

3.   Dissociative reactions (e.g., flashbacks) in which the individual feels or acts as if the traumatic event were recurring

4.   Intense or prolonged psychological distress or physiological reactivity at exposure to internal or external cues that symbolize or resemble an aspect of the traumatic event

Dissociation symptoms

5.   A subjective sense of numbing, detachment from others, or reduced responsiveness to events that would normally elicit an emotional response

6.   An altered sense of the reality of one's surroundings or oneself (e.g., seeing oneself from another's perspective, being in a daze, time slowing)

7.   Inability to remember at least one important aspect of the traumatic event (typically dissociative amnesia; not due to head injury, alcohol, drugs)

Avoidance symptoms

8.   Persistent and effortful avoidance of thoughts, conversations, or feelings that arouse recollections of the traumatic event

9.   Persistent and effortful avoidance of activities, places, or physical reminders that arouse recollections of the traumatic event

Arousal symptoms

10.   Sleep disturbance (e.g., difficulty falling or staying asleep, or restless sleep)

11.   Hypervigilance

12.   Irritable or aggressive behavior

13.   Exaggerated startle response

14.   Agitation or restlessness

APPENDIX 15A.   DSM-5 proposed criteria for DSM-IV-TR 308.3 acute stress disorder *(continued)*

C. The disturbance causes clinically significant distress or impairment in social, occupational, or other important areas of functioning.

D. Duration of the disturbance (symptoms described in Criterion B) is 3 days to 1 month after the traumatic event.

E. The disturbance is not due to the direct physiological effects of a substance (e.g., medication, alcohol) or a general medical condition (e.g., traumatic brain injury, coma), and the symptoms are not restricted to those of brief psychotic disorder.

Changes from DSM-IV-TR criteria: rationale

A1. Criterion criticized about definition of traumatic event.
A2. Criterion has no utility.

B. Symptoms have been collapsed into a single cluster, which requires endorsement of 8 or more symptoms. Symptoms have now been specified rather than appearing as general cluster descriptions as in DSM-IV. The data suggest that acute posttraumatic reactions may be varied and do not necessarily include dissociative or other DSM-IV acute stress disorder symptom clusters.

B1. Slight change of wording.
B2. Delete; rewording in new B2 makes the criterion more applicable across cultures.
B3/
B4. Combine.
B5. Slight change of wording.

C. Now itemized as four distinct **reexperiencing** symptoms that use the same wording as PTSD: 4, 5, 6, 7.

D. Now itemized as two distinct **avoidance** symptoms: 8 and 9.

E. Now now itemized as five distinct **arousal** symptoms: 10, 11, 12, 13, 14.

F. Unchanged.

G. Altered from minimum of 2 days to 3 days to reduce false positives.

H. Unchanged.

---

*An alternative option is to not include topic headings in Criterion B. In addition, the work group is further considering the number of symptoms that are required.

Source. American Psychiatric Association DSM-5 Development: Proposed Revision: 308.3 Acute Stress Disorder. Updated August 20, 2010. Available at: http://www.dsm5.org/ProposedRevisions/Pages/proposedrevision.aspx?rid=166#. Accessed September 15, 2010.

Discussion of rationale: Bryant RA, Friedman MJ, Spiegel D, Ursano R, Strain J: "A Review of Acute Stress Disorder in DSM-5." *Depression and Anxiety,* November 3, 2010 [Epub ahead of print]; Hinton DE, Lewis-Fernandez R: "The Cross-Cultural Validity of Posttraumatic Stress Disorder: Implications for DSM-5." *Depression and Anxiety,* December 13, 2010 [Epub ahead of print].

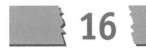

16

Psychopharmacology

Postacute Phase

Frederick J. Stoddard Jr., M.D.
Frank G. Dowling, M.D.

> *The foreign psychiatrists emphasize that they have found Haitians to be impressively resilient, but the disaster has nonetheless set off reactions ranging from anxiety through psychosis.... For those with a history of mental illness, the earthquake has been especially destabilizing. Many lost homes, caretakers and medication supplies, and the institutionalized were displaced too.... At the General Hospital, foreign psychiatrists say that they are seeing several new cases daily of psychosis, severe depression and other disorders.*
>
> *Sontag 2010*

Many psychiatrists and other physicians, often without disaster training, are consulted by survivors during the postacute phase of disaster. Like the psychiatrists mentioned in the quote above, who were treating victims of the Haiti earthquake more than 2 months after the disaster, psychiatrists working with survivors during the postacute phase have different considerations from those working with patients immediately following an incident.

Whereas the indications for psychopharmacotherapy are less clear in the acute phase (see Chapter 15 on acute phase psychopharmacology), they are clearer in the postacute phase, when DSM-IV-TR disorders (American Psychiatric Association 2000) become more the focus of clinical attention. A strong evidence base exists for use of medication as well as psychotherapy for patients with posttraumatic stress disorder (PTSD) and major depression (Rush and Nierenberg 2009). The evidence base is also strong for medication treatment for those survivors with psychoses (see Chapter 7, "Serious Mental Illness"), bipolar disorder (American Psychiatric Association 2002; Post and Altshuler 2009), substance abuse and withdrawal (American Psychiatric Association 2006), neuropsychiatric complications of medical-surgical conditions, and other disorders.

The postacute phase "spans from weeks to more likely months to years and refers to the period when a community may still suffer the longer-term effects of the catastrophe" (Berren et al. 1980; Disaster Psychiatry Outreach 2008). During this time, symptoms may resolve or syndromes may emerge. As people move into this phase, they become removed from the immediate threat or impact of the event, but its neurobiological impact may remain. They may have returned to family, school, work, and assisted living; reestablished housing; or become otherwise closer to "everyday life." This phase is remarkable for the clearer presence of psychiatric disorders and, for some individuals, a loss of or inability to function normally (Table 16–1). The triage approach of the acute phase transitions into short-term crisis interventions and then, during this postacute phase, into longer-term treatment. Some disaster survivors will require treatment for years (Terr 1979).

Unlike that in the acute phase, prescribing in the postacute phase is likely to be integrated into routine care, because practicing psychiatrists will normally see these patients near the survivors' homes and workplaces in clinics and private offices, in consultation with primary care physicians, and in hospital medical-surgical units. Patients may be seen for time-limited transitional periods before concluding acute treatment and being referred for longer-term care. Although a few psychiatrists, such as those working after the earthquake in Haiti, see patients near the site of the disaster, many others, after disasters such as 9/11, see patients far away from the site. This chapter provides an evidence base for integrating care for survivors of a disaster into psychiatrists' usual clinical practices.

In this chapter, we address the indications for use of anxiolytics, antidepressants, antipsychotics, α-adrenergic agonists and blockers, and mood stabilizers, and presume the availability of these resources for postacute pharmacological treatments. Pharmacotherapy recommendations must be adapted to the local realities of both the predisaster and postdisaster communities in which the disaster psychiatrist practices. Toward the end of the chapter is a special section on evaluation and treatment of traumatic brain injury.

TABLE 16–1.   Common postacute phase diagnoses and comorbidity

---

Common postacute diagnoses

PTSD

Major depressive disorder

Anxiety disorders other than PTSD (e.g., phobia, panic)

Substance abuse or withdrawal; drug-induced psychoses (see Chapter 8)

Personality disorders (see Chapter 9)

Child and adolescent disorders (see Chapter 17)

Also screen for

Prolonged grief

Psychotic disorders, including the following:

    Delirium or other cognitive disorders due to a medical condition

    Schizophrenia

    Bipolar disorder

Signs of impairment, especially functional disturbances (e.g., problems in acting on behalf of one's family or oneself following a disaster)}

Impairments in work and relationships; inability to care for self and family; inability to deal with benefit issues; inability to use supports such as family, friends, and social groups; marked anxiety and depression; psychosis; suicidal or homicidal ideations and behaviors

Inability to move on emotionally, preoccupation with event and its aftermath— with or without syndromal PTSD

Note.   PTSD = posttraumatic stress disorder.

Psychiatric Evaluation in the Postacute Phase

Whereas the focus in Chapter 5, "Psychiatric Assessment," is on evaluation of the acutely impacted survivor, the focus here is on postacute clinical evaluation of those exposed to disasters. In evaluating patients for continued or new treatment, it is important to differentiate psychiatric disorders from normal long-term responses by determining if patients meet the criteria for symptoms, severity, duration, and psychosocial impairment. Evaluation must address comorbid medical illnesses (Querques and Stern 2010), psychopharmacological interventions, longer-term care, and follow-up. Psychotherapeutic interventions are also likely to be indicated (see Chapter 14, "Psychotherapies"). In the postacute phase, psychiatrists should follow psychopharmacological treatment guidelines for specific disorders (American Psychiatric Association 1999, 2004; 2010).

Diagnostic Assessment

In the postacute phase, diagnostic assessment becomes more similar to that in traditional psychiatric care. Assessment is informed by the need to differentiate longer-term reactions from shorter-term ones, in a manner similar to evaluation of other patients with comorbid posttraumatic stress symptoms due to other types of traumatic stressors (Table 16–1). The following list includes recommendations particularly appropriate in the postacute phase.

- *History of present illness*—Elicit the narrative history of the patient's experience during and following the disaster. Obtain specific information about prior treatment, including medications prescribed during the acute phase. Evaluate the patient for safety, and consider the subjective experience of trauma as well as more objective evidence for the severity and nature of the trauma and/or injury, including experiences that are both related and unrelated to the disaster. Consider using an assessment tool for PTSD, such as the Clinician-Administered PTSD Scale (CAPS; Blake et al. 1990), Clinical Global Impressions—Improvement Scale (CGI-I; Guy 1956), Diagnostic Interview Schedule—PTSD module (DIS-PTSD; Robins et al. 1981), the PTSD module of the Structured Clinical Interview for DSM-IV (SCID-PTSD; First et al. 2002), Impact of Event Scale–Revised (IES; Weiss and Marmar 1997), or Davidson Trauma Scale (Davidson 1996).
- *Resilience*—Include an assessment of resilience when conducting a standard psychiatric interview, evaluating the patient's subjective experience of trauma as well as more objective evidence for the severity and nature of the trauma. As explained in Chapter 11, "Grief and Resilience," resilience may be assessed clinically as either the presence of positive traits, such as courage or humor, or the absence of pathological symptoms.
- *Key risk factors*—Review key risk factors as described in Chapter 5, "Psychiatric Evaluation." The neurobiology of risk factors is slowly being dissected, and may explain the degree of effectiveness and the importance of some drug treatments. Although the clinical relevance of genetic risk factors remains to be determined, studies of these factors include findings that risk of PTSD after trauma depends on traumatic load after disaster and the valine allele Val(158)Met COMT polymorphism (Kolassa et al. 2010). Caspi et al. (2003) showed that individuals who were homozygous for the short allele of 5-HTTLPR, the promoter region of the serotonin transporter gene, were more likely to respond to stress by becoming depressed and suicidal. A Finnish study found that stressful life events were linked to depression only in those who had the A2/A2 genotype of the dopamine receptor gene *DRD2* (Dimsdale et al. 2009).

- *Past medical and psychiatric history*—Screen for past medical and psychiatric history, "dose" of trauma exposure from the disaster and other causes, problems of living prior to the disaster, and availability of psychosocial supports. Where possible, obtain history from the medical team, family, and friends regarding the patient's prior and current traumas experienced. Multiple traumas add to risk for and increased severity of PTSD (see also Chapter 17, "Child and Adolescent Psychiatry Interventions").

- *History of substance use*—Screen for alcohol and drug use (see Chapter 8, "Substance Abuse"). Disaster exposure is linked to relapse of those with prior histories of abuse or dependence, and it is also associated with an overall increase in the use of addictive substances.

- *Subsyndromal symptoms*—Take into account normal themes and reactions, such as tormenting memories; fears of recurrence; questions such as "Were we really so lucky after all?"; survivor guilt; the rise and fall of "postdisaster utopias" (with idealization of the acute phase as a heroic period or a period with no conflicts); and intensification of the search for spiritual and other kinds of meaning in the face of overwhelming events (Disaster Psychiatry Outreach 2008). As in the acute phase, distress and symptoms, such as "partial" PTSD (Mylle and Maes 2004), that fall just short of full diagnostic criteria are important and deserve recognition, intervention, and treatment. Both disorders that meet full symptom criteria and subsyndromal symptoms (e.g., of PTSD or major depression) that are causing functional impairment should be treated in this phase, with the goal of remission of symptoms.

  Distress is ubiquitous in the postdisaster period, especially with the most severe events or intense exposure. In a study by North et al. (1999), 81% of directly exposed bombing survivors described themselves as "very upset," and 96% acknowledged at least one PTSD symptom. Although such findings might seem to suggest that almost everyone requires medication, this is not true. Many distressed people are resilient and therefore do not require treatment, and many others respond to psychotherapy alone (see Chapter 5, "Psychiatric Evaluation"; Chapter 11, "Grief and Resilience"; and Chapter 14, "Psychotherapies"). As a result, medications are appropriate only for a subpopulation of those impacted by a disaster.

Mental Status Examination

As in routine practice, the mental status examination provides the basis for determining target symptoms for pharmacotherapeutics. Withdrawn or impulsive behavior, depressed or manic mood, and cognition disturbed by amnesia or dissociation are among the symptoms that may be targets for monitoring effectiveness of drug treatment over time.

Physical Examination

The psychiatrist should consider the patient's neat or disordered appearance; the presence of a head injury or other injury; abnormal vital signs, especially elevated pulse rate (Zatzick et al. 2005); and abnormalities on neurological or cardiopulmonary examination. These observations or findings may suggest possible external (e.g., trauma, toxins) or internal (fight-or-flight response) responses to a disaster, which may affect the safe use or selection of drug classes. For instance, agents that may cause hypotension are inappropriate for someone with unstable vital signs.

Psychological Testing

Psychological or neuropsychological assessments should be done during the postacute phase to formally delineate abnormalities of executive function, attention, mood, intelligence, learning, memory, and other mental faculties. This type of assessment may be important both diagnostically and therapeutically following both natural and human-caused disasters, such as those due to an explosive, chemical, biological, or radiological event that may result in traumatic brain injury or subtle neuropsychological impairment (see section on traumatic brain injury later in this chapter). Testing may provide a comprehensive baseline for progress in recovery and for monitoring treatment progress with follow-up assessments (Blais et al. 2010).

Laboratory and Radiological Studies

During the postacute examination, laboratory tests should be performed to determine baseline liver function, thyroid-stimulating hormone, and thyroxine. Additionally, a delirium workup and electroencephalography (EEG) are important.

Where indicated, radiological studies should be conducted to detect possible injury or disease causing mental status change. Access to these studies may be limited due to the disaster, but much less so than during the acute phase.

Posttraumatic Stress Disorder

In light of the stronger evidence for short-term treatment, the decision of when to consider medication tapers may be partially informed by the expected course of PTSD (see Figure 16–1) and by any comorbidities. Research conducted 5–8 weeks after 9/11 showed a very high prevalence of PTSD after the attacks, with a 7.5% rate of PTSD among 1,008 adults liv-

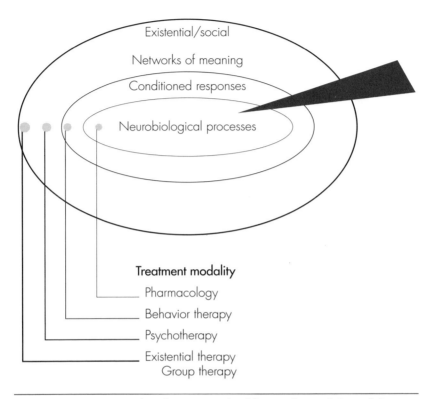

FIGURE 16–1. Levels of trauma: the biopsychosocial model.

Source. Shalev AY, Galai T, Eth S: "Levels of Trauma: A Multidimensional Approach to the Treatment of PTSD." *Psychiatry* 6:166–177, 1993.

ing south of 110th Street. Those at highest risk were those with the most severe exposure or personal loss (Galea et al. 2002). In a longitudinal study of 211 trauma survivors, Shalev et al. (1998) reported that at 4 months, 14.2% of subjects had major depression and 17.5% had PTSD (of whom 43.2% had comorbid major depression). In a study following 182 directly exposed survivors of the Oklahoma City bombing at 6 months and 1 year later, North et al. (1999) found that those at highest risk were those with the most severe and persistent avoidance symptoms. These and other studies provide insights and possible direction for assessment and management of PTSD and other psychiatric disorders (Benedek and Wynn 2009).

Overall, studies of PTSD suggest that PTSD starts quickly after traumatic events, tends to be chronic, and does not appear to be delayed in onset, and that Group C criteria of PTSD ("Persistent avoidance of stimuli associated with the trauma and numbing of general responsiveness") are of importance as markers or identifiers of PTSD meeting all criteria (listed in

---

TABLE 16–2.   DSM-IV-TR criteria for posttraumatic stress disorder

---

A.   The person has been exposed to a traumatic event in which both of the following were present:

  (1)   the person experienced, witnessed, or was confronted with an event or events that involved actual or threatened death or serious injury, or a threat to the physical integrity of self or others

  (2)   the person's response involved intense fear, helplessness, or horror. **Note:** In children, this may be expressed instead by disorganized or agitated behavior

B.   The traumatic event is persistently reexperienced in one (or more) of the following ways:

  (1)   recurrent and intrusive distressing recollections of the event, including images, thoughts, or perceptions.   **Note:** In young children, repetitive play may occur in which themes or aspects of the trauma are expressed.

  (2)   recurrent distressing dreams of the event.   **Note:** In children, there may be frightening dreams without recognizable content.

  (3)   acting or feeling as if the traumatic event were recurring (includes a sense of reliving the experience, illusions, hallucinations, and dissociative flashback episodes, including those that occur on awakening or when intoxicated).   **Note:** In young children, trauma-specific reenactment may occur.

  (4)   intense psychological distress at exposure to internal or external cues that symbolize or resemble an aspect of the traumatic event

  (5)   physiological reactivity on exposure to internal or external cues that symbolize or resemble an aspect of the traumatic event

C.   Persistent avoidance of stimuli associated with the trauma and numbing of general responsiveness (not present before the trauma), as indicated by three (or more) of the following:

  (1)   efforts to avoid thoughts, feelings, or conversations associated with the trauma

  (2)   efforts to avoid activities, places, or people that arouse recollections of the trauma

  (3)   inability to recall an important aspect of the trauma

  (4)   markedly diminished interest or participation in significant activities

  (5)   feeling of detachment or estrangement from others

  (6)   restricted range of affect (e.g., unable to have loving feelings)

  (7)   sense of a foreshortened future (e.g., does not expect to have a career, marriage, children, or a normal life span)

D.   Persistent symptoms of increased arousal (not present before the trauma), as indicated by two (or more) of the following:

  (1)   difficulty falling or staying asleep

  (2)   irritability or outbursts of anger

  (3)   difficulty concentrating

TABLE 16–2. DSM-IV-TR criteria for posttraumatic stress disorder *(continued)*

---

(4) hypervigilance

(5) exaggerated startle response

E. Duration of the disturbance (symptoms in Criteria B, C, and D) is more than 1 month.

F. The disturbance causes clinically significant distress or impairment in social, occupational, or other important areas of functioning.

Specify if:

Acute: if duration of symptoms is less than 3 months

Chronic: if duration of symptoms is 3 months or more

Specify if:

With Delayed Onset: if onset of symptoms is at least 6 months after the stressor

---

Source. Reprinted from the *Diagnostic and Statistical Manual of Mental Disorders,* 4th Edition, Text Revision. Washington, DC, American Psychiatric Association, 2000, pp. 467–468. Copyright © 2000, American Psychiatric Association. Used with permission.

Table 16–2), as distinct from normal reactions that include some symptoms but do not meet full criteria. North et al. (1999) found that improvement in Group C criteria parallels recovery from PTSD, and that in the absence of Group C criteria, Group B symptoms of PTSD ("The traumatic event is persistently reexperienced") and Group D criteria ("Persistent symptoms of increased arousal") are common, nonpathological responses. Not all researchers or clinicians agree with this, especially for children and adolescents. The North et al. (1999) study suggested that PTSD screening, diagnosis, and treatment should be of primary importance in response to populations affected by a disaster.

Postdisaster comorbidity with PTSD is also typical and important (see Table 16–1, earlier in chapter). In the North et al. (1999) study, rates of comorbidity with PTSD were as follows: major depression 55%, personality disorders 33%, panic or generalized anxiety disorder 29%, and alcohol abuse/ dependence 13%. The North et al. study implied a high rate of recurrence of preexisting major depressive disorder and exacerbation of preexisting drug and alcohol disorders (see also Chapter 8, "Substance Abuse"). In some studies, prevalence rates of depression were similar to those of PTSD (Breslau et al. 2000), highlighting the need to monitor for depressive symptoms as well as PTSD (Green et al. 1990). It is also important to screen for psychotic disorders such as bipolar disorder and schizophrenia (see Chapter 7, "Serious Mental Illness").

The fact that PTSD onset is noted to be early, and generally not late, is helpful both for making the diagnosis and for planning long-term treatment. Although the best epidemiological studies on PTSD either provide a snapshot in time or follow the course of the illness without controlling for medication management, these studies cannot provide definitive guidance for medication management. However, the rates of PTSD and rates of comorbidity can provide some guidance for when to expect the need for medication. It is clear that both medication and psychotherapy (see Chapter 14, "Psychotherapies") have a place in the treatment of PTSD (Cukor et al. 2009).

Expert panels have done meta-analyses of randomized controlled psychopharmacological studies of PTSD; on balance, the effectiveness of medication is modestly supported, although not by all panels and not for every patient. Stein et al. (2006), in their Cochrane review, determined that "although [PTSD is] traditionally treated with psychotherapy," there are both empirical and theoretical bases for medication management. In their review of 35 short-term randomized controlled trials to treat PTSD with medications, they were able to conduct a meta-analysis using 13 of these trials (with 1,272 participants) and concluded that "a significantly larger proportion of patients responded to medication (59.1%) than to placebo (38.5%)." A total of 17 trials involving 2,507 participants showed significant symptom reduction. Although different medications have been studied, the selective serotonin reuptake inhibitors (SSRIs) had greatest evidence for efficacy. The authors noted that medication also reduced comorbid depression and disability. As would be expected, active medication was less well tolerated than placebo. Their review of three maintenance trials supported long-term medication use, although meta-analytic techniques were not used to provide quantifiable levels of support for this conclusion. They concluded, "Medication treatments can be effective in treating PTSD, acting to reduce its core symptoms, as well as associated depression and disability. The findings of this review support the status of SSRIs as first-line agents in the pharmacotherapy of PTSD, as well as their value in long-term treatment. However, there remain important gaps in the evidence base, and a continued need for more effective agents in the management of PTSD" (Stein et al. 2006, abstract). An earlier review, by Stoddard (2000), yielded findings similar to those of Stein et al. (2006).

The Institute of Medicine (2007) found more limitations in a review of 37 randomized controlled trials of SSRIs (e.g., sertraline, fluoxetine, paroxetine, citalopram) in the treatment of PTSD. Seven of the 14 studies reviewed were weakly informative due to limitations such as "high or differential dropout rates across conditions and subpar handling of missing data." Of those seven studies, four were positive, three negative. The reviewers did not find adequate evidence to ascertain the efficacy of α-adrenergic blockers (e.g., prazosin; see Chapter 15 on psychopharmacology in the acute phase), anticonvulsants, atypical antipsychotics (e.g., olanzapine, risperidone), benzodiazepines, or monoamine oxidase inhibitors in PTSD.

Major Depressive Disorder

Some studies have found that major depressive disorder is almost as prevalent as PTSD after a disaster (Green et al. 1990) and is often comorbid with PTSD (North et al. 1999). Genetic risk factors, as discussed above in "Psychiatric Evaluation," help explain how genes appear to mediate the vulnerability to stress and increase the risk of depression after disasters. Table 16–3 presents the DSM-IV-TR criteria for major depressive episode.

Treatment in the Postacute Phase

The evaluation, including the overall diagnostic assessment in the postacute phase of presence or absence of the disorders described above as well as others, results in treatment goals (see Table 16–4) aiming to alleviate the core symptoms of the postacute phase disorders, lower risks, enhance resilience, improve the quality of life, decrease comorbidity, and reduce postdisaster disability. The biopsychosocial treatment plan is designed to meet those goals. The plan should include psychotherapeutic and psychosocial interventions described in prior chapters. For individuals with severe and persistent symptoms in the postacute phase, a pharmacotherapeutic treatment plan may be indicated as one core element of the overall treatment plan. Here we address pharmacotherapeutics for adult disaster survivors in the postacute phase. For pharmacotherapeutic recommendations for serious mental illness, substance abuse, children and adolescents, and the elderly, readers are referred to Chapters 7, 8, 17, and 18, respectively.

Pharmacotherapeutics

Pharmacological treatments that may be commonly used for the range of psychopathology after a disaster include anxiolytics, antidepressants, antipsychotics, α-adrenergic agonists, and mood stabilizers. Psychoeducation regarding the risks, side effects, benefits, and expected course of treatment for medications is an important part of the intervention and medicolegally necessary. The risk of contributing to addiction must be considered in prescribing after disasters, and practice should be adjusted to minimize that risk. The important components of a psychopharmacological treatment plan are described in Table 16–5.

It is helpful to consider two general categories of patients: 1) those with predisaster psychopathology requiring treatment for maintenance of eu-

TABLE 16–3.   DSM-IV-TR criteria for major depressive episode

A. Five (or more) of the following symptoms have been present during the same 2-week period and represent a change from previous functioning; at least one of the symptoms is either (1) depressed mood or (2) loss of interest or pleasure.

   Note: Do not include symptoms that are clearly due to a general medical condition, or mood-incongruent delusions or hallucinations.

   (1)   depressed mood most of the day, nearly every day, as indicated by either subjective report (e.g., feels sad or empty) or observation made by others (e.g., appears tearful).   **Note:** In children and adolescents, can be irritable mood.

   (2)   markedly diminished interest or pleasure in all, or almost all, activities most of the day, nearly every day (as indicated by either subjective account or observation made by others)

   (3)   significant weight loss when not dieting or weight gain (e.g., a change of more than 5% of body weight in a month), or decrease or increase in appetite nearly every day.   **Note:** In children, consider failure to make expected weight gains.

   (4)   insomnia or hypersomnia nearly every day

   (5)   psychomotor agitation or retardation nearly every day (observable by others, not merely subjective feelings of restlessness or being slowed down)

   (6)   fatigue or loss of energy nearly every day

   (7)   feelings of worthlessness or excessive or inappropriate guilt (which may be delusional) nearly every day (not merely self-reproach or guilt about being sick)

   (8)   diminished ability to think or concentrate, or indecisiveness, nearly every day (either by subjective account or as observed by others)

   (9)   recurrent thoughts of death (not just fear of dying), recurrent suicidal ideation without a specific plan, or a suicide attempt or a specific plan for committing suicide

B. The symptoms do not meet criteria for a mixed episode (see p. 365 in DSM-IV-TR).

C. The symptoms cause clinically significant distress or impairment in social, occupational, or other important areas of functioning.

D. The symptoms are not due to the direct physiological effects of a substance (e.g., a drug of abuse, a medication) or a general medical condition (e.g., hypothyroidism).

E. The symptoms are not better accounted for by bereavement, i.e., after the loss of a loved one, the symptoms persist for longer than 2 months or are characterized by marked functional impairment, morbid preoccupation with worthlessness, suicidal ideation, psychotic symptoms, or psychomotor retardation.

TABLE 16–4. Treatment goals in the postacute phase

Reduce the core symptoms of postacute phase disorders

Reduce risk of substance abuse, violence, suicide

Improve resilience

Improve quality of life

Reduce disability postdisaster

Reduce comorbidity

TABLE 16–5. Psychopharmacological treatment plan in the postacute phase

1. Obtain patient consent to treatment; request that patient contact clinician by phone to discuss medication benefits or problems between appointments

   - Identify target symptoms

   - Communicate positive expectation of response to treatment

2. Select primary medication and prescribe dosage regimen; select secondary medication(s) for comorbid conditions and prescribe dosage regimen

3. Evaluate response to treatment over time, with ratings of identified target symptoms, and monitor for adverse side effects and toxic effects

4. Adjust medication by dose or agent used, as indicated by response to treatment

---

thymia/control of symptoms or initiation of a new regimen, and 2) those without prior psychopathology who manifest symptoms of acute stress and require treatment for PTSD (Table 16–6), depression, or other disorders triggered or kindled by stress. This distinction between these two types of patients influences choice of medications. Survivors with both preexisting psychopathology and additional posttraumatic responses likely require re-institution of their prior drug treatment and possible additional medication, such as antianxiety agents (Table 16–7) or antidepressants (Table 16–8), for the posttraumatic effects of the disaster. In contrast, those with new disorders, such as PTSD or depression, require a trial of most likely only one or two medications for their condition and evaluation of treatment response.

Antidepressants are the standard psychopharmacological treatments for major depressive disorder. The evidence from a meta-analysis of randomized trials from 1980 to 2009 supports improved outcomes following treatment of patients meeting the severity criteria for the symptoms of major depressive disorder. According to Fournier et al. (2010), however, the benefits for patients with mild or moderate depressive symptoms may be minimal or nonexistent.

TABLE 16–6.   Pharmacotherapy for PTSD and comorbid conditions

For treatment of PTSD, emphasize the importance of consistent use of medication, and, with SSRIs, stress the idea of extended treatment to allow both for resolution of the syndrome and prophylaxis of relapse (might require 6–12 months or more of treatment, often 2+ years).

Classes of medication that might be considered for treatment of PTSD (and other comorbid conditions) include the full range of psychopharmacological treatments and should be targeted to diagnoses and/or symptoms as in any treatment:

Short-term low-dose sedatives (e.g., zolpidem, zaleplon, diphenhydramine, trazodone, mirtazapine) are useful for significant sleep symptoms.

Benzodiazepines (e.g., lorazepam, clonazepam, diazepam) are very useful but can cause dependence. The risk is higher with the shorter-acting benzodiazepines (e.g., alprazolam, which is also associated with greater risk of abuse and of rebound withdrawal symptoms), and with people who have a history of substance abuse or severe personality disorder (Kosten et al. 2000).

Note.   PTSD = posttraumatic stress disorder; SSRI = selective serotonin reuptake inhibitor.

TABLE 16–7.   Pharmacotherapy for anxiety

Benzodiazepines

β-adrenergic blockers (e.g., propranolol) (Pitman and Delahanty 2005)

α-adrenergic blockers (e.g., prazosin)

α-adrenergic agonists (e.g., clonidine, guanfacine)

Buspirone

Low-dose neuroleptics (e.g., haloperidol)

Gabapentin

Table 16–9 lists additional medications that may be useful in the treatment of postdisaster pathology. Although opiates are not a part of the standard treatment algorithm for any psychiatric diagnosis, this class of medication is helpful in postdisaster pharmacotherapy for patients whose pain from injury is worsening their psychiatric symptoms. In addition, some evidence suggests that opiates may reduce subsequent PTSD symptoms (Bryant et al. 2009; Stoddard et al., in press; also see Chapter 15 on psychopharmacology in the acute phase).

Psychopharmacological and psychotherapeutic treatments of PTSD and other syndromes require ongoing assessment. Discontinuation of medication is an important consideration. From the initial treatment agreement in the postdisaster phase, this topic should be discussed, including the risk of possibly relapsing or developing chronicity of the disorder. Side effects or

TABLE 16–8. Pharmacotherapy for depression

Selective serotonin reuptake inhibitors (SSRIs)—e.g., sertraline (FDA approved for treatment of PTSD), paroxetine (FDA approved for treatment of PTSD), citalopram, escitalopram, fluoxetine, fluvoxamine

Serotonin-norepinephrine reuptake inhibitors (SNRIs—e.g., venlafaxine, duloxetine

Antidepressants with alternative mechanisms of action—e.g., bupropion, mirtazapine, cyproheptadine, tricyclic antidepressants (TCAs), monoamine oxidase inhibitors (MAOIs)

Note. FDA=U.S. Food and Drug Administration; PTSD=posttraumatic stress disorder.

TABLE 16–9. Additional medications that may usefully augment treatment of postdisaster pathology

Mood stabilizers and anticonvulsants (e.g., lithium, divalproex, carbamazepine, lamotrigine, atypical antipsychotic medications)

Antipsychotic agents (e.g., risperidone, olanzapine, quetiapine, aripiprazole, ziprasidone, haloperidol, phenothiazines)

- "Typical" antipsychotics (e.g., haloperidol, phenothiazines) have adverse side effect of slowing of motor movements, and hence are called "neuroleptics."
- "Atypical" antipsychotics (e.g., risperidone, olanzapine, quetiapine, aripiprazole, ziprasidone) have less propensity to cause extrapyramidal side effects and tend to improve negative symptoms.

Noradrenergic agents (e.g., clonidine, propranolol, guanfacine)

Opiates: Evidence suggests that morphine may reduce subsequent posttraumatic stress disorder symptoms in children and adults requiring medical-surgical care for injuries (e.g., burns and other injuries) (Holbrook et al. 2010; Saxe et al. 2001; Stoddard and Saxe 2001; Stoddard et al. 2009).

D-cyloserine as an enhancement to prolonged exposure therapy (Cukor et al. 2009; Otto et al. 2010)

toxic effects of medications may increase impairment, such as with tardive dyskinesia, or be life threatening, such as with serotonin syndrome or a bipolar "switch," and therefore the patient should be monitored weekly or more often during and for several weeks following medication increases and decreases. Because follow-up may be especially challenging in a fluid postdisaster environment, the range of pharmacological options may be limited.

As treatment progresses through the postacute phase, those individuals who have developed—or have experienced relapses of—serious and persistent mental disorders such as bipolar illness, schizophrenia, chronic PTSD, or alcohol abuse (Zatzick et al. 2004a, 2004b) in the setting of the disaster experience will become distinct from those who are transiently symptomatic or whose symptoms have resolved. The patient's safety is the preeminent concern. When indicated, a patient should be immediately reevaluated and hospitalized if necessary. Appropriate referral to continuing outpatient treatment will be the next step in intervention. As in the disaster response phase, self-referral to one's own practice is usually not appropriate for psychiatrists who are certified disaster responders or volunteers. In addition, to preserve boundaries between professional and personal roles, referrals should be made as much as possible from the site at which treatment is being provided rather than through off-site contacts or phone conversations. Many states will have telephone help lines that may provide assistance with referrals. After a disaster, local district branches of the American Psychiatric Association may also generate referral protocols for their area.

Follow-up Plan

Unless a community had a significant lack of predisaster health care resources or has been unable to sufficiently reinstitute these services as it recovers, planning for follow-up care in the postacute phase is no different from that in routine nondisaster settings. Resourcefulness and creativity are demanded in cases where resources are limited, although it is unfortunate that guidance is scant for psychiatrists managing under conditions of scarcity. The psychiatrist who turns to the oft-cited book *Where There Is No Doctor: A Village Health Care Handbook* (Werner et al. 2009) will find no mention of mental health conditions but will at least find a model for the attitude and ways of making do with little. Therefore, the usual skills of the typical practitioner together with his or her less typically tapped flexibility are of great benefit to the disaster survivor during this postacute phase.

The disaster survivor's original treatment agreement should ideally include the plan for follow-up visits. The following topics should be covered in the agreement:

- Continuation of treatment if the patient has a positive response (lessening of target symptoms) without undue side effects. Psychiatrists may be tempted not to follow this commonsense approach due to the pressure to solve the problem quickly and therefore not try a treatment for enough time before switching.
- Compliance: Failure to take medication as prescribed is a very common reason that medications do not work.
- Consideration of alternative treatment options if symptoms do not improve or worsen, or if side effects or toxic effects, complications, noncompliance, or other treatment problems emerge.

Special Considerations for Assessment and Treatment of Traumatic Brain Injury

The psychiatrist responding to disaster should keep in mind the risk of traumatic brain injury (TBI), defined by the U.S. Department of Veterans Affairs/Department of Defense (2009) in their practice guideline for management of concussion and mild TBI as "a traumatically induced structural injury and/or physiological disruption of brain function as the result of an external force" that results in at least one of the following immediately after the event: loss of or a decreased level of consciousness; memory loss for events immediately before or after the injury (posttraumatic amnesia); alteration of consciousness at the time of the injury (e.g., confusion, disorientation, slowed thinking); neurological deficits (e.g., weakness, loss of balance, change in vision, praxis, paresis/plegia, sensory loss, aphasia) that may or may not be transient; or intracranial lesion.

In the general population, the most common causes of TBI are motor vehicle accidents, falls, and violence (Rao and Lyketsos 2000). Natural disasters such as earthquakes, hurricanes, tsunamis, and floods can cause TBI, or acts of terrorism and warfare can result in TBI from blast-induced injuries. Whereas moderate and severe TBI are associated with clear neurological signs that facilitate making the diagnosis, mild TBI is more common, difficult to diagnose, and results in long-term neuropsychiatric sequelae in about 10%–15% of cases. Because moderate or severe TBI usually results in more obvious neurological sequelae, this discussion will focus on mild TBI. In mild TBI or concussion, there may be brief or even no loss of consciousness. Common symptoms experienced immediately after the injury include feeling dazed or confused; "seeing stars"; and not remembering the event/injury. Three categories of common symptoms observed later on, which may last briefly or for several days, might include

- *Physical*—headache, nausea, vomiting, dizziness, fatigue, blurry vision, sleep disturbance, sensitivity to light or noise, balance problems, transient neurological abnormalities
- *Cognitive*—attention, concentration, memory, speed of processing, judgment, executive function
- *Behavioral/emotional*—depression, anxiety, agitation, irritability, impulsivity, aggression

Confusion or altered level of consciousness at the time of the injury can be difficult to differentiate from the intense fear, helplessness, confusion, or dissociative symptoms that can be experienced as an immediate psychological reaction to the event itself. In addition, many signs of TBI overlap symptoms seen in common postdisaster stress or psychiatric difficulties such as PTSD, depression, panic disorder, or generalized anxiety disorder. In most instances, neurological examination and neuroimaging may yield nonspecific or no findings and are not helpful in making the diagnosis (Rogers and Read 2007). Neuropsychological testing is a luxury in normal circumstances and will likely be unavailable in the postdisaster setting. Persistent symptoms such as headaches, dizziness, light and sound sensitivity, and memory deficits that do not seem to correlate with PTSD or mood symptoms may raise the suspicion of persistent sequelae of TBI. In addition, confusion or forgetfulness during routine tasks or activities that are not usually anxiety producing may raise suspicion of TBI. Symptoms are compared against an individual's norm or baseline, as best as that can be determined. Observations of family or friends may be helpful.

In treating patients with known or suspected TBI, the following general principles (U.S. Department of Veterans Affairs/Department of Defense 2009) are useful:

- Avoid medications that may lower the seizure threshold (e.g., bupropion).
- The rule of thumb is "start low, go slow," because a patient with TBI may respond to—or experience more side effects at—lower doses of medications.
- Because the full range of doses of psychiatric medications may be needed to achieve a therapeutic response, avoid the mistake of underdosing if medication is well tolerated.
- Consider giving limited supplies of medication for a patient who is impulsive or a significant suicide risk.
- Advise patients to minimize the use of caffeine, herbals, supplements, and energy products that can cause or worsen agitation or irritability.
- When possible, avoid or use with caution medications that can cause confusion, cognitive slowness, fatigue, or drowsiness (e.g., benzodiazepines, anticholinergics, lithium).

Controlled data on the efficacy of psychiatric medications in TBI are lacking. The Department of Defense and Department of Veterans Affairs (2009) have perhaps the most experience in treating patients with TBI and psychiatric difficulties. Their clinical guideline recommends consideration of the following:

- *For concentration or memory difficulties*—an SSRI or cautious use of a stimulant.
- *For anxiety*—short-term (cautious) use of an anxiolytic or an SSRI.

- *For depression*—an SSRI.
- *For irritability, mood lability, or poor frustration tolerance*—an anticonvulsant or an SSRI.
- *For insomnia*—cautious use of a nonbenzodiazepine hypnotic such as zolpidem or zaleplon.
- *For nightmares, violent outbursts, or agitation during sleep*—prazosin.

Conclusion

Psychopharmacological treatment in the postacute phase poses many challenges. Many psychiatrists and other physicians without disaster training are consulted by survivors months later and far from the disaster site. Consequently, considerations differ from those in the acute phase. Clinical evaluation and biopsychosocial treatment planning in the postacute phase are more similar to those in conventional psychiatric care. Diagnostic assessment is more likely to result in recognition of a major psychiatric disorder such as PTSD, major depression, panic disorder, substance abuse, or TBI, although normal responses, especially bereavement, are common. The evaluation results in treatment goals to reduce symptoms, reduce risks, improve resilience, improve the quality of life, and reduce disability. The treatment plan to meet these goals may include psychotherapy and psychosocial interventions together with medication if indicated. The psychopharmacological treatment plan for the postacute phase includes obtaining informed consent, identifying target symptoms, selecting medications and prescribing them, monitoring the patient's response and adjusting medications as needed, initiating ongoing reassessment, and scheduling planned follow-ups. Among the candidate medications are anxiolytics, antidepressants, sedatives, mood stabilizers, antipsychotics, prazosin, and D-cyloserine. If symptoms do not improve, alternative treatment options should be considered. If symptoms do improve, treatment should be maintained to ensure long-term remission.

▨ Teaching Points

- Psychiatric disorders diagnosed in the postacute phase are potentially disabling conditions requiring prompt treatment, but only rarely with medication alone.
- Psychoeducation regarding the risks, side effects, benefits, and expected course of medication treatment is an important part of the intervention and medicolegally necessary.
- The patient's safety is paramount. When indicated, patients should be immediately reevaluated and hospitalized if necessary.

- Comorbidity is common during the postdisaster phase, especially involving PTSD, affective disorders, and substance use disorders.
- The SSRIs are effective for treating PTSD and major depression.
- Other agents that show promise for alleviating suffering after disasters include analgesics, mood stabilizers (anticonvulsants), other antidepressants, and sedatives.
- The risk of contributing to addiction must be considered when prescribing medications after disasters, and practice must be adjusted to minimize that risk.
- Multimodal treatment should be provided for each diagnosed disorder.
- Failure to take medication as prescribed is a common reason that medications do not work.
- From the time of the initial treatment agreement in the postdisaster phase, discontinuation of medication should be discussed, including the risk of possibly relapsing or developing chronicity of the disorder.

Review Questions

16.1 Among disaster survivors, which of the following groups are likely to be at the highest risk for developing chronic PTSD?

    A. Those with no acute stress disorder.
    B. Those meeting full PTSD diagnostic criteria, including Group C symptoms.
    C. Those with prior history of psychological trauma.
    D. A, B, and C.
    E. B and C only.

16.2 The evidence base for medication treatment of PTSD is strongest for which of the following?

    A. Atypical antipsychotics.
    B. SSRIs.
    C. Mood stabilizers.
    D. Benzodiazepines.
    E. Prazosin.

16.3 The psychiatric disorders most commonly seen during the postacute phase are

A. PTSD and dementia.
B. Delirium, PTSD, and dysthymic disorder.
C. Panic disorder, substance abuse, and bipolar disorder.
D. PTSD, major depression, panic disorder, and substance abuse.
E. PTSD, personality disorders, and overanxious disorder.

16.4 Patients with depression who are most likely to respond to antidepressant treatment are those with

A. All symptoms and criteria required for the diagnosis of major depressive disorder.
B. Injuries.
C. Mild or moderate depressive symptoms.
D. Resilience.
E. The ability to return to school or work.

16.5 Before prescribing medication for a survivor during the postacute phase, which of the following should be obtained?

A. History of prior disaster experience.
B. Chief complaint, family history, and work history.
C. Referral information, history of present illness, mental status examination, and physical examination.
D. Referral information, prior response to treatment, and magnetic resonance imaging (MRI) findings.
E. Screening tests for PTSD, electrocardiogram, and laboratory tests, including liver function and electrolytes.

References

American Psychiatric Association: Practice Guideline for the Treatment of Patients With Delirium. Washington, DC, American Psychiatric Association, May 1999 with August 2004 update (revision pending). Available at: http://www.psychiatryonline.com/pracGuide/pracGuideChapToc_2.aspx. Accessed January 2011.

American Psychiatric Association: Diagnostic and Statistical Manual of Mental Disorders, 4th Edition, Text Revision. Washington, DC, American Psychiatric Association, 2000

American Psychiatric Association: Practice Guideline for the Treatment of Patients With Bipolar Disorder, 2nd Edition. Washington, DC, American Psychiatric Association, April 2002 with November 2005 update (revision pending). Available at: http://www.psychiatryonline.com/pracGuide/pracGuideChapToc_8.aspx. Accessed January 2011.

American Psychiatric Association: Practice Guideline for the Treatment of Patients With Acute Stress Disorder and Posttraumatic Stress Disorder. Washington, DC, American Psychiatric Association, November 2004 with March 2009 update (revision pending). Available at: http://www.psychiatryonline.com/pracGuide/pracGuideTopic_11.aspx. Accessed January 2011.

American Psychiatric Association: Practice Guideline for the Treatment of Patients With Substance Use Disorders, 2nd Edition. Washington, DC, American Psychiatric Association, May 2006 with April 2007 update (revision pending). Available at: http://www.psychiatryonline.com/pracGuide/pracGuideChapToc_5.aspx. Accessed January 2011.

American Psychiatric Association: Practice Guideline for the Treatment of Patients With Major Depressive Disorder, 3rd Edition. Washington, DC, American Psychiatric Association, 2010. Available at: http://www.psychiatryonline.com/pracGuide/pracGuideTopic_7.aspx. Accessed January 2011.

Benedek DM, Wynn GH: Clinical Manual for Management of PTSD. Washington, DC, American Psychiatric Publishing, 2009

Berren MR, Beigel A, Ghertner S: A typology for the classification of disasters. Community Ment Health J 16:103–111, 1980

Blais MA, O'Keefe SM, Norman DK: Psychological and neuropsychological assessment, in Massachusetts General Hospital Handbook of General Hospital Psychiatry, 6th Edition. Edited by Stern TA, Fricchione GL, Cassem NH, et al. Philadelphia, PA, Saunders Elsevier, 2010, pp 53–60

Blake DD, Weathers FW, Nagy LN, et al: A clinician rating scale for assessing current and lifetime PTSD: the CAPS-1. Behavior Therapist 18:187–188, 1990

Breslau N, Davis GC, Peterson EL, et al: A second look at comorbidity in victims of trauma: the posttraumatic stress disorder-major depression connection. Biol Psychiatry 48:902–909, 2000

Bryant RA, Creamer M, O'Donnell, et al: A study of the protective function of acute morphine administration on subsequent posttraumatic stress disorder. Biol Psychiatry 65:438–440, 2009

Caspi A, Sugden K, Moffitt TE, et al: Influence of life stress on depression: moderation by a polymorphism in the 5-HTT gene. Science 301:386–389, 2003

Cukor J, Spitalnick J, DiFede J, et al: Emerging treatments for PTSD. Clin Psychol Rev 29:715–726, 2009

Davidson JRT: Davidson Trauma Scale (DTS). North Tonawanda, NY, Multi-Health Systems, 1996

Davidson JRT, Stein DJ, Shalev AY, et al: Posttraumatic stress disorder: acquisition, recognition, course, treatment. J Neuropsychiatry Clin Neurosci 16:135–147, 2004

Dimsdale JE, Irwin MR, Keefe FJ, et al: Stress and psychiatry, in Comprehensive Textbook of Psychiatry. Edited by Sadock BJ, Sadock VA, Ruiz P. Philadelphia, PA, Lippincott Williams & Wilkins, 2009, pp. 2410–2423

Disaster Psychiatry Outreach: The Essentials of Disaster Psychiatry: A Training Course for Mental Health Professionals (Course Syllabus). New York, Disaster Psychiatry Outreach, 2008. Available as DPOCourseSyllabus_052108.pdf at: https://sites.google.com/a/disasterpsych.org/blog/File-Cabinet. Accessed December 21, 2009.

First MB, Spitzer RL, Gibbon M, et al: Structured Clinical Interview for DSM-IV-TR Axis I Disorders (SCID-I). New York, Biometrics Research, New York State Psychiatric Institute, 2002

Fournier JC, DeRubeis RJ, Hollon SD, et al: Antidepressant drug effects and depression severity. JAMA 303:47–53, 2010

Galea S, Ahern J, Resnick H, et al: Psychological sequelae of the September 11 attacks in New York City. N Engl J Med 346:982–987, 2002

Green LG, Grace MC, Lindy, JD, et al: Buffalo Creek survivors in the second decade: comparison with unexposed and nonlitigant groups. J Appl Soc Psychol 20:1033–1050, 1990

Guy W: ECDEU Assessment Manual for Psychopharmacology Revised (DHEW Publ No ADM 76-338). Rockville, MD, U.S. Department of Health, Education and Welfare, Public Health Service, Alcohol, Drug Abuse, and Mental Health Administration, National Institutes of Mental Health Psychopharmacology Branch, Division of Extramural Programs, 1956

Holbrook TL, Galarneau MR, Dye JL, et al: Morphine use after combat injury in Iraq and posttraumatic stress disorder. N Engl J Med 362:168–170, 2010

Institute of Medicine: Treatment of PTSD: An Assessment of the Evidence. Consensus Report. Washington, DC, Institute of Medicine of the National Academies, October 17, 2007. Available at: http://www.iom.edu/Reports/2007/Treatment-of-PTSD-An-Assessment-of-The-Evidence.aspx. Accessed January 2011.

Kolassa IT, Kolassa S, Ertl V, et al: The risk of posttraumatic stress disorder after trauma depends on traumatic load and the catechol-o-methyltransferase Val(158)Met polymorphism. Biol Psychiatry 67:304–308, 2010

Kosten TR, Fontana A, Sernyak MJ, et al: Benzodiazepine use in posttraumatic stress disorder among Vietnam veterans with substance abuse. J Nerv Ment Dis 188:454–459, 2000

Mylle J, Maes M: Partial posttraumatic stress disorder revisited. J Affect Disord 78:1:37–48, 2004

North CS, Nixon SJ, Shariat S et al: Psychiatric disorders among survivors of the Oklahoma City bombing. JAMA 282:755–762, 1999

Otto MW, Tolin DF, Simon NM, et al: Efficacy of D-cycloserine for enhancing response to cognitive-behavior therapy for panic disorder. Biol Psychiatry 67:365–370, 2010

Pitman RK, Delahanty DL: Conceptually driven pharmacological approaches to acute trauma. CNS Spectr 10:99–106, 2005

Post RM, Altshuler LL: Mood disorders: treatment of bipolar disorders, in Comprehensive Textbook of Psychiatry. Edited by Sadock BJ, Sadock VA, Ruiz P. Philadelphia, PA, Lippincott Williams & Wilkins, 2009, pp. 1743–1812

Querques J, Stern TA: Approach to consultation psychiatry: assessment strategies, in Massachusetts General Hospital Handbook of General Hospital Psychiatry, 6th Edition. Edited by Stern TA, Fricchione GL, Cassem NH, et al. Philadelphia, PA, Saunders Elsevier, 2010, pp. 7–14

Rao V, Lyketsos C: Neuropsychiatric sequelae of traumatic brain injury. Psychosomatics 41:95–103, 2000

Robins LN, Helzer JE, Croughan J, et al: National Institute of Mental Health Diagnostic Interview Schedule. Its history, characteristics, and validity. Arch Gen Psychiatry 38:381–389, 1981

Rogers JM, Read CA: Psychiatric comorbidity following traumatic brain injury. Brain Injury 21:1321–1333, 2007

Rush AJ, Nierenberg AA: Mood disorders: treatment of depression, in Comprehensive Textbook of Psychiatry. Edited by Sadock BJ, Sadock VA, Ruiz P. Philadelphia, PA, Lippincott Williams & Wilkins, 2009, pp. 1734–1742

Saxe G, Stoddard F, Courtney D, et al: Relationship between acute morphine and course of PTSD in children with burns: a pilot study. J Am Acad Child Adolesc Psychiatry 40:915–921, 2001

Shalev AY, Galai T, Eth S: Levels of trauma: a multidimensional approach to PTSD. Psychiatry 6:166–177, 1993

Shalev AY, Freedman S, Peri T, et al: Prospective study of PTSD and depression following trauma. Am J Psychiatry 155:630–637, 1998

Sontag D: Mental care in Haiti goes from bad to horrid: quake's aftermath reveals a system in collapse. The New York Times, March 20, 2010, pp 1, 7

Stein DJ, Ipser JC, Seedat S: Pharmacotherapy for post traumatic stress disorder (PTSD). Cochrane Database of Systematic Reviews 2006, Issue 1. Art. No.: CD002795. DOI: 10.1002/14651858.CD002795.pub2.

Stoddard FJ: Psychopharmacology of PTSD. Annual Psychopharmacology Course, Massachusetts Psychiatric Society, Waltham, MA, November 2000

Stoddard F, Saxe G: Ten-year research review of physical injuries. J Am Acad Child Adolesc Psychiatry 40:1128–1145, 2001

Stoddard FJ, Sorrentino EA, Ceranoglu TA, et al: Preliminary evidence for the effects of morphine on PTSD symptoms in one- to four-year-olds with burns. J Burn Care Res 30:836–843, 2009

Stoddard FJ, Sheridan RL, Martyn JAJ, et al: Pain management, in Combat and Operational Behavioral Health. Edited by Ritchie EC. Textbooks of Military Medicine (Lenhart MK, ed). Department of the Army, Office of the Surgeon General, Borden Institute (in press)

Terr L: Children of Chowchilla: a study of psychic trauma. Psychoanal Study Child 34:552–623, 1979

U.S. Department of Veterans Affairs/Department of Defense: VA/DoD Clinical Practice Guideline for Management of Concussion/Mild Traumatic Brain Injury (mTBI). Prepared by the Management of Concussion/mTBI Working Group, April 2009. Available at: http://www.healthquality.va.gov/management_of_concussion_mtbi.asp. Accessed March 30, 2010.

Weiss D, Marmar C: The Impact of Event Scale—Revised, in Assessing Psychological Trauma and PTSD. Edited by J. Wilson J, Keane T. New York, Guilford, 1997, pp 399–411

Werner D, Thuman C, Maxwell J: Where There Is No Doctor: A Village Health Care Handbook. Berkeley, CA, Hesperian, 2009

Zatzick DF, Jurkovich G, Russo J, et al: Posttraumatic stress, alcohol disorders, and recurrent trauma across level 1 trauma centers. J Trauma 57:360–366, 2004a

Zatzick DF, Roy-Byrne P, Russo J, et al: A randomized effectiveness trial of stepped collaborative care for acutely injured trauma survivors. Arch Gen Psychiatry 61:498–506, 2004b

Zatzick DF, Russo J, Pitman RK, et al: Reevaluating the association between emergency department heart rate and the development of posttraumatic stress disorder: a public health approach. Biol Psychiatry 57:91–95, 2005

Child and Adolescent Psychiatry Interventions

Heather L. Shibley, M.D.
Frederick J. Stoddard Jr., M.D.

> *International relief workers discovered a two year old child trapped beneath a collapsed building two days following the massive earthquake in Haiti. He had been all alone and without food and water. Working desperately hard, they were able to free him from wreckage. The relief workers described his facial expression changing from one of shock to one of relief and joy after they were able to reunite him with his parents.*

> "Haiti Earthquake: Stories From the Survivors" 2010

Millions of children and adolescents are impacted by the effects of disasters and wars throughout the world. During disasters, children are one of the most vulnerable populations due to their limited communication skills, immature cognitive abilities, and high dependency on their parents and other adults (National Commission on Children and Disasters 2010). Children are impacted by both the specific nature of the disaster and the emotional distress experienced by their parents, their teachers, and the people in their community (Pine and Cohen 2002). Vulnerability is increased for children experiencing the cumulative impact of traumas, such as children in Sri Lanka whose functioning was impacted by three event types: tsunami and disaster, war, and family violence (Catani et al. 2010). Children and adolescents have distinct needs predisaster, as well as during the acute and postacute phases of a disaster. Mental health professionals specializing in child psychiatry, child psychology, and nursing, together with pediatricians, are in a unique position to meet these needs because of their understanding of childhood development, childhood disorders, and family dynamics. Research on the mental health effects of disasters on children is increasing, and is helping to inform and improve interventions to lessen the trauma of disasters (Masten and Osofsky 2010). In this chapter, we focus on interventions for infants, children, and adolescents, and present relevant empirical literature, professional guidelines, and evidence-informed interventions.

Predisaster Phase

Predisaster planning is an integral piece of disaster psychiatry. The first stage in predisaster planning for children is developing personal and family preparedness plans. In addition, psychiatrists and other mental health professionals should be trained in the mental health needs of children prior to the disaster and updated by just-in-time training. In their core curricula, disaster training programs include lectures on disaster mental health, including Psychological First Aid (PFA) for children. Methods of communication and rapid activation should be planned ahead. Relationships should be established beforehand with agencies that deal with children—such as local schools; hospitals; obstetric, pediatric, and child mental health clinics; the juvenile courts; and police—to enable psychiatrists to help after a disaster strikes with children, adolescents, and families, including with assessment and treatment where indicated. Forming relationships with the media prior to disasters is important to ensure that public health announcements are helpful to schools and parents (see Chapter 2, "Communicating Risk Before, During, and After a Disaster"). Additionally, collaboration with media representatives is needed to plan helpful, rather than traumatic, announcements; warnings to families about forthcoming graphic images to allow time for them to encourage their children to leave the room; and guidance for parents who may need to seek professional help for their children. Also, because traumatized children normally express their feelings though play and art rather than verbal communication, it is important to have a supply kit ready with art supplies, hand puppets, emergency vehicles, doctor's kits, and a dollhouse with dolls of different ethnic backgrounds (Disaster Psychiatry Outreach 2008).

Acute Phase

Immediately after a disaster strikes, mental health professionals serve many different roles, including implementing PFA, screening the population to obtain a rough estimate of the number of children at risk, assisting with establishing telephone hotlines, and developing public health education programs (Laor and Wolmer 2007). Mental health clinicians serving children and families are most effective when they are well-integrated members of the larger emergency disaster response. Psychiatrists and other members of the disaster team may be significantly impacted by working with children who are physically and emotionally suffering from the effects of a disaster. Good self-care and supervision by or consultation with experienced disaster workers are critical to disaster work. Although in this chapter we do not cover all of the complicated scenarios that psychiatrists and allied professionals may face, we provide basic guidelines for interventions with children in disaster settings.

Psychological First Aid for Children

Contrary to common belief, no data support debriefing for children in the immediate aftermath of a disaster. The potential risks of exposing children to peers with more extreme emotional responses and experiences outweigh any of the potential benefits (Brymer et al. 2006; Cohen et al. 2006a). PFA for children is different from that for adults (see Chapter 12, "Psychological First Aid"). Whereas the focus for adult survivors is on assuring safety and securing food, water, shelter, and first aid, the focus for children also involves more developmentally targeted interventions (Schreiber and Gurwitch 2006; Stoddard and Menninger 2004). PFA for children incorporates a series of strategies focusing on children and their families, in which parents, teachers, and community resources give basic psychological support for infants, children, and adolescents. PFA should be adapted to fit the cultural and religious beliefs of the people impacted by the disaster. As discussed in the following list, the basic goals of PFA include listening, protecting, connecting, modeling calm and optimistic behavior, and teaching.

1. **Listen**—Allow children the opportunity to share their experiences and express their feelings. Pay attention to what they say and do, because children often express their feelings nonverbally. Provide time and space for children to tell their stories creatively through playing or drawing. However, if a child is reluctant to share or discuss feelings, respect his or her disinclination (to avoid retraumatization), while remaining available to discuss feelings when the child is ready. Acknowledge and validate children's feelings while giving reassurance that adults will provide protection and care as much as possible. Also, observe any changes in sleep, appetite, play, mood, physical complaints, school achievements, and peer interactions, because these may be clues as to how a child is dealing with the disaster.

2. **Protect**—When possible, reestablish structure, routines, and stability for children, such as returning to school and after-school activities. Provide honest, age-appropriate information regarding recent events as well as what adults are doing to keep them safe, but avoid too much detail or overexposure. Educate parents, teachers, and children about the typical reactions that infants, children, and adolescents experience during the acute disaster phase. For example, parents of young children should be reassured that some regression and clinginess is normal in the acute phase following a disaster. In addition, young children may have guilty thoughts and need to be reassured that the disaster is not their fault.

3. **Connect**—Reestablish children's normal social relationships and connections with family, friends, neighbors, teachers, and other community resources. Whenever possible, children should be immediately reunited with their parents after a disaster. When they cannot be reunited, they should be reassured that they will be with caring adults for as long as necessary (Cohen et al. 2006a). Supportive caregivers have been shown to foster resilience and mitigate the risk of developing posttraumatic stress symptoms in children and adolescents. Parental presence during and directly following the disasters, as well as positive parental coping, are among the most critical protective factors for children (Laor and Wolmer 2007; Masten et al. 1990).

4. **Model calm and optimistic behavior**—Particularly in times of crisis, children and adolescents observe adults' reactions, learn from their cues, and follow their lead. Adults should be encouraged to acknowledge their personal distress while demonstrating a positive, optimistic (yet realistic) approach toward individual, family, and community recovery. Parental assessment is an integral part of the child evaluation, so the psychiatrist can support their resilience and recognize any psychopathology or poor family functioning that may place the child at higher risk for psychological sequelae (Pine and Cohen 2002).

5. **Teach**—Help children and adolescents and the adults who care for them to understand the range of common stress reactions, and the ways that such reactions may affect them in school or other settings. In addition, teach children to understand some ways to cope with stress, and provide the opportunity for them to participate, even peripherally, in recovery efforts. Examples of how children can be involved while minimizing the risks of injury or retraumatization include letter or card writing, bake sales, and replanting bushes or trees after fires or floods. Emotional coping and recovery are enhanced by decreasing initial distress and uncertainty and increasing self-efficacy, hope, and adaptive skills.

A special intervention for children is establishing a defined space for them to play, designated with a sign, such as "Kids' Corner." It should be an inviting and comfortable space where the pediatric mental health team can observe and interact with children and their families (Disaster Psychiatry Outreach 2008). Providing children the opportunity to tell their stories to supportive family or to child health professionals is therapeutic and allows the mental health team the chance to identify and correct cognitive distortions.

In contrast to the typical child and adolescent psychiatric evaluation, which can last two or three sessions, the disaster psychiatry evaluation is brief. This evaluation focuses on assessing individual risks and serves to screen and identify acute symptoms and identify those children who require more thorough evaluation and disposition. It is a form of triage. Children at higher risk include those who display intense anxiety, depressed mood, hypervigilance, anger, dissociation, complicated grief, disturbed sleep, and disorientation, as well as those with predisaster psychopathology, including prior traumatic exposures, which can increase cumulative risk (Becker-Blease et al. 2010; Young 2006). More thorough screening and possibly treatment are necessary for children who have physical injuries; whose family members have been injured or killed; who were proximally exposed to the disaster; who were separated from their parents or caregivers; and who experienced major losses, such as destruction of their home or school (Laor and Wolmer 2007; Shaw et al. 2007). Children who have lost a loved one or close friend in the disaster may experience traumatic grief, which occurs when the trauma interferes with and compounds the normal grief process (Cohen et al. 2006b). These children may require specialty counseling, when available, in which both the trauma and the death can be processed. Further information, as well as training, on childhood traumatic grief is available through the National Child Traumatic Stress Network (www.nctsnet.org).

Promoting Positive Coping Skills for Acute Distress Responses

While normal resilience and distress reactions are frequent after disasters, it is common to think only of posttraumatic stress disorder (PTSD) as the principal response to traumatic events such as disasters. It is important to identify PTSD (Cohen et al. 1998) and to recognize that certain symptoms, such as reexperiencing, effortful avoidance, and dysphoria, appear to signal ongoing impairment (Kassam-Adams et al. 2010). However, children and adolescents may display a wide range of normal emotional reactions, psychopathology, and risky behaviors. Frequently, they show mild signs and symptoms of distress that are not clinically significant, but some meet the DSM-IV-TR criteria for adjustment disorders, separation anxiety disorder, other anxiety disorders, depressive disorders, bereavement, substance use disorders, and disruptive behavior disorders (American Psychiatric Association 2000).

Mental health professionals should educate children and their families about potential emotional and behavioral responses to a disaster. They should teach stress reduction strategies and healthy coping techniques, as well as review red-flag symptoms that indicate the need for parents to seek further evaluation for themselves or their children. Normalizing certain postdisaster reactions increases survivors' sense of self-efficacy and self-control and decreases anxiety in both parents and children. Emphasis should be placed on the self-limited nature of the acute distress response. Mental health professionals should also focus on teaching parents how to encourage children to express their feelings and thoughts and to reassure children that the disaster was not their fault. Parents and teachers should provide age-appropriate factual information regarding the disaster and recovery response, because children often imagine worse scenarios if they are uninformed or misinformed (Cohen et al. 2006a). Parents should also be encouraged to assign small help-giving roles to children to allow them to achieve a sense of mastery and to counter feelings of helplessness and passivity (Flynn and Nelson 1998). Evidence suggests that parents should limit children's television viewing because the graphic pictures and stories can easily overwhelm them and can exacerbate the severity of PTSD (Pfefferbaum et al. 1999).

Distribution of Handouts

Preprinted materials that convey succinct information in bulleted format can be very useful in times of disaster. These can be distributed via schools or at the disaster site. Many people will be distracted and inattentive, and written material enables them to look back over the information when the situation is less chaotic. The American Academy of Child and Adolescent Psychiatry has disaster-related handouts in their "Facts for Families" series, including "Children and Grief," "Being Prepared: Knowing Where to Find Help for Your Child," "Helping Children After a Disaster," and "Posttraumatic Stress Disorder (PTSD)" (www.aacap.org). Providing guidance to parents on how to talk with, listen to, support, and reassure their children in the acute aftermath of a disaster is often very useful and increases parents' confidence (Cohen et al. 2006a). Information about community mental health and school-based clinics should also be distributed.

Postacute Phase

During disasters, children may sustain multiple losses, including loss of family members and friends, loss of school and daytime routines, and loss of basic human assumptions such as safety and security (Laor and Wolmer 2007). Therefore, during the postacute phase in the first few weeks after a disaster, children do best with a quick return to structure and routine (Shaw et al. 2007). Families can help restore this sense of normalcy by implementing mealtime and bedtime routines. Reopening schools, churches, and community after-school programs also creates a sense of structure, routine, and support.

Disasters impact not only individuals, families, and schools, but also entire communities. Community-based interventions following a disaster include creating jobs and specialty training, restoring youth sports, organizing memorials, and creating community programs in the arts and humanities (Laor and Wolmer 2007). Sustaining, restoring, and building mental health and substance programs are important for children and adolescents, as well as their families, who are having difficulty after disasters.

Recommendations for Schools

Because trust is difficult to build in the postacute phase, and because parents generally trust teachers, who have frontline access to the children, schools have been identified as a good place to initiate recovery efforts (Klingman 1993). Schools are very important acutely because children are likely to be in school, and schools may be directly impacted by the disaster (as demonstrated following earthquakes in China, Turkey, and Haiti). Unfortunately, in major disasters, school systems may be disrupted or destroyed.

Traumatized parents, experiencing their own grief, may not be reliable reporters of their children's mental health problems, may not seek mental health evaluation for their children, and may be unable to provide the intense support their children require. Hence, many children who are impacted do not receive any treatment (Cohen et al. 2006a). Therefore, widespread screenings at schools accessing a broad range of symptoms with standardized measures can detect many children who otherwise would go unnoticed. In addition to being sites for screening, schools can serve as treatment centers. Child mental health professionals should first meet with school administrators and with teachers alone to ensure that the teachers are adjusting well and are not directly traumatized themselves. Then, mental health professionals may be asked to teach and assist administrators and teachers with how to deal with their students' responses to the disaster and associated traumas. The teachers may assist with communicating and educating their students about normal responses to disasters, by modeling healthy ways of coping, and by instilling self-efficacy, hope, and the expectancy of a return to normalcy. The teachers may also learn how to identify those children who may benefit from evaluation or treatment (Laor and Wolmer 2007; Schreiber and Gurwitch 2006).

School-based interventions can be targeted as focus groups for administrators and counselors (Kataoka et al. 2009) or for a whole class or smaller groups of high-risk children (Klingman 1993). One example of a teacher-led class activation program consisted of one parent session and eight 2-hour sessions focusing on safety, psychoeducation, emotions following death and disaster, and future-oriented planning. It demonstrated that combined therapeutic techniques (cognitive-behavioral therapy [CBT], psychoeducation, and play techniques) soon after a disaster reduced children's dissociation and posttraumatic symptoms, and improved adaptation 3 years later (Wolmer et al. 2003, 2005). Cognitive Behavioral Intervention for Trauma in Schools (CBITS; Jaycox 2003) is an evidence-based, brief, manualized group CBT program that also includes four parent sessions and one teacher psychoeducation session. In a randomized controlled study, students who had received CBITS reported significantly lower posttraumatic stress and depressive symptoms (Wong et al. 2002).

Specialized Treatment Postdisaster

Although most children and adolescents will respond well to the natural support systems in their community and to PFA, a minority will require more specialized mental health treatment (Cohen et al. 2006a) or substance abuse treatment (Chemtob et al. 2009; Saxe et al. 2006). Those with continued evidence of distress should be enrolled in a more structured, culturally informed, brief, crisis-intervention–focused supportive psychotherapy that typically lasts one to six sessions. The focus is on psychoeducation, relaxation exercises, cognitive reframing, coping mechanisms including distraction, physical and social activities, and problem solving (Goenjian et al. 1997). A randomized study comparing meditation and relaxation to a narrative exposure therapy in Sri Lanka during the first months after the tsunami revealed that the brief six-session treatment was effective in both treatment groups (Catani et al. 2009). This study is noteworthy because it targeted a population that was already heavily traumatized secondary to the civil war and other disasters. Sri Lanka is also culturally distinct from many of the populations studied previously. It is imperative that planned mental health interventions be culturally and religiously informed.

Children who display continued psychopathology, such as sustained posttraumatic stress symptoms, following a brief treatment typically require a more intensive, formal psychotherapy. CBT has the largest evidence base and has been used in individual and group formats, including school programs (Wethington et al. 2008). CBT usually lasts approximately 10–16 weeks. Chemtob et al. (2002) showed a decrease in PTSD symptoms in a randomized controlled trial using CBT in both individual and group formats compared with a wait-list control group. Goenjian et al. (1997) performed a study in Armenian adolescents following a major earthquake. They compared a group of adolescents receiving CBT focused on both trauma and grief with a control group that received no intervention. The control group demonstrated worsening of both PTSD and depression symptoms, whereas the treatment group displayed an improvement in PTSD and no change in depression symptoms.

Trauma-focused CBT (TF-CBT) is one type of specialized CBT treatment that has proved to be effective in trauma survivors (Cohen et al. 2006b). The focus is on reconstructing the traumatic experience to desensitize the child to the trauma and to allow the child to achieve mastery over the situation. TF-CBT consists of psychoeducation, stress management and relaxation exercises, affect identification and modulation, cognitive restructuring, exposure therapies such as trauma narratives and drawings, identification of themes such as guilt and revenge, conjoint child and family sessions, and safety enhancement (Cohen et al. 2006). Web-based TF-CBT training is available at http://tfcbt.musc.edu.

Play psychotherapy is a type of psychodynamic psychotherapeutic treatment that is effective in treating children exposed to trauma, and is particularly appropriate for young children (Ablon 1996). One of the most widely practiced forms of child psychotherapy, it utilizes play as a way for a child to create or use objective soothing experiences with the therapist (e.g., play with dolls, drawings, storytelling, songs) to overcome the emotional effects of trauma, providing a positive transitional experience or mental space ("transitional object") and thereby aiding continuation of normal development (Winnicott 1951). Even as the psychotherapeutic environment provides safety, so does the creative play, which the child retains after the formal therapeutic relationship is over. Through the use of therapeutic play, children can safely share and reenact the trauma in displacement with an empathic therapist, in a private and protected therapeutic setting, and eventually gain understanding, as well as the sense of mastery that was lacking in the real-life experience. The attentive therapist will listen to the child's own language, observe the child's spontaneous play, label the child's feelings with words the child understands, and interpret the child's thoughts, helping the child to work through the original feelings of anxiety and helplessness, gain a greater sense of self-awareness, and learn healthier coping mechanisms (Terr 1990). This method can also be effective in small groups of children hospitalized with a variety of traumas, including those traumatized by the pain, fears, and surgeries associated with burns or other injuries (Stoddard 2002). Although play psychotherapy is for the child, occasionally parents or guardians attend sessions, and providing information and helpful feedback to them about the child's progress in therapy is essential to its success.

Pediatric Psychopharmacology After Disasters

In general, most children do not require psychotropic medications in the acute aftermath of a disaster because they respond well to therapeutic interventions and family support. Interventions that provide nurturance and comforting, such as breastfeeding, holding, and reassuring of young children, and providing age-appropriate adult-supervised structure and play opportunities in older children's environments, may be as calming as or more calming than medication. Providing opportunities for children to be of help in age-appropriate ways (e.g., collecting funds for children who have been hurt) may both satisfy altruistic yearnings and relieve feelings of helplessness.

Acute Phase: On Site at Schools, Clinics, Offices, and Hospitals

Due to the lack of research in pediatric psychopharmacology in the acute stages following a disaster, most information is derived either from emergency pediatric or acute pediatric and surgical care settings (Lorberg and Prince 2010) or from studies of adults after disasters. Consultation with child and adolescent psychiatrists in person or via telepsychiatry is advised if possible.

Before medications are prescribed, a child psychiatric history should be obtained, which includes the history of present illness, developmental history, pediatric history, current physical health, allergies, medications used, substance abuse, family history, school history, and social history including relationships within the family. Physical and mental status examinations should accompany the history gathering.

Although most children do not require medication, some children, especially those requiring hospitalization for injuries or other illness, may manifest symptoms or diagnoses that are likely to improve with medication. In the following discussion of psychopharmacological treatment of pediatric patients, we address medications that may be required in the acute and postacute phases following a disaster. When prescribing for children and adolescents, the practitioner calculates dosages according to a milligram per kilogram scale. It is safest to start with the lowest possible dosages and titrate upward to minimize and monitor any side effects or toxic effects; in other words, the recommendation is to "start low, go slow." (Additional cautions regarding prescribing for children following disasters are listed in Table 17–1.) When children are unlikely to be available for follow-up or are unable to call regarding questions or problems, medications with significant side effects or toxicity should either not be prescribed or be prescribed with only a 2- to 3-day supply.

Psychopharmacological agents are often prescribed for preexisting comorbidities, such as antidepressants for depression or stimulants for attention-deficit/hyperactivity disorder (ADHD). Whereas medication used for these indications may be approved by the U.S. Food and Drug Administration (FDA), most other medications used after a disaster are prescribed off-label. Occasionally, children display acute symptoms of distress, such as insomnia, agitation, delirium, behavioral dysregulation, and mood symptoms, that interfere significantly with their functioning. When there is acute risk, hospitalization is indicated if possible. Although the topic here is postdisaster pediatric psychopharmacology, not pediatric intensive care, there are parallels, and after a disaster some injured or ill children will require inpatient care.

TABLE 17–1. Prescribing for children after disasters: extreme caution is advised

The prescribing of psychotropic medications for children after disasters is significantly limited by the following:

1. The use of psychotropic medications is discouraged in socially disorganized disaster settings because the recommended follow-up monitoring may be impossible. For antidepressants, the U.S. Food and Drug Administration recommends *weekly* check-ins for the first month after a new prescription or dosage change, then follow-up visits *every 2 weeks* for the next month, with *monthly* meetings thereafter. For monitoring treatment, it is also helpful to have the patient complete a symptom inventory for the condition being treated before each meeting.

2. Although it may be indicated to prescribe psychotropic medications acutely in a hospital setting, as described in Tables 17–2, 17–3, and 17–4, it is usually not indicated to prescribe during a disaster in a community setting where specialized follow-up is impossible. The later tables in this chapter are primarily appropriate for use in the hospital, and not to encourage physicians in the community to simply prescribe when it is impossible to pay proper attention to what is required for safe use of medication.

3. After disasters, drugs such as analgesics, benzodiazepines, and stimulants are sometimes diverted for illegal purposes.

4. Prescribing psychotropic medications when no child psychotherapy is available is discouraged. Optimally, antidepressants should be prescribed in conjunction with therapy and closely monitored, but psychotherapy is often not available in rural or postdisaster settings.

5. Antipsychotic medications may be prescribed by physicians in hospital settings where follow-up is possible. However, children should not be given antipsychotic medications without baseline blood tests or without close monitoring of blood tests and Abnormal Involuntary Movement Scale exams by physicians (Guy 1976; Munetz and Benjamin 1988).

The recommendations that follow address psychopharmacological treatment of children ages 7 years and older, although with child psychiatric or pediatric consultation, treatment for younger children may be cautiously initiated on a milligram per kilogram basis.

Pain

Management of pain in infants, children, and adolescents is essential, and psychiatrists contribute both to the assessment of factors contributing to pain and to its treatment. Interventions to reduce even very severe pain and associated symptomatology vary from psychological interventions (e.g., hypnosis and relaxation), to physical interventions (e.g., surgery treating an injury, positioning), to medications of many types (antibiotics, analgesics, antipsychotics, anxiolytics) for which benefits must be balanced against any risks of side effects or toxic effects (Stoddard et al. 2002). Breast-feeding may rapidly reduce pain, as well as associated anxiety, in the nursing infant. Acetaminophen or ibuprofen may be remarkably effective for severe pain, and these two medications are the only available analgesics after some major disasters. Pharmacological management of severe pain is the treatment of choice if analgesics are available in the postdisaster care setting (Schechter et al. 2003; Stoddard and Saxe 2001; Stoddard et al., in press). Evidence is increasing that pain is an important predictor of later posttraumatic symptomatology in people with severe injuries, and that these symptoms are reduced by early administration of opiates (Holbrook et al. 2010; Saxe et al. 2001).

Insomnia

Disrupted sleep is common after a disaster and may be an early symptom of stress and anxiety. Psychopharmacological intervention may be indicated if the insomnia is persistent and causes functional daytime impairment. If that is the case, young children may benefit from low-dose diphenhydramine on a milligram per kilogram basis for 5–7 days (Disaster Psychiatry Outreach 2008; Donnelly 2003). Children should be closely observed, because a small subset may experience paradoxical disinhibition. If this occurs, diphenhydramine should be discontinued. If low-dose diphenhydramine is not effective and insomnia continues or is accompanied by significant anxiety, a short-term trial of a low-dose benzodiazepine, such as lorazepam, on a milligram per kilogram basis may be tried (see Table 17–2). Again, the patient should be monitored for paradoxical disinhibition. If insomnia is associated with symptoms of acute stress disorder or PTSD and follow-up is possible as recommended, an antidepressant such as sertraline may be considered and titrated to effect.

TABLE 17–2. Selected benzodiazepines used in pediatric critical care

Drug	Routes of administration	Onset (minutes)	Half-life (hours)	Metabolism
Clonazepam	po	30–60	Adult data: 20–80 (Wozniak et al. 2001)	CYP3A
Diazepam	iv (painful), im, po, pr (gel)	iv: 1–3 pr: 7–15 po: 30–60	Child data: 15–21 (Cassem et al. 2004)	CYP2C19* CYP3A
Lorazepam	iv, im, po	iv: 1–5 im: 10–20 po: 30–60	Child data: 10.5±2.9 (Chess and Thomas 1984)	Phase II glucuronidation only
Midazolam	iv, im, po, pr	iv: 1–3 im: 5–10 po/pr: 10–30	Child data: 0.8–1.8 (Kovacs 1985)	CYP3A

Note. im=intramuscular; iv=intravenous; po=oral; pr=rectal.
*15%–20% of Asians and 3%–5% of whites are poor metabolizers of cytochrome P450 (CYP) 2C19 substrates.

Source. Adapted from Stoddard F, Usher C, Abrams A: "Psychopharmacology in Pediatric Critical Care." *Child and Adolescent Psychiatric Clinics of North America* 15:611–655, 2006. Copyright © 2006, Elsevier, Inc. Used with permission.

Anxiety and Depression

In the acute stages of a disaster, many children and adolescents experience anxiety. Numerous disaster workers report experiencing helplessness and a longing to take away all of the children's distress. However, most anxiety resolves without psychotropic medications, and therefore antianxiety medication such as lorazepam should be reserved for only severe, persistent, functionally impairing anxiety. In the weeks after a disaster, if a child continues to display signs or symptoms of depression or anxiety and follow-up is possible as recommended, selective serotonin reuptake inhibitors (SSRIs) may be helpful (Donnelly 2003). Sertraline, fluoxetine, and imipramine are three agents that have been found to be effective for acute stress disorder, PTSD, and depression in school-age children (Stoddard et al. 2006). Sertraline can be started at dosages of 6.25 mg for young children and 12.5 mg for older children and adolescents. Dosages frequently are titrated up to 25–50 mg and can be increased further as needed. Fluoxetine can be initiated at dosages of 2.5 or 5 mg, depending on the child's weight, and subsequently titrated up to 10–20 mg. Imipramine has more side effects, including rare cardiac arrhythmias, and is lethal in overdose; therefore, it is no longer first-line treatment for anxiety or depression. Imipramine can be started at 10 or 25 mg at bedtime. Table 17–3 lists antidepressants commonly prescribed for children. All antidepressants carry a black box warning for suicidality in children and adults younger than age 25 and therefore should be prescribed in conjunction with therapy and close medication management monitoring (U.S. Food and Drug Administration 2007). The FDA recommends weekly appointments for the first month, every other week for the second month, and then monthly appointments thereafter. When follow-up as recommended is possible, the black box warning should not prevent providers from prescribing effective medications for depression, which can be life-threatening. Antidepressants are typically continued at the therapeutic dosage for approximately 9–12 months and then slowly tapered if tolerated.

Agitation

If a child is displaying intense aggression, severe mood dysregulation, psychotic symptoms, or self-injurious behavior, or is a threat to self or others, he or she should be evaluated for hospitalization. Agitation may be associated with delirium—a medical emergency involving a disturbance of consciousness, a change in cognition (that is often dramatic), a fluctuating disturbance over hours to days, and evidence of a medical etiology (e.g., medication or substance, injury, infection, malnutrition, mania) (American Psychiatric Association 2000). (See Table 17–4.)

CHILD AND ADOLESCENT PSYCHIATRY INTERVENTIONS

TABLE 17–3. Selected antidepressants used in pediatric critical care

Drug	Formulation	Initiating dose	Side effects
Fluoxetine	Tablet, oral disintegrating tablet	5–20 mg po daily	Irritability Akathisia Insomnia
Sertraline	Tablet, solution, intramuscular injection	12.5–25 mg po daily	Appetite decrease (acute use) or increase (chronic) Gastrointestinal symptoms
Citalopram	Tablet, oral solution	10–20 mg po daily	Platelet dysfunction Sexual side effects
Escitalopram	Tablet, oral solution	2.5–5 mg po daily	Suicidality*

Note.   The dosages and side effect profiles are general guidelines and are not intended to be definitive. Medication selection and dosing should be individualized and accompanied by appropriate clinical and laboratory monitoring. po=oral.
*U.S. Food and Drug Administration black box warning applies to all antidepressants in children and adolescents.

Source.   Adapted from Stoddard F, Usher C, Abrams A: "Psychopharmacology in Pediatric Critical Care." *Child and Adolescent Psychiatric Clinics of North America* 15:611–655, 2006. Copyright © 2006, Elsevier, Inc. Used with permission.

TABLE 17–4.   Selected neuroleptics used in pediatric critical care

Drug	Formulation	Initiating dose[a]	Side effects and toxic effects[b]
Aripiprazole	Tablet	2.5–5 mg po qd	* Occasional agitation, anxiety + Hypotension 0 Hyperprolactinemia 0 Glucose intolerance 0 Weight gain + EPS + NMS
Haloperidol	Tablet, im injection, iv	0.2–0.5 mg iv tid for 1–2 days	* QT$_c$ prolongation + Hypotension ++ Hyperprolactinemia + Glucose intolerance 0 Weight gain +++ EPS +++ NMS
Olanzapine	Tablet, oral disintegrating tablet, im injection	2.5 mg po bid	* Anticholinergic effects ++ Hypotension + Hyperprolactinemia ++ Glucose intolerance +++ Weight gain + EPS + NMS

TABLE 17–4. Selected neuroleptics used in pediatric critical care *(continued)*

Drug	Formulation	Initiating dose[a]	Side effects and toxic effects[b]
Quetiapine	Tablet	25 mg po bid	* Sedation ++ Hypotension 0 Hyperprolactinemia + Glucose intolerance ++ Weight gain 0 EPS + NMS
Risperidone	Tablet, solution, im injection	0.25 mg po qd	* Hepatotoxicity +++ Hypotension ++ Hyperprolactinemia + Glucose intolerance ++ Weight gain ++ EPS + NMS
Ziprasidone	Tablet, im injection	20 mg po/im qd	* QT_c prolongation + Hypotension + Hyperprolactinemia + Glucose intolerance 0 Weight gain + EPS + NMS

Note. The dosing guidelines provided are for general guidance and are not intended to be definitive. Medication selection and dosing should be individualized and accompanied by appropriate clinical and laboratory monitoring. bid=twice a day; EPS=extrapyramidal symptoms; im=intramuscular; iv=intravenous; NMS=neuroleptic malignant syndrome; po=oral; qd=every day; tid=three times a day.
[a]Not approved for children younger than 18 years; [b]Key for side effects and toxic effects of concern (Gardner et al. 2005): *=slightly less common side effect; +++=high risk; ++=moderate risk; +=low risk; 0=negligible risk.

Source. Adapted from Stoddard F, Usher C, Abrams A: "Psychopharmacology in Pediatric Critical Care." *Child and Adolescent Psychiatric Clinics of North America* 15:611–655, 2006. Copyright © 2006, Elsevier, Inc. Used with permission.

When recommended baseline and follow-up laboratory studies and monitoring are possible for school-age children with severe agitation or delirium, psychiatrists may consider off-label use of atypical antipsychotics, such as risperidone 0.25–0.5 mg, quetiapine 25 mg at bedtime or twice daily, olanzapine 2.5 mg at bedtime or twice daily, or aripiprazole 2.5–5 mg/day (see Table 17–4); for younger children, diphenhydramine or low-dose benzodiazepines are recommended (Stoddard et al. 2006). When prescribing atypical antipsychotics, the psychiatrist needs to obtain baseline and follow-up laboratory studies, including complete blood count, liver function tests, and fasting glucose and fasting lipid panel, as well as to record height, weight, vital signs, and body mass index. In addition, the Abnormal Involuntary Movement Scale (AIMS; Guy 1976) should be conducted at baseline and monitored monthly, because dystonias and tardive dyskinesia are known risks of antipsychotics (Lane et al. 1985).

Although β-blockers (e.g., propranolol) were once thought to have benefit in preventing PTSD, further studies have not supported their use, and they are not recommended in children (see Chapter 15, "Psychopharmacology: Acute Phase"). Likewise, whereas α_2-adrenergic agonists such as clonidine are occasionally used in children for hyperarousal and impulsivity, these have potential adverse cardiovascular side effects (hypotension, arrhythmia), rendering them inappropriate for use after a disaster except in a hospital setting (Donnelly 2003).

Inattention and Distractibility

Children often present with inattention, hyperactivity, and high levels of distraction following a trauma or disaster. These behavior changes are more likely secondary to the hyperarousal of a traumatic reaction to the disaster than signs of a new diagnosis of ADHD. Screening should focus on identifying any additional symptoms of PTSD, depression or anxiety, and premorbid functioning. Stimulants are often indicated for children who were on these medications but do not have their medication secondary to the disaster, or who have an independently confirmed prior history of ADHD. Children and adolescents with ADHD may be significantly disruptive when forced to live in temporary shelters without their stimulant medications. If possible, pharmacies should be contacted to confirm prior dosing, and clinicians should be aware of the high rate of abuse of these medications. Stimulants are prescribed on a milligram per kilogram basis, with low dosages being immediate-release methylphenidate 2.5–5 mg twice daily and longer-acting methylphenidate (e.g., Concerta) 18 mg each morning (see Table 17–5). Prior to prescribing stimulants, the psychiatrist should obtain the family's and individual's cardiac history, and the individual's

TABLE 17–5. Selected stimulants for attention-deficit/hyperactivity disorder

Generic name	Brand name	Initiating dose, mg	Usual daily dosage, mg (mg/kg)
Methylphenidate IR	Ritalin (tablets)	2.5 or 5 qd or bid	10–60 (0.3–1.5)
	Methylin (chewable)	2.5 or 5 qd or bid	10–60 (0.3–1.5)
Methylphenidate ER	Ritalin LA (capsules)	10–20 qd	20–60 (0.6–1.5)
	Metadate CD (capsules)	10–20 qd	20–60 (0.6–1.5)
Methylphenidate OR	Concerta (OROS)	18 qd	18–72 (0.4–1.8)
Mixed amphetamine IR	Adderall (tablets)	2.5 or 5 qd	5–40 (0.2–1)
Mixed amphetamine ER	Adderall XR (capsules)	5 qd	5–40 (0.2–1)
Amphetamine sulfate IR	Dexedrine (tablets)	5 qd	5–30 (0.2–0.7)
Dexmethylphenidate IR	Focalin (tablets)	2.5 bid	5–30 (0.2–0.7)
Dexmethylphenidate ER	Focalin XR (capsules)	5 qd	5–30 (0.2–0.7)

Note. Stimulants are approved by the U.S. Food and Drug Administration for children >6 years old. bid=twice a day; ER=extended release; IR=immediate release; OR=osmotic release; qd=every day.

Caveats for clinicians prescribing stimulants:

- Contraindications to stimulant use include known hypersensitivity to the medication and glaucoma.
- Stimulants may cause insomnia, sleep disturbances, decreased appetite, nausea, abdominal pain, headaches, tachycardia, blood pressure changes, irritability, and rebound symptoms such as lability of mood. Also, may cause small decreases in height and weight.
- Stimulants may have the potential to be abused, particularly in disaster settings.
- Stimulants may exacerbate/aggravate symptoms of anxiety, tension, and agitation and may cause tics or psychosis in individuals predisposed to these illnesses.
- Stimulants should not be used in combination with monoamine oxidase inhibitors.
- Stimulants may cause cardiovascular problems, including sudden cardiac death, in people with preexisting cardiac structural abnormalities.

Source. Green 2007; Spetie and Arnold 2007.

heart rate, blood pressure, height, and weight should be recorded and monitored regularly. See Table 17–5 for more detailed information regarding the side effects of stimulants.

Postacute Phase: At School, as Outpatients, and in Hospitals

The preceding section addresses mainly acute-phase psychiatric symptoms and diagnoses. During the postacute phase, parents may take their children (or teachers or pediatricians may refer them) for treatment in conventional practice settings for these and other conditions. In this phase, the evidence base is clear in children for FDA-approved pharmacological treatments of PTSD, major depression, ADHD, and most other medication-responsive child psychiatric disorders (see also Chapter 16, "Psychopharmacology: Postacute Phase"). Nevertheless, it is essential to evaluate and take into consideration the impact of the disaster on, and the degree of its contribution to, the child's presenting symptoms.

Conclusion

In preparing to meet the postdisaster needs of children, it is important to evaluate and consider their developmental needs, as well as the needs of their parents, families, and schools. Pediatric services, other child services, and schools should have specific plans and staff disaster training to anticipate and meet the needs of children and staff, and should coordinate their planning with other disaster agencies in the community. Children's mental health needs range from support utilizing PFA for acute conditions, such as acute distress, to psychotherapeutic treatment of disorders that may persist, such as PTSD or depression, which require ongoing evaluation and treatment whenever possible. Psychopharmacological treatment may be indicated in hospital settings, where recommended baseline laboratory tests, ongoing monitoring, and child psychiatric consultation (e.g., telepsychiatry) may be possible. Effective preparation, including staff training, may mitigate the impact of disaster trauma for infants, children, adolescents, and their families.

■ Teaching Points

- Infants, children, and adolescents are among the most vulnerable populations following a disaster.
- It is important in anticipation of possible disasters to plan psychoeducational points for the media, which may help children and families cope better.

- After a disaster, reunification of children separated from their families is a priority wherever possible.
- Interventions to assist children in schools and their teachers are critical.
- Evidence indicates that parental PTSD impacts children, and therefore interventions that support parents benefit their children.
- Postdisaster responses seen in children include a normal range of distress reactions and resilience, PTSD, other anxiety disorders, adjustment disorders, bereavement, and depression, as well as substance use disorders in adolescents.
- For children severely impacted by a disaster, psychotherapy, including play psychotherapy, TF-CBT, or family therapy, may be indicated.
- In the acute phase, a few school-age children may require psychopharmacological treatment, primarily anxiolytics for acute stress. In the postacute phase, other medications may be indicated in hospital settings, where laboratory tests and recommended follow-up monitoring is possible.
- Interventions after disasters should be sensitive to the varying impacts of trauma and loss during the developmental stages from infancy through adolescence.
- Disaster plans and effective disaster preparation in children's agencies, schools, and health care facilities, including staff training, may mitigate the impact of disaster trauma for infants, children, adolescents, and their families.

Review Questions

17.1 How is Psychological First Aid for children different from that for adults?

    A. It focuses on ensuring safety.
    B. It targets decreasing initial distress.
    C. It emphasizes self-efficacy.
    D. It is developmentally focused.
    E. It focuses on securing staples such as food and water.

17.2 Children with which of the following risk factor(s) are the most vulnerable to developing psychopathology following exposure to a disaster?

    A. Those who have been personally injured or who have sustained losses.

    B. Those who have been separated from caregivers or whose caregivers are suffering from posttraumatic distress.

    C. Those with predisaster psychopathology.

    D. Those with prior traumatic experiences.

    E. All of the above.

17.3 Relationships with the media, schools, and community organizations should be developed during which disaster phase?

    A. Predisaster.

    B. Acute disaster.

    C. Subacute disaster.

    D. Postacute disaster.

    E. Recovery phase.

17.4 Which type of therapy has the largest evidence base for children who continue to display psychopathology and sustained posttraumatic symptoms?

    A. Play therapy.

    B. Dialectical behavioral therapy.

    C. Cognitive-behavior therapy.

    D. Supportive therapy.

    E. A and C.

17.5 What is the role of psychopharmacology during and following disasters?

    A. Medications should be prescribed for the majority of children who have experienced a disaster.

    B. Medications can be useful for a select minority of children in both the acute and postacute phases, and range from antidepressants to anxiolytics to antipsychotics.

    C. Medications should not be prescribed to children in the disaster setting.

    D. Selective serotonin reuptake inhibitors are the only class of medication that has a role in disaster psychiatry.

    E. Medications should be rapidly titrated upward.

References

Ablon SL: The therapeutic action of play. J Am Acad Child Adolesc Psychiatry 35:545–549, 1996

American Psychiatric Association: Diagnostic and Statistical Manual of Mental Disorders, 4th Edition, Text Revision. Washington, DC, American Psychiatric Association, 2000

Becker-Blease KA, Turner HA, Finklehor D: Disasters, victimization, and children's mental health. Child Dev 81:1040–1052, 2010

Brymer M, Jacobs A, Layne C, et al. (National Child Traumatic Stress Network/National Center for PTSD): Psychological First Aid: Field Operations Guide, 2nd Edition. July 2006. Available at: http://www.naccho.org/topics/HPDP/infectious/upload/PsyFirstAid-2.pdf. Accessed February 8, 2011.

Cassem NH, Papakostas GI, Fava M, et al: Massachusetts General Hospital Handbook of General Hospital Psychiatry, 5th Edition. Edited by Stern TA, Fricchione, Cassem NH, et al. Philadelphia, PA, CV Mosby, 2004, pp 69–92

Catani C, Kohiladevy M, Ruf M, et al: Treating children traumatized by war and tsunami: a comparison between exposure therapy and meditation-relaxation in North-East Sri Lanka. BMC Psychiatry 9:22, 2009

Catani C, Gewirtz AH, Wieling E, et al: Tsunami, war, and cumulative risk in the lives of Sri Lankan schoolchildren. Child Dev 81:1176–1191, 2010

Chemtob CM, Nakashima J, Hamada RS: Psychosocial intervention for postdisaster trauma symptoms in elementary school children: a controlled community field study. Arch Pediatr Adolesc Med 156:211–216, 2002

Chemtob CM, Nomura Y, Josephson L, et al: Substance use and functional impairment among adolescents directly exposed to the 2001 World Trade Center attacks. Disasters 33:337–352, 2009

Chess S, Thomas A: Origins and Evolution of Behavior Disorders: From Infancy to Early Adult Life. Cambridge, MA, Harvard University Press, 1984

Cohen JA, Burnet W, Dunne JE, et al: Practice parameters for the assessment and treatment of children and adolescents with posttraumatic stress disorder. J Am Acad Child Adolesc Psychiatry 37 (suppl):4S–26S, 1998

Cohen JA, Mannarino AP, Gibson LE, et al: Interventions for children and adolescents following disasters, in Interventions Following Mass Violence and Disasters: Strategies for Mental Health Practice. Edited by Ritchie EC, Watson PJ, Friedman MJ. New York, Guilford, 2006a, pp 227–256

Cohen JA, Mannarino AP, Deblinger E: Treating Trauma and Traumatic Grief in Children and Adolescents. New York, Guilford, 2006b

Disaster Psychiatry Outreach: The Essentials of Disaster Psychiatry: A Training Course for Mental Health Professionals (Course Syllabus). New York, Disaster Psychiatry Outreach, 2008. Available as DPOCourseSyllabus_052108.pdf at: https://sites.google.com/a/disasterpsych.org/blog/File-Cabinet. Accessed December 28, 2009.

Donnelly CL: Pharmacologic treatment approaches for children and adolescents with posttraumatic stress disorder. Child Adolesc Psychiatr Clin North Am 12:251–269, 2003

Flynn BW, Nelson ME: Understanding the needs of children following large scale disasters and the role of government. Child Adolesc Psychiatr Clin North Am 7:211–227, 1998

Gardner DM, Baldessarini RJ, Waraich P: Modern antipsychotic drugs: a critical overview. CMAJ 2005;172:1703–1711, 2005

Goenjian AK, Karayan I, Pynoos RS, et al: Outcome of psychotherapy among early adolescents after trauma. Am J Psychiatry 154:536–542, 1997

Green WH: Sympathomimetic amines and central nervous system stimulants, in Child and Adolescent Clinical Psychopharmacology. Philadelphia, PA, Lippincott Williams & Wilkins, 2007, pp 55–90

Guy W: Abnormal Involuntary Movement Scale (AIMS), in ECDEU Assessment Manual for Psychopharmacology—Revised (DHEW Publ No ADM 76-338). Washington, DC, U.S. Department of Health, Education and Welfare, 1976. Available at: http://flmedicaidbh.fmhi.usf.edu/pdf/AIMS_Quest.pdf. Accessed July 7, 2010.

Haiti earthquake: stories from the survivors. Times Online, January 15, 2010. Available at: http://www.timesonline.co.uk/tol/news/world/us_and_americas/article6987620.ece. Accessed July 6, 2010.

Holbrook TL, Galarneau MR, Dye JL, et al: Morphine use after combat injury in Iraq and post-traumatic stress disorder. N Engl J Med 362:110–117, 2010

Jaycox LH: CBITS: Cognitive-Behavioral Intervention for Trauma in Schools. Frederick, CO, Sopris West, 2003

Kassam-Adams N, Marsac ML, Cirilli C: Posttraumatic stress disorder symptom structure in injured children: functional impairment and depression symptoms in a confirmatory factor analysis. J Am Acad Child Adolesc Psychiatry 49:616–625, 2010

Kataoka SH, Nadeem E, Wong M, et al: Improving disaster mental health care in schools: a community-partnered approach. Am J Prev Med 37(suppl):S225–S229, 2009

Klingman A: School based interventions following a disaster, in Children and Disasters. Edited by Saylor CF. New York, Plenum, 1993, pp 165–186

Kovacs M: The natural history and course of depressive disorders in childhood. Psychiatric Annals 15:387–389, 1985

Lane RD, Glazer WM, Hansen TE, et al: Assessment of tardive dyskinesia using the Abnormal Involuntary Movement Scale. J Nerv Ment Dis 173:353–357, 1985

Laor N, Wolmer L: Children exposed to disaster: the role of the mental health professional, in Lewis's Child and Adolescent Psychiatry. Edited by Martin A, Volkmar FR. Philadelphia, PA, Lippincott Williams & Wilkins, 2007, pp 727–739

Lorberg BA, Prince JB: Psychopharmacological management of children and adolescents, in Massachusetts General Hospital Handbook of General Hospital Psychiatry, 6th Edition. Edited by Stern TA, Fricchione GL, Cassem NH, et al. Philadelphia, PA, Saunders Elsevier, 2010, pp 467–498

Masten AS, Osofsky JD: Disasters and their impact on child development: introduction to the special section. Child Dev 81:1029–1039, 2010

Masten AS, Best KM, Garmezy N: Resilience and development: contributions from the study of children who overcome adversity. Dev Psychopathol 2:425–444, 1990

Munetz MR, Benjamin S: How to examine patients using the Abnormal Involuntary Movement Scale. Hosp Community Psychiatry 39:1172–1177, 1988

National Commission on Children and Disasters: 2010 Report to the President and Congress (AHRQ Publ No 10-M037). Rockville, MD, Agency for Heathcare Research and Quality, October 2010

Pfefferbaum B, Nixon SJ, Krug RS, et al: Clinical needs assessment of middle and high school students following the 1995 Oklahoma City bombing. Am J Psychiatry 156:1069–1074, 1999

Pine DS, Cohen JA: Trauma in children and adolescents: risk and treatment of psychiatric sequelae. Biol Psychiatry 51:519–531, 2002

Saxe G, Stoddard F, Courtney D, et al: Relationship between acute morphine and course of PTSD in children with burns: a pilot study. J Am Acad Child Adolesc Psychiatry 40:915–921, 2001

Saxe GN, Ellis BH, Kaplow J: Collaborative Treatment of Traumatized Children and Teens: The Trauma Systems Therapy Approach. New York, Guilford, 2006

Schechter N, Berde CB, Yaster M (eds): Pain in Infants, Children and Adolescents. Baltimore, MD, Williams & Wilkins, 2003, pp 128–141

Schreiber M, Gurwitch R: Listen, protect, and connect: psychological first aid for children and parents. Washington, DC, Ready.gov, 2006. Available at: http://www.ready.gov/kids/_downloads/PFA_SchoolCrisis.pdf. Accessed March 15, 2008.

Shaw JA, Espinel Z, Shultz JM (eds): Children: Stress, Trauma and Disasters. Tampa, FL, Disaster Life Support Publishing, 2007

Spetie L, Arnold EL: Attention deficit/hyperactivity disorder, in Lewis's Child and Adolescent Psychiatry. Edited by Martin A, Volkmar FR. Philadelphia, PA, Lippincott Williams & Wilkins, 2007, pp 430–454

Stoddard FJ: Care of infants, children and adolescents with burn injuries, in Child and Adolescent Psychiatry, 3rd Edition. Edited by Lewis M. Philadelphia, PA, Lippincott Williams & Wilkins, 2002, pp 1188–1208

Stoddard FJ, Menninger EW: Guidance for parents and other caretakers after disasters or terrorist attacks, in Disaster Psychiatry Handbook. Edited by Hall RCW, Ng AT, Norwood AE. Washington, DC, American Psychiatric Association, 2004, pp 44–56

Stoddard F, Saxe G: Ten-year research review of physical injuries. J Am Acad Child Adolesc Psychiatry 40:1128–1145, 2001

Stoddard FJ, Sheridan RL, Saxe G, et al: Treatment of pain in acutely burned children. J Burn Care Rehabil 23:135–156, 2002

Stoddard F, Usher C, Abrams A: Psychopharmacology in pediatric critical care. Child Adolesc Psychiatr Clin North Am 15:611–655, 2006

Stoddard FJ, Sheridan RL, Martyn JAJ, et al: Pain management, in Combat and Operational Behavioral Health. Edited by Ritchie EC. Textbooks of Military Medicine (Lenhart MK, ed). Department of the Army, Office of the Surgeon General, Borden Institute (in press)

Terr LC: Too Scared to Cry: Psychic Trauma in Childhood. New York, Basic Books, 1990

U.S. Food and Drug Administration: Antidepressant Use in Children, Adolescents, and Adults. May 2, 2007. Available at: http://www.fda.gov/drugs/drug-safety/informationbydrugclass/ucm096273.htm. Accessed January 16, 2011.

Wethington HR, Hahn RA, Fuqua-Whitley DS, et al: The effectiveness of interventions to reduce psychological harm from traumatic events among children and adolescents: a systematic review. Am J Prev Med 35:287–313, 2008

Winnicott DW: Transitional objects and transitional phenomena, in Collected papers: Through Paediatrics to Psycho-Analysis 41:585–595, 1951

Wolmer L, Laor N, Yazgan Y: School reactivation programs after disaster: could teachers serve as clinical mediators? Child Adolesc Psychiatr Clin North Am 12:363–381, 2003

Wolmer L, Laor N, Dedeoglu C, et al: Teacher-mediated intervention after disaster: a controlled three-year follow-up of children's functioning. J Child Psychol Psychiatry 46:1161–1168, 2005

Wong M, Stein B, Jaycox L, et al: Cognitive behavioral intervention for trauma in schools. Los Angeles, UCLA Health Services Research Center, 2002. Available at: http://www.hsrcenter.ucla.edu/research/cbits.shtml. Accessed January 16, 2011.

Wozniak J, Biederman J, Richards JA: Diagnostic and therapeutic dilemmas in the management of pediatric-onset bipolar disorder. J Clin Psychiatry 62 (suppl 14):10–15, 2001

Young BH: The immediate response to disaster: guidelines for adult psychological first aid, in Interventions Following Mass Violence and Disasters: Strategies for Mental Health Practice. Edited by Ritchie EC, Watson PJ, Friedman MJ. New York, Guilford, 2006, pp 134–154

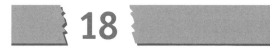

18

Geriatric Psychiatry Interventions

Kenneth Sakauye, M.D.

Disasters cause disproportionately high rates of morbidity and mortality in the elderly population (Fernandez et al. 2002). For elderly people, the most common psychiatric outcomes are anxiety, depression, and memory complaints rather than posttraumatic stress disorder (PTSD) (Galea et al. 2008). Interventions in the elderly are largely based on evidence from Class III (nonexperimental study) or Class IV (committee reports or opinions and/or clinical experience of respected authorities), and the strength of recommendations is largely Level D (directly based on Class IV evidence or extrapolated from Class I [randomized controlled trial or meta-analysis of randomized controlled trials], Class II [controlled study without randomization or other type of quasi-experimental study], or Class III evidence).

General Evaluation of Risk

General issues in acute evaluation are discussed in Chapter 5, "Psychiatric Evaluation." In addition, the American Association for Geriatric Psychiatry (AAGP) Disaster Preparedness Task Force reviewed the existing literature and prepared a position statement about the needs of the elderly population (Sakauye et al. 2009). Underreporting about, lack of attention to, and lack of statistics specific to this age group were evident in the Haiti earthquake in January 2010, although virtually all geriatric organization blogs and Web sites, as well as some news stories, highlighted the unique problems facing frail elderly survivors. A key variable that is not well addressed in current research is the appraisal of the postdisaster stress (sense of control vs. hopelessness) felt by elderly persons.

The dominant current view rests on the dose-response hypothesis for identifying who has the greatest risk for negative outcomes. The Substance Abuse and Mental Health Services Administration (SAMHSA) outlined six broad groups in decreasing order of risk for psychiatric sequelae after a disaster. This list applies equally to the elderly population (U.S. Department of Health and Human Services 2003). As shown in Table 18–1, this hierarchy roughly corresponds to the Severity of Psychosocial Stressors Scale (Axis IV) in DSM-III-R (American Psychiatric Association 1987), which rates severity of stress from no stress to catastrophic stress. The revised Axis IV classification (Psychosocial and Environmental Problems) in DSM-IV and DSM-IV-TR (American Psychiatric Association 1994; 2000) does not include ratings for severity of stress.

Although SAMHSA risk groups 5 and 6 are considered to be at lower risk, even those individuals may perceive their stress as extreme because of uncertainty about the future; insecurity; loss of a supportive community, infrastructure, or essential services; having no doctors, churches, stores, phone or Internet service, transportation, or mail; interruption of treatment; and seeing little or no progress toward recovery. The following case exemplifies a typical elderly person's response in the absence of direct exposure to trauma.

> Mrs. J, an 85-year-old woman, was living in a life care community when Hurricane Katrina hit New Orleans. The residents relocated to Baton Rouge and did not experience any direct trauma. Mrs. J showed no problems until 2 months after returning to her residence, when staff noticed moderate depression with anxiety, as well as cognitive impairment. Her family had not returned, she had lost touch with many of her old friends, there was no telephone service, 90% of the staff members were new, and news reports left her convinced that it would take 10 years to even remove the debris from the city. Mrs. J felt hopeless and was mourning the loss of her city.

Unique Risks for Elderly People

An unexpected finding by the AAGP Disaster Preparedness Task Force (Sakauye et al. 2009) included the fact that older adults typically request less disaster financial aid than younger groups. This is possibly related to the perceived stigma about receiving aid, increased self-reliance, concern about loss of other entitlements, and lower reading skills or language barriers that increase difficulty navigating bureaucratic systems; whatever the

TABLE 18–1. Dose-response hypothesis of risk

SAMHSA risk group hierarchy[a] (from most to least at risk)	DSM-III-R Severity of Psychosocial Stressors Scale (Axis IV)[b]
1. Seriously injured victims; bereaved family members	Code 6: Catastrophic stressor
2. Victims with high exposure to trauma; evacuees	Codes 4–5: Extreme or severe stress
3. Bereaved extended family members and friends; rescue/recovery workers; service providers involved with death notifications and bereaved families	
4. People who lost homes, jobs, pets, valued possessions; mental health providers; clergy, chaplains; emergency health care providers; school personnel involved with survivors, families of victims; media personnel covering the disaster	
5. Government officials; groups that identify with target victim group; businesses with financial impacts	Code 3: Moderate stress
6. Community at large	

Note. SAMHSA=Substance Abuse and Mental Health Services Administration.
[a]U.S. Department of Health and Human Services (2003).
[b]American Psychiatric Association (1987).

reason, older persons have greater difficulty achieving economic recovery after a disaster (Kaniasty and Norris 1995). Outreach and direct offers of assistance are often required rather than waiting for a call for help. Social supports, which are a primary buffer against stress, are often lost after a disaster and compound the impact of loss.

Elderly persons seem to have a higher propensity not to heed governmental warnings to evacuate (Gladwin and Peacock 1997). In part, their choice may be due to prior successful disaster experiences, which may give them a false sense of security and result in an increased tendency to refuse to leave their home in the face of a pending disaster.

Elderly people who are at highest risk for negative outcomes are those who are of advanced age; who are frail or have complex medical illness; who have cognitive impairment (e.g., elderly with dementia), severe mental illness or chronic disability due to mental illness (e.g., schizophrenia, affective disorder, and depression), impaired mobility, or sensory impairment; and who lack close family caregivers or local social supports. Dementia is a special issue, because elderly individuals with dementia lack the capacity to understand or cope with stress, have an inability to communicate needs, and have a much higher risk for developing delirium during illness.

Alexithymia, which may be seen at a higher rate in the elderly, is another unique factor. Alexithymia is defined as having "no words for feelings" and encompasses a lack of awareness of affect and an inability to generate "signal anxiety." It has been associated with somatization and may have a neurobiological basis in a dysfunction in the anterior cingulate nucleus and amygdala (Henry et al. 2006; Paradiso et al. 2008; Taylor et al. 1999). It is unclear whether alexithymia constitutes a risk factor that increases somatization (because patients cannot cope well or anticipate needs) or represents a protective factor (because such individuals are less able to perceive emotional change and seem more resilient). For healthy older adults, life experience leading to better knowledge and coping abilities, as well as the protective effect of alexithymia, may make them, as a group, more resilient to trauma, with marginally lower rates of PTSD (Huang et al. 2010; Norris et al. 2002) (see Table 18–2).

Neurobiological Risk Factors

Little has been explored about the possible neuroendocrine or genetic vulnerability factors in elderly people. A general stress-related finding for all age groups has been mild elevation of cortisol with loss of diurnal variability, which has been observed in patients with depression, PTSD, Alzheimer's disease, and chronic stress. Inhibited neurotrophin response, such as a decrease in brain-derived neurotrophic factor or TrkB tyrosine kinase ac-

TABLE 18–2. Factors that influence vulnerability in the elderly population during disasters

Factors that increase vulnerability

    Decreased sensory awareness (cognitive impairment)

    Preexisting medical conditions (frailty)

    Impaired physical mobility

    Socioeconomic limitations (low income, low reading skills, language barriers)

    Preexisting psychiatric morbidity

    Social isolation

Factors that serve as buffers

    Positive social supports

    Expectability (anticipation)

Factors with bidirectional influence

    Alexithymia

Source. Sakauye et al. 2009.

tivity, has also been found in patients with a variety of psychiatric disorders, affecting neuronal mitochondrial activity and protein production. It is known that neurotrophin response is reduced in older adults (Ziegenhorn et al. 2007), making them more likely to be vulnerable to stress effects. In addition, preventing adrenergic flooding is speculatively a way to reduce evolution to PTSD. β-Adrenergic blockers (e.g., propranolol; Pitman et al. 2002), α-adrenergic blockers (e.g., prazosin; Peskind et al. 2007), and selective serotonin reuptake inhibitors (SSRIs) have all been studied for their potential to prevent the autonomic hyperarousal that is thought to lead to progression of anxiety disorders or depression. As detailed in Chapters 15 and 16 on acute psychopharmacology and postacute psychopharmacology, respectively, the efficacy of these agents has not yet been conclusively demonstrated in younger patients, and their safety and tolerability in older patients have not been tested.

Psychiatric Outcomes

The hierarchy of responses first described by Lindemann (1944) after the Cocoanut Grove nightclub fire is still the most commonly used conceptual framework for estimating the mental health effects of disasters. In response to acute trauma, people may experience a range of reactions. The majority of people will cope well, many will have immediate minor stress responses, some will experience delayed responses of anxiety and depression, and a few will develop persistent PTSD. This model can be graphed as illustrated in Figure 18–1, with increasingly fewer people showing persisting problems over time. In general, most people are resilient, including the elderly.

Estimates of rates of specific mental illnesses following a disaster differ widely by the type of disaster, extent of destruction, speed of recovery from the disaster, and individual factors. The Community Advisory Group (CAG) surveyed 815 adults who had lived in the areas hit by Hurricane Katrina and who had requested help from the Red Cross. Interviews were conducted 5–8 months after the disaster and again 1 year after that. Although an age breakdown was not provided for the sample, 41.8% showed serious mental illness or PTSD 18 months after the hurricane, and 6.4% showed persisting suicidal ideation (Kessler et al. 2008). In general, in the geriatric population, mood, anxiety, and PTSD symptoms that are seen in younger adults occur less reliably, and acute stress may be expressed in a somatic way (Amore et al. 2007). A rise in substance abuse does not appear to be as much of a problem as in younger populations.

Mild memory impairment following trauma has been an underrecognized problem in the elderly population. After Hurricane Katrina, this was commonly referred to as "Katrina brain" by the locals. It has been a general finding that anxiety often leads to a memory disorder. In older persons under extreme stress, one often sees entrenched memories, such as in PTSD, or the converse of amnesia or thought blocking. The neurobiological basis has been speculated to be a disruption of frontocingulate circuits due to hypothalamic-pituitary-adrenal axis (HPA) and cortisol dysfunction causing disruption of cholinergic and frontal dopamine circuits. Interconnections among the thalamus, amygdala, and hippocampus suggest a reason for the strong association between memory and stress (Sakauye 2008a). The main reasons to be aware of the association of stress and memory impairment are to avoid overdiagnosing dementia in elderly persons after a disaster and to try to avoid making cognitive impairment worse through use of benzodiazepines and other tranquilizers.

Intervention Strategies

Disaster response can be conceptually divided into three phases: immediate response (first week or so), early or acute response (1 week to 2 months), and late or postacute response (2 months and longer). In all phases, care providers must be alert to the risk of negative psychiatric outcomes after a disaster and know the signs of emotional distress (Substance Abuse and Mental Health Services Administration, "The Spirit of Recovery: All Hazards Behavioral Health Preparedness and Response—Building on the Les-

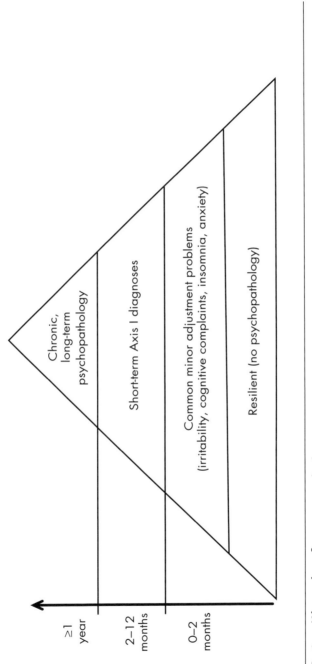

FIGURE 18–1. Hierarchy of responses to trauma.

This schematic illustrates that many people cope well after a trauma, although most will show mild adjustment difficulties early on. Intermediate effects after 2 months demonstrate that many (approximately one-third) will develop some Axis I diagnosis. Some will experience long-term problems, but not the majority of trauma victims.

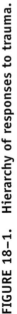

sons of Hurricanes Katrina, Rita, and Wilma"; unpublished notes from a meeting held in New Orleans, LA, May 22–24, 2006).

In general for the elderly, at any phase of response, it is important to do the following:

- Triage for patients at risk
- Check for prior psychiatric history
- Avoid interruption of psychotropic medication treatment
- Screen for depression, anxiety, cognitive impairment, and psychosis
- Check for substance use
- Avoid medications on the Beers Criteria for potentially inappropriate medications in older adults (Fick et al. 2008)

Patients with known psychiatric illness or cognitive problems need additional support, as well as continuation of existing medications. Due to compromised health or cognitive impairment, elderly people are more likely to need social support to mitigate the effects of stress. In addition, responses to each phase emphasize different issues.

Immediate Response

Psychological First Aid (PFA; see Chapter 12) should be provided as an immediate response. PFA involves addressing immediate needs, ensuring immediate physical safety, attending to physical comfort, promoting social engagement, protecting from additional trauma or trauma reminders, attending to grief and spiritual issues, helping with finding family if separated from them, attending to traumatic grief, and stabilizing emotionally overwhelmed survivors. Continuation of medical treatment regimens must be assured, and psychotropic medication may be needed for anxiety or sleep. PFA has been provided in both group and individual venues (Brymer et al. 2006). Strategically, the goal of psychological first response is aimed at providing a sense of control and mastery over the trauma.

PFA for patients with dementia is qualitatively different from that for other individuals. One can anticipate agitation in most dementia patients after a trauma. Even minor life changes can feel catastrophic to a patient with dementia and cause agitation. Having an attachment figure to reassure and protect the individual in times of stress is far more beneficial than taking medication. However, if medications are needed, the main guideline in dementia care after a disaster is to avoid using medications listed in the Beers Criteria for potentially inappropriate medication use in the elderly (Fick et al. 2008). Medications that are usually inappropriate include sedative psychotropics or antihistamines, or medications with high anticholinergic potential. Starting dosages for elderly patients should be 50% less than the usual starting dosages for younger patients.

Acute Response

Screening high-risk patients and doing evaluations on the high-risk group are important in the acute response phase. A triage tool for vulnerable older adults was developed after Hurricane Katrina to identify compromised elders without family help. Developed by Dyer et al. (2008), this simple screening instrument taps three main areas: 1) not having any social support or being separated from social supports; 2) existing health, memory, or activities of daily living (ADL) limitations; and 3) need for case management. In addition, it is essential to avoid interruption of psychiatric and medical treatment to minimize the risk of relapse. After high-risk or symptomatic individuals are identified, they should be referred for treatment or further evaluation. Appropriate response is impossible to achieve if a large geographic area has been devastated and the social infrastructure has been destroyed. In the absence of hospitals, gas, water, electricity, roads, food distribution, housing, sewage, medical supplies, telephone, and professionals, patients cannot receive help locally. Arrangements must be available for evacuation to intact service areas if needed.

The most common needs in this phase are primarily social and environmental. Important goals are to reunify families, rebuild the infrastructure to make life livable, provide reliable information, continue medications, and evacuate the most severely impaired to a place where hospital care can be provided.

Dementia care requires a stable and expectable environment, preferably with familiar people or family. Adding psychotropic medications should be avoided, but if patients need them, they should not be given highly sedating medications, benzodiazepines, or highly anticholinergic medications. Restraints should also be avoided because they often increase agitation. Behavioral management techniques include stimulus control, cognitive-behavioral techniques such as skill elicitation or differential reinforcement, reorientation, structured social activities, and staff training on improving communication techniques (Sakauye 2008b).

Postacute Response

In the postacute phase, some patients will need formal psychiatric treatment. Psychotherapy and psychotropic medications may be needed.

There is no best treatment approach for anxiety disorders, partly because there are many subtypes of anxiety disorders, and most studies focus only on generalized anxiety disorder or PTSD. Also, few outcome studies have specifically addressed elderly people. Typically, the psychotherapy choice consists of eclectic models that are matched with the person. According to a review of the literature, the following treatment hierarchy is applied: First, patients are taught palliative or distraction techniques (relaxation exercises, meditation, soothing thoughts). If symptoms persist, cognitive-behavioral therapy (CBT) is tried. The goal is to help the patient gain control over specific symptoms through problem-solving skills, guided imagery, or psychoeducation. Some patients will need more time-intensive, insight-oriented therapies that focus on developing awareness and understanding of unconscious influences on present behaviors and unconscious resistances (Sakauye 2008a). Medication approaches have shifted to use of antidepressants—namely SSRIs or serotonin-norepinephrine reuptake inhibitors (SNRIs)—as the initial trial. In older adults, treatment of major psychiatric disorders, such as major depression or psychosis, does not differ from traditional approaches.

Dementia patients may seem worse after a disaster. It is unclear whether the apparent deterioration in cognition and ADL functions is permanent or whether the patient can recover. The appearance of psychiatric symptoms, such as psychosis, depression, or agitated behaviors, is assumed to be reversible.

Preparation

Because of the nearly global lack of attention to elderly issues in the literature to date, it is imperative to designate elderly people as a special population within state disaster plans (see Chapter 6, "Special Populations," for discussion of other groups). The AAGP Disaster Preparedness Task Force (Sakauye et al. 2009) recommends the following:

- Modify state disaster plans to include special plans for frail elderly and dementia patients that address communication needs to ensure that the elderly are warned of impending disasters when possible.
- Have special precautions for the frail elderly, such as safe houses; train care providers on unique population needs (e.g., dementia management).
- Have MedicAlert jewelry or microchip implants, as well as electronic medical records that can be accessed from distant sites, to avoid interruption of treatment.
- Train first responders to deal with frail elderly.
- Establish services for frail elderly or dementia patients and contingency plans in the event the primary plan falls short.
- Develop plans to prevent separation from family and pets.

- Identify programs that deal with the elderly; make prior arrangements with the state or federal agencies in charge to involve these programs in recovery efforts.

In *Geriatric Mental Health Disaster and Emergency Preparedness,* Toner et al. (2010) address many of the issues listed above in more detail. The authors describe several examples of model disaster response programs, including the collaborative Geriatric Emergency Preparedness and Response initiative and the Canadian model. They emphasize the importance of team management and training. One model involved special training using character role-play cards to teach how to deliver care to special populations. The dissemination of similar training through the Red Cross might be an important first step in improving geriatric disaster care.

Conclusion

It is important to recognize that most elderly are survivors but are still at risk for psychiatric problems after a trauma, especially if they are frail or have a cognitive or health disability. Activities of daily living (ADL) limitations and cognition should be assessed in all elderly, and family support should be assessed if there are any limitations. It is crucial to continue existing treatment to prevent potential relapse of any preexisting illness. It is also important to avoid benzodiazepines, sedative antihistamines, anticholinergic medications, and polypharmacy because of known risks for falls and confusion.

■ Teaching Points

- Proximity to the disaster is only one risk factor. How one views the disaster and the degree of helplessness engendered are probably more salient in determining which people will show psychiatric sequelae after a disaster.

- Elderly people may actually be better prepared than younger people for a disaster because they often have previously experienced milder disasters and scares; however, they may be least willing to heed advice to evacuate or move.

- The most vulnerable elderly are those who have a physical or mental disability or prior psychiatric history.

- Lack of social supports is a major challenge in care determinations.

- Psychiatrists should be careful not to overdiagnose dementia, because mild cognitive impairment is quite common for elderly persons who are under stress.

- Major goals of Psychological First Aid (PFA) are to give hope, provide physical comfort, promote social engagement, reunify families, and provide accurate information about what to expect and what is happening. An additional goal of PFA is making sure that an attachment figure is available to guide an elderly patient.

Review Questions

18.1 Which of the following circumstances may pose the highest risk for developing postdisaster psychiatric problems?

A. Having lost a pet or valued possession.
B. Having been bereaved of a friend.
C. Owning a business severely impacted by the disaster.
D. Being a rescue worker.
E. Having the trait of alexithymia.

18.2 The most common psychiatric condition in elderly people 2 months after a disaster is

A. Panic disorder.
B. Major depressive disorder.
C. Memory impairment.
D. Somatoform disorder.
E. PTSD.

18.3 A class of psychiatric medications that may help prevent PTSD after a disaster is

A. α-Adrenergic blockers (e.g., prazosin).
B. Sedative antihistamines (e.g., diphenhydramine).
C. Atypical antipsychotics (e.g., quetiapine).
D. Benzodiazepines (e.g., clonazepam).
E. Anticonvulsants (e.g., valproic acid).

18.4 An especially important component of Psychological First Aid for dementia patients is

A. Institutional care.
B. An attachment figure.
C. Sensory reduction (quiet time, isolation).
D. Reorientation.
E. Sensitivity to culture and diversity.

18.5 In treating chronic anxiety after a trauma, the most commonly used psychotherapy approach with elderly people is

 A. Validation therapy.
 B. Cognitive-behavioral therapy.
 C. Psychodynamic psychotherapy.
 D. Reminiscence therapy.
 E. Cognitive enhancement therapy.

References

American Psychiatric Association: Diagnostic and Statistical Manual of Mental Disorders, 3rd Edition, Revised. Washington, DC, American Psychiatric Association, 1987

Amore M, Tagariello P, Laterza C, et al: Beyond nosography of depression in elderly. Arch Gerontol Geriatr 44 (suppl):13–22, 2007

Brymer M, Jacobs A, Layne C, et al. (National Child Traumatic Stress Network/National Center for PTSD): Psychological First Aid: Field Operations Guide, 2nd Edition. July 2006. Available at: http://www.naccho.org/topics/HPDP/infectious/upload/PsyFirstAid-2.pdf. Accessed February 8, 2011.

Dyer CB, Regev M, Burnett J, et al: SWiFT: a rapid triage tool for vulnerable older adults in disaster situations. Disaster Med Public Health Prep 2 (suppl):S45–S50, 2008

Fernandez LS, Byard D, Chien-Chih L, et al: Frail elderly as disaster victims: emergency management strategies. Prehosp Disaster Med 7:67–74, 2002

Fick DM, Cooper JW, Wade WE, et al: Updating the Beers criteria for potentially inappropriate medication use in older adults: results of a US consensus panel of experts. Arch Intern Med 163:2716–2724, 2008

Galea S, Tracy M, Norris F, et al: Financial and social circumstances and the incidence and course of PTSD in Mississippi during the first two years after hurricane Katrina. J Trauma Stress 21:357–368, 2008

Gladwin H, Peacock WG: Warning and evacuation: a night for hard houses, in Hurricane Andrew: Ethnicity, Gender, and the Sociology of Disasters. Edited by Peacock WG, Morrow BH, Gladwin H. London, UK, Routledge, 1997, pp 52–74

Henry JD, Phillips LH, Maylor EA, et al: A new conceptualization of alexithymia in the general adult population: implications for research involving older adults. J Psychosom Res 60:535–543, 2006

Huang P, Tan H, Liu A, et al: Prediction of posttraumatic stress disorder among adults in flood districts. BMC Public Health 10:207, 2010

Kaniasty K, Norris FH: In search of altruistic community: patterns of social support mobilization following Hurricane Hugo. Am J Community Psychol 23:447–477, 1995

Kessler RC, Galea S, Gruber MJ, et al: Trends in mental illness and suicidality after Hurricane Katrina. Mol Psychiatry 13:374–384, 2008

Lindemann E: Symptomatology and management of acute grief. Am J Psychiatry 101:141–148, 1944

Norris FH, Kaniasty K, Conrad ML, et al: Placing age differences in cultural context: a comparison of the effects of age on PTSD after disasters in the United States, Mexico, and Poland. J Clin Geropsychol 8:153–173, 2002

Paradiso S, Vaidya JG, McCormick LM, et al: Aging and alexithymia: association with reduced right rostral cingulate volume. Am J Geriatr Psychiatry 16:760–769, 2008

Peskind ER, Bonner LT, Hoff DJ: Prazosin reduces trauma-related nightmares in older men with chronic posttraumatic stress disorder. J Geriatr Psychiatry Neurol 164:1693–1999, 2007

Pitman RK, Sanders KM, Zusman RM, et al: Pilot study of secondary prevention of posttraumatic stress disorder with propranolol. Biol Psychiatry 51:189–192, 2002

Sakauye KM: Anxiety disorders, in Geriatric Psychiatry Basics. Edited by Sakauye KM. New York, WW Norton, 2008a, pp 160–172

Sakauye KM: Treating behavioral disturbances associated with dementia, in Geriatric Psychiatry Basics. Edited by Sakauye KM. New York, WW Norton, 2008b, pp 98–119

Sakauye KM, Streim JE, Kennedy GJ, et al: AAGP position statement: disaster preparedness for older Americans: critical issues for the preservation of mental health. Am J Geriatr Psychiatry 17:916–924, 2009

Taylor GJ, Bagby RM, Parker JDA: Disorders of Affect Regulation: Alexithymia in Medical and Psychiatric Illness. New York, Cambridge University Press, 1999

Toner JA, Meirswa TM, Howe JL (eds): Geriatric Mental Health Disaster and Emergency Preparedness. New York, Springer, 2010

U.S. Department of Health and Human Services: Mental Health All-Hazards Disaster Planning Guidance (DHHS Publ No SMA 3829). Rockville, MD, Center for Mental Health Services, Substance Abuse and Mental Health Services Administration, 2003. Available at: http://store.samhsa.gov/product/SMA03-3829. Accessed September 2009.

Ziegenhorn AA, Schulte-Herbruggen O, Danker-Hopfe H, et al: Serum neurotrophins: a study on the time course and influencing factors in a large old age sample. Neurobiol Aging 28:1436–1445, 2007

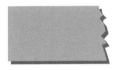

PART IV

EMERGING AND OTHER TOPICS

Frederick J. Stoddard Jr., M.D.,
Anand Pandya, M.D., and
Craig L. Katz, M.D.,
Section Editors

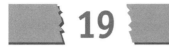

Psychiatrists as Ambassadors

Grant H. Brenner, M.D.

When people think of mental health professionals, they may often imagine private office and hospital settings and related traditional treatment models. However, in acute and ongoing disaster preparedness and response, professionals work in other roles, which may involve no direct clinical care. These roles include formal and informal consultation to various groups and organizations, ongoing professional involvement through expert opinion and collaborative work on various projects, ongoing involvement in maintaining readiness between disasters, advocacy and policy making, consultation with public health authorities, and on-site and remote work providing training, supervision, and support.

In all of these roles, it is of paramount importance for mental health professionals to comport themselves in a professional, amiable, and helpful manner in the service of providing assistance, increasing recognition of mutual interdependence with other responders, and mitigating stigma directed against mental health. They must strive to maintain standards of excellence and advocacy without compromising on important issues. The balance between diplomacy and upholding standards is a delicate and difficult one to achieve, requiring great patience and perspective. Creating a self-sustaining collaborative process requires the thoughtful nurturing of an atmosphere of safety and mutual respect and, furthermore, the balancing of frequently competing needs of diverse individuals and groups to accomplish broader overlapping goals (Brenner 2009; Disaster Psychiatry Outreach 2008).

This chapter begins with examination of key issues related to taking up nontraditional roles, typically outside of the professional office and hospital setting, under the rubric of "psychiatrist as ambassador." An overview of organizational consulting follows, focusing on the basics of group relations and group dynamics, the importance of taking on roles and adopting the consulting stance, and the benefits and challenges inherent in wearing many hats. The basic issues involved in interdisciplinary collaboration among religious, spiritual care, and mental health disaster workers are discussed, as well as the importance of maintaining self-care and the relevance of considering how traumatic experiences are opportunities for growth. The chapter ends with conclusions and future directions.

Ambassadorship

In the fourth edition of *The American Heritage Dictionary of the English Language* (2006), one definition of *ambassador* is "an unofficial representative: *ambassadors of goodwill.*" In various senses, the disaster mental health professional serves as an emissary and representative of the field, entering into literal and metaphorical foreign territory where mental health perspectives are not necessarily native. The intent is to be an ambassador of goodwill whenever possible, while also pursuing myriad other goals. Developing the skills and experience to balance so many competing forces requires sustained effort and a solid understanding of multiple areas of expertise.

Each professional must take up ambassadorship uniquely and individually, making use of himself or herself as a person across roles. There is no one recipe for doing this, only heuristic guidelines and complementary frameworks for understanding that are not within the usual purview of psychiatric training. A specific factor that is important to note is the (often accurate) perception that psychiatrists tend to "overpathologize," identifying disease and disorder where none is present. Considering that in the acute phases of disasters, the majority of survivor responses are normal (Disaster Psychiatry Outreach 2008), it is important for the mental health professional to be aware of this perception and to exercise tact, both to avoid alienating colleagues and to provide appropriate care and consultation, free from over- and underpathologizing and from excessive medicalization of experience.

Group relations theory furnishes useful tools for the disaster mental health professional in unfamiliar settings. The important concepts of person in role, core elements of psychoanalytic theory, viewing the group as an entity unto itself ("group as a whole"), and other key considerations (expanded below) are the foundations of group relations theory. Because each disaster is unique and disasters expand the boundaries of ordinary experience, working as an ambassador presents gratifying creative challenges, demanding artfulness and subtlety. Simultaneously, the same psychiatrist must be able to make optimal use of himself or herself—tuning into intuition, common sense, the basic ability to keep a level head, and other skills that take long years to polish—to accomplish various, often shifting, goals.

Collaboration

One of the most important functions that a disaster psychiatrist can serve is to facilitate the development of short- and long-term collaborative processes for the groups with whom the professional is working. In the acute phases of disaster, collaboration is comparatively easy to achieve because the sense of immediacy and urgency demands a pragmatic focus. This situation parallels an acute care setting (e.g., operating room, emergency department, intensive care unit) in which people temporarily set aside differences to work on clear tasks. As time wanes and passes into the postacute phases, the sense of acuity dissipates, interorganizational agendas begin to predominate, and individual burnout increases, leading to the erosion of existing collaborative processes and preventing their ongoing development. Several strategies can be employed in an effort to sustain collaboration under such circumstances, including but not limited to regular meetings that incorporate an ongoing discussion of how to continue to work collaboratively; a clear delineation of different groups' goals and responsibilities (including areas of overlap and areas of differentiation); and the use of organizational strategies to explicitly manage work flow (Brenner 2009). In an important sense, collaborative practice for the group is akin to maintaining routines of self-care for the individual, which are essential to maintain, costly when resources are scarce, and easy to neglect.

A potential problem arises when outside disaster psychiatrists enter into an affected community, offering assistance out of genuine goodwill, but potentially alienating and marginalizing local professionals. Important tasks such as identifying and coordinating with local psychiatrists may fall through the cracks. Even when such efforts are made, a variety of influences (e.g., competition, the effects of traumatic experience on interpersonal relationships, a lack of need for additional help) may create difficulties when local and outside groups respond to the same situation. (These considerations are addressed in greater depth in Chapter 1, "Preparation and Systems Issues.") The following case vignette demonstrates some problems that can result from lack of collaboration.

> Following Hurricane Katrina, a large group of outside responders descended on New Orleans to offer assistance. Among this group were disaster mental health professionals, including psychiatrists from distant health

care systems and from national professional organizations. While their help was appreciated and useful, some local psychiatrists reported that although they themselves had the requisite skills and willingness to offer assistance, they were not contacted by the outside organizations and were left out of planning and response. Several years later, these local psychiatrists continue to report significant feelings of resentment.

Such dynamics create difficulties beyond the time of the disaster. Persisting negative feelings are impediments to future collaborative efforts. Lack of collaboration not only sets in motion personal bad feelings but also sows the seeds for systemic inefficiency.

Group and Systems Perspectives: Group Relations Theory

A brief review of group relations theory is helpful for the psychiatrist intending to work within the milieu of disaster response. Wilfred Bion, an object relations–oriented psychoanalyst and military psychiatrist, developed group therapy approaches to be able to work with large numbers of soldiers in the absence of sufficient individual therapists after World War II. He chronicled his findings in his book *Experiences in Groups* (Bion 1961).

Subsequent thinkers, notably with the A. K. Rice Institute for the Study of Social Systems and the Tavistock Institute of Human Relations, have expanded Bion's work. The perspective they describe is psychoanalytically informed. The object of study is the group as a whole; the individual group member is not viewed exclusively as an individual. Whatever the individual gives voice to is understood as coming both from his or her individual personality and experience as well as, importantly, from what he or she is "holding" on behalf of the group. The group, like an individual, is influenced by powerful unconscious forces of which it is only peripherally aware. For example, in a process group, the work of the group is directed toward understanding and articulating these unconscious forces, reflecting on them as they unfold within the group ("reflection-in-action").

Because unconscious forces are even more powerful in the context of disaster response, conceptualizing the group as a whole and seeing oneself as voicing aspects of group experience, in the service of the group, is a powerful lens. Similarly, it is important to listen to what others say in the same way. This perspective provides information about what is going on, which can be used to positively influence the process and to more effectively situate oneself in relation to the work. Doing so requires a high level of reflective function and a willingness to look diligently beneath the surface. Primitive psychological processes, such as splitting, projective identification, and scapegoating, among others, predominate in a group that is not functioning well (Wells 1985).

Bion (1961), through his work with many groups, developed the perspective that groups exist in two essential states—the *working group* and the *basic assumption group*. Groups oscillate between these states, which often also overlap, occurring simultaneously. In the working group, the group cohesively addresses its stated task(s). It is minimally mired down in destructive dynamics that interfere with work. In the basic assumption group, the group is caught up in maladaptive defenses and repetitive destructive interpersonal patterns that interfere with its working effectively on its stated task(s).

Although subsequent thinkers have described additional basic assumption configurations, Bion (1961) initially described three basic assumption groups: fight-flight, pairing, and dependency groups. In the *fight-flight group,* the group is controlled by fear and vacillates between avoidance and conflict. The worst-case scenario for this group, at either end of the spectrum, is to completely fall apart and stop meeting or to be constantly preoccupied with internal fighting. In the *pairing group,* varying dyads form powerful relationships, with the unconscious and sometimes conscious motivation to rescue the group, and the presumption that the group has unconsciously "put them up to it." These pairings may seem hopeful, and may be productive at times, but generally prevent the group from focusing collectively on its work by displacing the focus onto different pairs. Finally, in the *dependency group,* the group and its members become de-skilled, and look to one member to do all the work or depose the group leader, in effect electing an imaginary savior who keeps the group from the difficult and painful process of getting to work (Bion 1961).

Role and Consulting Stance

Although it is not useful or appropriate to take on the role of therapist while working with nontherapeutic groups, elements of the therapist role may be useful to the psychiatric ambassador. The disaster psychiatrist may take on many roles, sometimes more than one role simultaneously. Therefore, it is of utmost importance to have a conceptual framework to help manage the many hats one may wear.

"Role" is a foundational notion. A role is neither a rigid position nor an inauthentic "act" one plays. Rather, taking on a particular role provides an organizing framework for interfacing effectively with other people and the context. Roles translate and mediate among selves and contexts. According to Shapiro and Carr (1991), awareness of specific role(s) provides a "holding environment that allows for containment of impulses and affirmation of individual experience as it interacts with the experiences of others" (p. 77). Likewise, "membership in an organization creates a shared notion of task that sustains individuals in their roles. So long as we have a sense of what we belong to, we can struggle to discover the task the organization is performing in the roles we have in relation to that task" (p. 77). Consultants are defined as "individuals who, in using and interpreting their feelings in their roles, stand both inside and outside themselves, and both inside and outside their organizations. Such consultants become immersed in the dynamics of the organization and consciously try to discover within themselves and through their own experiences a sense of the issues that are important to the organization. They consider how their feelings generated in their roles reflect both organizational process and an outside perspective" (p. 81).

In the consulting stance, one adopts an essential reflective attitude toward group process and content, and toward one's own internal individual processes as they interact with the context. Several elements are requisite for taking the consulting stance: 1) one should have a basic awareness of group dynamics and group process (as noted above); 2) one should be aware of one's role(s) and internal responses; 3) one should be aware of how others may perceive oneself; and 4) one should be aware of one's own countertransferential responses. A challenge to the consultant's professional role is the necessity to manage and contain chaotic forces (e.g., anger, seductiveness) in order to be effective and avoid getting drawn into destructive enactments (e.g., taking sides, giving favors). Destructive enactments result from the loss of self-reflection and the use of dissociative defenses (e.g., distancing, overinvolvement) in the face of the overwhelming experience encountered by the consultant. The hazards of destructive enactments are present in ordinary treatment settings—such as in process groups, inpatient wards, hospital administrations, and emergency departments—and may be much amplified in the charged atmosphere of disaster preparedness and response. The consultant in the stress of disaster consultation can face a reflective balancing act between urges to self-protectively retreat away from and wishes to rapidly engage in helping.

Several key elements are required to be an effective consultant. In addition to having awareness of the substance or content of the work at hand, it is essential for the consultant to be aware of his or her responsibilities (which depend on the context); his or her own and others' feelings; the importance of trust and of effectively speaking to distrust when it is present; and his or her own goals and needs, as well as the goals and needs of the organization(s) he or she represents. It is necessary to thoughtfully approach the above considerations in any specific piece of work while maintaining authenticity and being aware of what expertise may appropriately be offered. This is especially true for the psychiatrist working outside of familiar settings, in which comfortable forms of authority (e.g., offering recommendations as a physician) may not be suitable. In the role of consultant-ambassador, the mental health professional is generally not directing others as to what they should do; this is a managerial role (Block 1981). As consultants, therefore, mental health professionals may provide insight, information, and the benefit of experience to guide the process and often help others to make better decisions. This theme may also be conceptualized as a shift from "interventionist" to "empowerment" approaches, in which the disaster mental health practitioner enables communities and other groups to make full use of their potential for the long haul, rather than exclusively providing direct care in the short term (Gist et al. 1998).

Finally, the nature of authority relations has arguably shifted, particularly in contemporary Western cultures, leading to a leveling of authority, greater consumerism regarding health care, and at times mistrust of traditional authority figures such as physicians (Eisold 2009). It is incumbent upon the disaster psychiatrist to take this shift into consideration when serving in multiple roles, while recognizing that in some cultures, physicians may be seen as traditionally authoritative. Adaptively flexible approaches are required, and it is often necessary to shift one's authority stance dynamically in relation to changing contextual factors, thereby adopting a pluralistic, rather than singular, approach.

Wearing Many Hats

Disaster psychiatry draws upon, integrates, and expands beyond other psychiatric areas of expertise. The disaster psychiatrist has to move fluidly among many roles. These areas of expertise include consultation-liaison psychiatry, community psychiatry, emergency psychiatry, international psychiatry, traumatology, child psychiatry, and preventive medicine, and often basic Psychological First Aid (see Chapter 12) and medical care, when required (Disaster Psychiatry Outreach 2008). Few people are expert in all of these areas, but all disaster psychiatrists must have some familiarity with each.

Furthermore, the disaster psychiatrist may also wear other hats (Disaster Psychiatry Outreach 2008): therapist, educator, supervisor, co-organizer (e.g., of conferences or work groups), expert consultant, administrator, media liaison, author, social/professional networker, activist, and anthropologist. These additional roles are as important as being skilled in providing direct care. In all of these roles, the psychiatrist must maintain an awareness of being the representative of the profession and take special note of how his or her bearing, demeanor, and conduct are perceived by others. At times, it may be difficult to keep this overarching framework in mind, especially when there are more pressing needs and work to be done. However, because of the collaborative nature of disaster work, which spans over many years, not just for the duration of one disaster, it is extremely important to continually work toward maintaining an atmosphere of thoughtful mutual respect conducive to effective collaboration.

Charged and sometimes adversarial and heated emotions get stirred up in different phases of disaster, and these emotions may threaten working relationships and interorganizational alliances (Brenner 2009; Disaster Psychiatry Outreach 2008). Therefore, to be an effective consultant, the disaster psychiatrist must maintain professionalism and a collaborative stance. By keeping this stance in mind, the psychiatrist facilitates the short- and long-term development of the field and, thereby, furthers the goal of following multiple pathways to help people in need. These pathways may include direct care of survivors and responders, effective functioning by wearing the "many hats" (taking on multiple roles), and serving as an organizational consultant in encouraging better interagency cooperation.

Disaster Mental Health, Religion, and Spiritual Care

In the aftermath of a disaster, the majority of people initially seek help from their community and from religious groups (Milstein and Manierre 2009). For instance, after the 9/11 attacks on New York City, 90% of people turned to faith-based sources for help in coping (Schuster et al. 2001). These sources of support may include personal spiritual-based practices, but such practices most often occur in the context of congregational religion and with the support of community and clergy within that faith community. It is important to note that psychiatric training and practice have traditionally neglected the importance of spirituality and religion (although there are important exceptions). Current World Psychiatric Association recommendations suggest that mental health providers should develop a more nuanced understanding of spiritual and religious practices to best serve the needs of the populations with whom they work (Cox and Gray 2009). Furthermore, some authors emphasize the need for emergency mental health responders to be aware of their own spiritual and religious perspectives when providing services (Nardi 2009), both to facilitate self-care and to avoid common pitfalls related to failure to attend to key differences.

The same issues are relevant when working with multiple disaster response groups, which in addition to including faith-based organizations, will also include individuals with diverse spiritual and religious backgrounds. As an ambassador, the disaster psychiatrist must develop an awareness of how to work effectively with religious and spiritual care–based disaster responders. Because of reluctance to appreciate religious and spiritual dimensions, mental health professionals often overlook the role of religion and spirituality. It is easy to emphasize unidirectional referrals from clergy to mental health, without recognizing the importance of working collaboratively with clergy. Disaster psychiatrists need to assess affected populations, including themselves, for how a disaster may be interfering with faith practices and routine participation in communities of faith (with family, friends, pastoral caretakers). However, for many, such interference does not occur, and a disaster bolsters faith and community cohesiveness (Milstein and Manierre 2009).

The consultant's role as an ambassador to a postdisaster community has its risks. As in any relationship, in the heated emotional setting surrounding disasters, the danger of an unwitting faux pas is magnified. Survivors, including community leaders and responders, may be especially sensitive, and if the consultant is not careful, he or she may disrupt a therapeutic and/or working alliance, which often encompasses spiritual and religious affiliations and practices. Discussion here of appropriate consideration of spiritual and religious factors in disaster work can be thought of as a proxy for other community characteristics, including cultural, ethnic, and gender differences. Creating collaborative and mutually reciprocal relationships between mental health and faith-based/spiritual-care individuals and organizations may be the single most effective way to ensure optimal resource allocation for assisting populations in need. This effort is enhanced when the disaster mental health professional is aware of how his or her own attitudes and beliefs regarding religion, spirituality, and culture affect his or her role as a consultant.

Self-Care and Growth Following Adversity

Disaster response and traumatology have traditionally focused on the concept of recovery—that is, returning to predisaster function. However, there is a growing emphasis on the importance of benefiting from the experience of disaster and trauma, going beyond recovery to what different authors have termed "posttraumatic growth" (Zoellner and Maercker 2006), "growth following adversity" (Park and Helgeson 2006), and "vicarious resilience" (Hernandez et al. 2007). These concepts are related to self-care; in focusing on growth-oriented potentialities, the individual is likely to be more resilient. When psychiatrists or other mental health professionals convey this perspective both in words and in deeds, they may positively influence the group and enhance their impact as ambassadors.

A Successful Collaboration

In early 2009, a mental health work group was charged with systematizing that part of the City of New York Family Assistance Center Plan pertaining to mental health services provision (I was a member, representing Disaster Psychiatry Outreach). The final document totaled some 250 pages, subsuming multiple levels of function essential to a coordinated disaster response involving innumerable groups. Of these 250 pages, approximately 5 are devoted to mental health and spiritual care services. These services include medical first aid, Psychological First Aid, spiritual first aid, mental health needs assessment, spiritual triage, psychiatric assessment, affected persons medical support, basic medical care, provision of medications, crisis intervention, casualty support, ministry of presence, facilitating rituals, advocacy, medical needs efficacy, medical outreach, mental health/spiritual care outreach, disaster psychiatry consultation/liaison, psychiatric treatment, faith community referrals, staff support, and postaction staff support. The various services are provided by at least six separate groups with overlapping and distinct functionalities. For each of these services, the work group developed a description of the services rendered, designated the lead agency for the service, and explicitly identified the potential agencies that might provide those specific services (City of New York 2009).

Participation in this relatively calm working group required careful attention to all of the factors reviewed in this chapter. For example, it was important to recognize who was in charge of leading the work group and to effectively follow their lead, while at the same time giving input and making suggestions as required. Furthermore, because this work group included groups with potentially different perspectives and goals, such as mental health and faith-based orientations, it was very important to bear these differences in mind during planning meetings and while crafting specific pieces of work. At the same time, as a representative of the disaster psychiatry volunteer organization, I had the responsibility of ensuring that this group's perspective was included in a respectful manner in the form of key elements that otherwise would have been omitted. Successfully accomplishing the task of the work group was facilitated by several factors: 1) a strong desire to collaborate, 2) the presence of a clear unmet need to have a systematic plan in place that unified disparate interest groups, 3) skillful leadership, 4) a history of the groups and individuals involved having worked together successfully for many years in the crucible of acute disaster response and other related activities (e.g., planning, conferences, professional networking, etc.), and 5) an atmosphere of mutual respect and appreciation of difference as well as commonality. Awareness of personal factors, emotional and psychological responses, individual past history, and so on, provided a firm unifying foundation to engage with and complete a successful project.

Conclusion

This chapter has focused on several key factors involved in disaster psychiatry ambassadorship. Given the need to enter into the alien setting of a disaster, the importance of some disaster training, and the need to adapt existing psychiatric skills, it would be easy for a disaster mental health professional to decide not to try to learn to reflect on oneself as an emissary, in order to represent psychiatry to those who are not familiar with it. Although most other disaster workers are welcoming and eager to work side by side, this is not always the case. Sometimes, this is due to stigma surrounding mental health, and in particular psychiatry. Some people have had bad experiences with psychiatry. It is important to be aware of this possibility, rather than becoming defensive, and to maintain respect and integrity. By cultivating relationships and consciously striving to be diplomatic and respectful, the disaster mental health worker stands the best chance of creating sustainable collaborative relationships and opportunities for effective intervention, empowerment, consultation, and working cooperatively by wearing those "many hats" through multiple stages of disaster. Given the multifaceted nature of disaster mental health, it is helpful to conceptualize the role of ambassador as a metarole—an overarching role that subsumes many fluidly shifting subroles.

Disaster mental health is a young field. As such, it is still inventing itself and forging new paths. In the future, the role of psychiatrist as ambassador will continue to take on greater relevance. Areas of knowledge not traditionally taught in mental health training are of growing relevance, such as building an alliance with a community over time, diplomacy, public health perspectives, conflict resolution, business and consulting models, advocacy and policy-making skills, and interface with governmental and nongovernmental groups. Failure to take on these challenges diminishes the potential contributions of the field of disaster mental health. Given the long-standing inattention and stigma toward mental health needs in society, disaster mental health advocacy is of paramount importance. By successfully engaging with the challenges inherent in disaster mental health ambassadorship, the field can expand its impact.

■ Teaching Points

- Regardless of the context, when working as a disaster mental health professional, one should always bear in mind the importance of diplomatically being a representative of the field, maintaining standards of professionalism, and acting as an ambassador of goodwill.

- Collaboration may occur easily under some circumstances, but sustaining a collaborative atmosphere generally requires ongoing effort and attention.
- Disaster mental health professionals must develop competence in many areas and learn to shift among many roles based on the demands of the context.
- Developing the capacity to maintain reflective function in spite of stress prevents disaster mental health professionals from becoming reactive and engaging in destructive enactments that interfere with working effectively.
- Paying attention to and cultivating good self-care habits, especially in stressful work environments, will both prevent negative consequences for the individual and provide a reference point for other individuals and groups.
- Mental health professionals and religious and spiritual care providers work side by side in disasters. They must be familiar with one another's perspectives and approaches in order to best serve populations in need and to work collaboratively with one another.
- A potential important outcome of disasters is not only recovery but also growth as a result of effective response to adversity.
- Developing ambassadorship skills across multiple settings and phases of disaster work is likely to facilitate positive advocacy and policy change.

Review Questions

19.1 Who developed the theory of basic assumption and working group dynamics?

    A. Fairbairn.
    B. Winnicot.
    C. Klein.
    D. Rice.
    E. Bion.

19.2 Which of the following statements regarding how psychiatrists may use authority in disaster work is *false*?

    A. It is important to recognize and assess for variations in how different individuals and groups relate to authority figures.

B.　One may generally assume that most people will view psychiatrists as trusted representatives of authority with a solid base of expertise.

C.　Authority relations are thought to have shifted significantly in the past several decades.

D.　Psychiatrists must recognize that in disaster response, there are multiple authority figures, all of whom must work together collaboratively.

E.　The disaster psychiatrist must take an adaptively flexible approach to authority relations, adjusting his or her stance to accommodate changing contextual factors.

19.3　Good reasons to refrain from pathologizing most survivors' acute reactions to disaster include all of the following *except*

A.　It is not possible to make a diagnosis of posttraumatic stress disorder based on a few days of symptoms.

B.　Most survivor responses are normal, and assigning inappropriate pathological labels may do harm.

C.　Psychiatry is seen as overpathologizing, and a persistent, inappropriate focus on identifying abnormality or dysfunction will erode goodwill and impede collaboration.

D.　It is better to routinely conceal potentially distressing clinical information from people in an effort to protect them.

E.　All of the above are good reasons.

19.4　Which of the following is *not* a key element of effective collaboration?

A.　Listening to others and respecting their skills.

B.　Having familiarity with individuals prior to working together during distressing circumstances.

C.　Knowing how to convince others that they must listen to you, the psychiatrist, because as a physician you are best qualified to be in charge.

D.　Working within preexisting frameworks based on an understanding of how different groups interrelate with one another.

E.　Having an awareness of one's own interior processes and countertransferential responses, as well as of how others may perceive oneself.

19.5 To which of the following are affected individuals likely to turn first for help and support following disasters?

    A. Mental health providers.

    B. Police and fire department personnel.

    C. Politicians.

    D. Clergy and community support.

    E. Public health officials.

References

The American Heritage Dictionary of the English Language, 4th Edition. Boston, MA, Houghton Mifflin, 2006

Bion WR: Experiences in Groups. London, Tavistock, 1961

Block P: Flawless Consulting: A Guide to Getting Your Experience Used. San Francisco, CA, Pfeiffer, 1981

Brenner G: Fundamentals of collaboration, in Creating Spiritual and Psychological Resilience: Integrating Care in Disaster Relief Work. Edited by Brenner G, Bush D, Moses J. New York, Routledge, 2009, pp 3–17

City of New York: Family Assistance Center Plan. New York, City of New York, April 17, 2009

Cox J, Gray A: Psychiatry for the person. Curr Opin Psychiatry 22:587–593, 2009

Disaster Psychiatry Outreach: The Essentials of Disaster Psychiatry: A Training Course for Mental Health Professionals (Course Syllabus). New York, Disaster Psychiatry Outreach, 2008. Available as DPOCourseSyllabus_052108.pdf at: https://sites.google.com/a/disasterpsych.org/blog/File-Cabinet. Accessed December 28, 2009.

Eisold K: What You Don't Know You Know. New York, Other Press, 2009

Gist R, Lubin B, Redburn BG: Psychosocial, ecological, and community perspectives on disaster response. J Loss Trauma 3:1, 25–51, 1998

Hernandez P, Gangsei D, Engstrom D: Vicarious resilience: a new concept and work with those who survive trauma. Fam Proc 46:229–241, 2007

Milstein G, Manierre A: Normative and diagnostic reactions to disaster: clergy and clinician collaboration to facilitate a continuum of care, in Creating Spiritual and Psychological Resilience: Integrating Care in Disaster Relief Work. Edited by Brenner G, Bush D, Moses J. New York, Routledge, 2009, pp 219–225

Nardi TJ: Religious/spiritual beliefs: a hidden resource for emergency mental health providers. Int J Emerg Ment Health 11:37–41, 2009

Park C, Helgeson V: Introduction to the special section: growth following highly stressful life events. Current status and future directions. J Consult Clin Psychol 74:791–796, 2006

Schuster MA, Stein BD, Jaycox LH, et al: A national survey of stress reactions after the September 11, 2001, terrorist attacks. N Engl J Med 345:1507–1512, 2001

Shapiro ER, Carr AW: Lost in Familiar Places: Creating New Connections Between the Individual and Society. New Haven, CT, Yale University Press, 1991, pp 75–88

Wells L Jr: The group-as-a-whole perspective and its theoretical roots, in Group Relations Reader 2. Edited by Colman AD, Geller MH. Washington, DC, AK Rice Institute, 1985

Zoellner T, Maercker A: Posttraumatic growth in clinical psychology: a critical review and introduction of a two component model. Clin Psychol Rev 26:626–653, 2006

20

Legal and Ethical Issues

Anand Pandya, M.D.

In September 1998, Swissair Flight 111 crashed in Canadian waters after taking off from JFK Airport in New York City. Dr. Ramos was working in a New York City emergency room when he received a call from the city's Department of Mental Health informing him that family members were gathering at JFK and that psychiatrists might be helpful there. At the airport, Dr. Ramos quickly became aware that many agencies felt competitive and distrustful of other agencies. He felt doubly isolated because the stigma against psychiatry seemed quite strong. Realizing that very few would spontaneously reach out to him to inform him of psychiatric needs, Dr. Ramos worked to reduce the barriers between different agencies. He humbly offered to help others with a variety of nonclinical tasks. With the help of his modeling, the guardedness and territoriality between agencies broke down.

A social worker from the Red Cross initially felt threatened by Dr. Ramos, but she eventually developed enough trust to inform Dr. Ramos about a flight attendant who had lost several colleagues on the flight. The social worker arranged for Dr. Ramos to work alongside the flight attendant so that he could talk to her. After a few minutes, the flight attendant acknowledged that she was getting light-headed because she had not taken a break to eat a meal or even get some water since the moment she heard of the crash. Dr. Ramos identified a Salvation Army volunteer nearby who was able to get the flight attendant some food and water. While eating and drinking, the flight attendant became less guarded, eventually acknowledging that she had bipolar disorder and was afraid that this disaster was going to cause her to attempt suicide again. He learned that the flight attendant had forgotten both of her psychiatric medications, lorazepam and lithium, when she rushed to the airport that morning, but she would not leave to get them because she worried that she would lose her job if anyone knew that she had a mental illness. Dr. Ramos asked enough questions to feel confident that the flight attendant was not suicidal now. He prescribed the medication and

informed the Red Cross social worker of the situation so that she could pro-
cure the lorazepam and lithium for the flight attendant. By the time Dr. Ramos went home, he felt proud that he was able to be helpful in some small
way. But then he began to worry about the ethical and legal risks of the
work that he had just done.

What if the flight attendant took an overdose on the medication he prescribed? Should he have written a note in a chart to explain why he did not
hospitalize her? And what if the Red Cross social worker told someone else
about the medications? He knew that the flight attendant would feel be-
trayed if anyone from the airlines discovered her diagnosis because of his
"loose lips."

Disaster psychiatry may be perceived initially as a low-liability practice
with a clear ethical imperative. However, there are a variety of reasons why
disaster psychiatry may pose significant legal liability and ethical challenges.
Some of these challenges are highlighted in the fictionalized vignette above,
including the fluidity of roles that is often required in disaster psychiatry, the
imperative for collaboration that may conflict with the mandates of confidentiality, the lack of charting, the urge to ignore the possibility of malingering, and the intense emotional reactions that can make it tempting to
blur boundaries. In addition, if Dr. Ramos worked long enough as a disaster
psychiatrist, he might eventually respond to disasters in other states and he
might attempt to do research to contribute to the collective understanding
of this field. These practices would force Dr. Ramos to consider further legal
and ethical issues involving licensure, malpractice coverage, and human subject protections.

Conflicting Roles and Flexibility

Dr. Ramos exemplifies how effective disaster psychiatrists switch roles frequently, serving alternately as a doctor, a general humanitarian responder,
and a consultant to help others understand or manage the psychiatric consequences of the disaster. With this flexibility of roles, it may be difficult to
pinpoint the moment when a doctor-patient relationship begins.

The demand for role flexibility in disaster psychiatry can become particularly tricky when one is serving in a role as a consultant to an organization (see Chapter 19, "Psychiatrists as Ambassadors," for further details
about this common and valuable role). In such a capacity, one may con-
ceive of one's work as serving as a consultant to a specific leader who is
seeking input. Alternatively, one may consider one's job to be pursuing the
best interests of the whole agency or set of agencies that one is observing
after a disaster—for instance, the city fire department or all state agencies
gathered at JFK Airport. Some experienced disaster psychiatrists would see

their job in a broader context and consider it their obligation to serve the best interests of the whole disaster response system and the best interests of all of the survivors and first responders who need help. Each of these different perspectives creates a different set of obligations. What may be in the best interests of an individual leader may not be in the best interests of the whole agency, and what may be in the best interests of an organization may not be in the best interests of the larger disaster response. Table 20–1 provides a summary of some of the differences and similarities in a psychiatrist's obligations depending on who is the identified client for his or her services.

For example, because of the stigma against mental illness, if an individual or organization is perceived as requiring psychiatric attention, his, her, or its role in the disaster response may be negatively affected. Each agency and each individual may have a complex set of reasons for wanting to serve in the disaster response. Ongoing participation in a disaster may represent, aside from the emotional investment, a significant financial or career opportunity for some organizations or individuals. In such situations, ethical issues arise when a psychiatrist becomes aware of issues that may impair a person's or an organization's ability to contribute effectively to the disaster response. Of course, it is optimal when a psychiatrist can successfully address an individual's psychopathology or an organization's dysfunction. However, if a psychiatrist is unable to effectively intervene with an individual whose alcoholism endangers others or an agency that has developed a culture of distrust, indignation, or competitiveness that is subverting the work of other disaster responders, at what point does the psychiatrist shift to a higher level of responsibility to remove this individual or organization from the larger response effort?

Merlino (2010) describes one common ethical pitfall: the request for "fitness for duty" evaluation. To be a flexible and helpful member of a larger disaster response team, the mental health professional may be tempted to evaluate whether specific responders are fit to do their job; however, a fitness-for-duty evaluation is a specialized service that requires an awareness of the employee's legal rights. When a psychiatrist serves in the role of performing a fitness-for-duty evaluation for an agency, it is a specific, reimbursed role on behalf of the agency, which is distinct from any consultative or treatment relationship to individuals working in the disaster setting. It must be clear that the psychiatrist performing a fitness-for-duty evaluation does not establish a treatment relationship with the patient, or else the psychiatrist would place himself or herself in an ethical bind because an honest evaluation may require the psychiatrist to betray his or her responsibility to "first, do no harm." To avoid misleading the subject of a fitness evaluation into thinking that he or she is engaging in the usual confidential dialogue

TABLE 20–1.   Ethical psychiatric roles defined by the identified client

Individual patient as client	Organizational leader as client	Organization as client	Whole disaster response as client
Treat the distress and dysfunction of the individual	Advise the leader on how to best manage the disaster response	Advise the leader on how to best manage the disaster response	Treat the distress and dysfunction of any individual
Do not betray confidentiality even if in the better interests of others	Inform the leader about observed psychopathology so that he or she can address this and/or remove individuals who are not helping the organization	Inform the leader about observed psychopathology so that he or she can address this and/or remove individuals who are not helping the organization	Work to reduce organizational dysfunction
Work to reduce organizational dysfunction to the degree that it adversely affects an individual patient	Work to reduce organizational dysfunction	Work to reduce organizational dysfunction	When it is not possible to treat the dysfunction of any individual, work to reduce his or her role in the disaster response
	Treat the distress and dysfunction of the leader	Treat the distress and dysfunction of the leader	When organization is working in a way that is counterproductive to the disaster response as a whole, work to reduce the role of that organization
	Do not betray the leader by informing others of the leader's distress and dysfunction	When it is not possible to treat the dysfunction of a leader, work to reduce his or her role	

with a doctor, a psychiatrist is required to have an explicit discussion about the lack of confidentiality and the purpose of the evaluation before beginning an assessment, as described by the American Psychiatric Association (2004). Such clarity about one's role is difficult to achieve in the chaos of postdisaster response. It is therefore prudent to defer such evaluations to specialists who are not part of the disaster response.

Confidentiality

In the opening case vignette, Dr. Ramos wisely worked to open communication with other agencies, but when he discussed the flight attendant's medications with the Red Cross social worker, he was unintentionally violating confidentiality. Although psychiatrists can serve an important role in developing productive relationships between agencies while collaborating on the care of individuals in distress, it is important to remember that this team of disaster responders differs dramatically from a multidisciplinary team in hospitals. Health care systems such as hospitals usually form a circle of confidentiality where there is permission to share medical information, with explicit policies and with laws (such as the Health Insurance Portability and Accountability Act of 1996, commonly called HIPAA) to protect such confidential information from being shared outside of this setting. This is generally understood by patients. At a disaster site, however, a psychiatrist cannot assume that individuals who share their psychiatric and medical information are giving their permission to share that information with anyone else.

Obtaining written consent to discuss confidential information is often impractical when developing impromptu psychiatric services and may be awkward and off-putting in situations where the doctor-patient relationship is established through gradual outreach. In the case study, Dr. Ramos may never have considered himself the flight attendant's psychiatrist, but by the end of the vignette, when Dr. Ramos has prescribed medications for the flight attendant, he was engaging in a professional service that is generally considered the basis for a doctor-patient relationship. Documenting what was discussed in an impromptu chart may be the only practical way to document what was and was not discussed with a patient. As with all of psychiatry, the degree of detail to be maintained in a medical record can vary tremendously depending on the level of service provided. If one simply provides general psychoeducation and a list of referrals to an individual, the documentation does not need to be as detailed as in cases where one prescribes medications. In some circumstances, even such rudimentary documentation as maintaining a log of individuals who received any sort of professional help may be sufficient. To the degree that such a log consistently documents a clinician's recommendations, this can serve as evidence in case of a bad outcome or a later claim of malpractice.

Charting

Documentation of services fulfills other medicolegal purposes aside from reducing liability (Disaster Psychiatry Outreach 2008). It can be used in legal proceedings, such as attempts to seek compensation for pain and suffering from a party that is accused of being responsible for the disaster, whether due to malice or negligence. In human-made disasters, the potential for subsequent lawsuits is obvious, but even in cases of natural disasters, litigation may be necessary to obtain funds from insurance companies or governmental relief programs. In such cases, although a psychiatrist may have no responsibility to provide financial recompense to survivors, he or she still may be subpoenaed to provide information that supports the survivors' claims against others. In such situations, some psychiatrists may feel a fiduciary responsibility to advocate for a patient, and adequate contemporaneous documentation will be considered stronger evidence than recollections months or years after the event. Psychiatrists who are aware of this possibility, who experience positive feelings toward their patients, or who feel indignation or anger about the disaster may be tempted to exaggerate the degree of pain and suffering in their clinical documentation. Such attempts to tailor the chart are unethical and pose risks of unintended consequences (Dwyer and Shih 1998). For example, if a psychiatrist does not provide a balanced and objective picture of the patient's presentation in the chart by emphasizing the degree of distress and impairment that the patient is experiencing, this same chart could work against the patient if there is a subsequent question of fitness for duty.

Malingering

In the opening case vignette, Dr. Ramos appears to take the flight attendant's word that she has been taking a controlled substance, without considering whether she may be fabricating her story with the intent to receive a substance with abuse potential. He does not appear to have asked her about her history of substance abuse. Despite a lack of data regarding the rates of malingering after disasters, the literature on malingering after traumas in general suggests that at least some disaster survivors are likely to engage in this behavior. After the 9/11 attacks, Disaster Psychiatry Outreach encountered some cases in which individuals appeared to be exaggerating their psychiatric symptoms so they could obtain controlled substances. To avoid being an accessory to malingering, psychiatrists are challenged to remain objective in the context of a disaster that can and will stir up strong feelings. To maintain maximum objectivity in charting, they should be careful to differentiate observations from patients' reports (e.g., by avoiding writing, "Patient had multiple bruises from the train crash," when it would be more accurate to say, "Patient had multiple bruises that she reports were caused by the train crash").

Cases of exaggerating or feigning a posttraumatic illness have been described for over a century (Resnick 1995). Some of the atypical presentations that are suggestive of malingering of posttraumatic stress disorder (PTSD) include claims that one is incapable of work while not reporting an inability to engage in recreational activity; reports that nightmares are an exact replaying of the trauma; and more general signs of malingering, such as evasiveness, inconsistency in symptoms reported, or antisocial personality traits. By contrast, individuals with PTSD tend to report a decrease in both recreational and work functioning, and civilians with PTSD tend to report that their nightmares contain some recurrent themes from the traumatic event but that the details vary over time (Resnick 1995).

Clinicians' Psychological Reactions to a Disaster as a Legal and Ethical Pitfall

Alongside the pitfalls described above that relate to the external disaster environment, which requires flexibility and encourages informal services, internal psychological factors also contribute to the risks for unethical behavior and legal liability. Such factors include the strong emotional reactions to disasters from which psychiatrists are not immune. Many readers may identify with Dr. Ramos in the case study, even after learning about the many ethical and liability issues raised by his actions. Dr. Ramos's intense urge to be helpful is a normal reaction to the dramatic and chaotic circumstances. A range of "countertransferences" have been described that make it especially difficult for psychiatrists to maintain their usual clinical distance (Pandya 2010). Although the blurring of professional boundaries through the "identification, idealization, enmeshment, and advocacy" spectrum is the most obvious manifestation, other feelings include anger and frustration toward patients who do not get better or who overwhelm psychiatrists with their neediness (Disaster Psychiatry Outreach 2008).

To avoid problems, psychiatrists should consider their own motivations for doing disaster work. Upon reflection, they may recognize their own anger or anxiety about the disaster, an urge to escape from the routine, or the satisfaction and sense of worth that comes from being part of a historical event or a media event. Such motivations can skew clinical judgment and may make it harder to set limits. Because idealization of patients and an inability to set limits are recognized risk factors for boundary problems (Norris et al. 2003), the high value placed on flexibility in disaster settings and the countertransferences described above can combine to increase the risk of boundary violations. Such boundary violations may be mistaken as relatively benign boundary crossings in a context where it may seem artificial and withholding to maintain the usual clinical distance. In this context, clinicians may not recognize the legal and ethical consequences until it is too late. The following are some potential boundary violations that may be especially tempting after a disaster:

- Accommodating a patient's request for a change of time even when this interferes with the treatment of one's prior patients
- Referring patients that one encounters during outreach at a disaster site into one's own private practice
- Revealing too many details about a specific patient's treatment to others because one is so moved by the experience
- Embellishing or minimizing the degree of disability that a patient is experiencing to accommodate the preference of the patient
- Avoiding a patient who needs help but who induces a sense of hopelessness

Licensure and Liability Coverage

Given the risks described above, it is important to confirm that one has adequate malpractice coverage for one's work in a disaster response. Good Samaritan laws cannot be assumed to apply to all disaster psychiatry work (Disaster Psychiatry Outreach 2008). Such laws vary from state to state, and traditionally these laws were not developed to cover services provided days and weeks after a disaster when the situation no longer qualifies as an emergency (Kantor 2010). A variety of laws have expanded the situations in which responders to disasters may be covered for their services, especially if they are provided under the auspices of governmental agencies (Kantor 2010). In addition, the Volunteer Protection Act of 1997 may cover many health care professionals who provide volunteer services. However, this act requires that the health care professional is "licensed, certified or authorized by the appropriate authorities for the activities or practice in the state" where the harm was done (Kantor 2010, p. 196). This suggests that volunteer psychiatrists who "self-deploy" (go to a disaster site to provide services outside of the auspices of an established disaster response organization) are less likely to be covered for services that they provide. In addition to satisfying the requirement "authorized by the appropriate authorities," larger organizations are also more likely to have addressed the liability and licensure issues, especially if they have prior experience providing health care. The licensure issue is important for any out-of-state psychiatric service. The Emergency Management Assistance Compact (2009), a congressionally ratified organization that has all 50 states as members, created a framework so that when a governor declares a state of emergency, personnel deployed by other states will have their credentials honored across state lines and will get liability coverage for their work at the disaster site. This system, however, applies to personnel deployed by the state, not to individuals who self-deploy.

Psychiatrists often become involved in disaster response through the American Red Cross or the district branches of the American Psychiatric Association (APA). Although the APA and its district branches are valuable sources of information about disasters, they are not structured to be direct providers of medical services. Therefore, when psychiatrists arrange to go to a disaster through the APA, they should plan to have their own malpractice coverage and should not assume that the APA has arranged coverage for them. The American Red Cross is structured to provide direct care, but their mental health care service works on a nonmedical model, which allows psychiatrists and other types of mental health providers only to provide generic mental health services (North et al. 2000). These generic mental health services are consistent with the principles of Psychological First Aid, which are described in Chapter 12. Therefore, if a psychiatrist is deployed by the American Red Cross, he or she would be acting outside the scope of his or her designated role in that organization when engaging in such medical activities as hospitalizing a patient, making diagnoses, and writing prescriptions. As a result, psychiatrists would not be insured against medical malpractice claims by the American Red Cross for the practice of these essential psychiatric activities.

Ethical Issues in Disaster Psychiatry Research

Given the limitations in the available research on disaster psychiatry, there is a strong need for psychiatrists to systematically acquire and analyze data that can inform subsequent disaster responses. However, several ethical issues are raised by disaster psychiatry research. To conduct such research ethically, a psychiatrist must consider the decisional capacity of participants, their vulnerability, the balance of risks and benefits, and the adequacy of the informed consent (Collogan et al. 2004). In reviewing the limited data on the degree to which disaster survivors have capacity to consent to research, Rosenstein (2004) concluded that although there is reason to suspect that decision-making capacity will be compromised in some survivors of disasters, there is insufficient evidence to show that they have a lower capacity than the general public. He noted that institutional review boards may have limited experience with reviewing protocols for this setting, and he suggested that some of the concerns about diminished decisional capacity can be addressed by using the acute setting only to obtain consent for future contact at a time when subjects will be better able to understand the risks and benefits. Based on the available data, survivors of disasters should not in general be considered a "vulnerable population" in the technical sense, but processes should be in place to ensure adequacy of informed consent when there is any doubt (Collogan et al. 2004). In a review of the experience of individuals who have participated in research after experiencing trauma, Newman and Kaloupek (2004) noted that although a few subjects experience intense distress, most have a positive view of their participation in research. Future research that better helps determine which subjects are more likely to experience distress could better inform the prospective planning of research and could also inform clinical practice. North et al. (2002) made a variety of suggestions to maximize subject protection. These include maximizing the degree of predisaster planning for research and using local psychiatrists to monitor for issues requiring clinical attention. The literature suggests that there is a way to conduct valuable, ethical research and that although the logistical challenges of postdisaster research remain daunting (North 2004), it is important to balance this against an ethical imperative to help ensure that future psychiatrists are better equipped with research that can help survivors of disasters (Kilpatrick 2004).

Conclusion

The array of issues outlined in this chapter are intended to overcome any assumptions that noble intentions are sufficient to ensure that disaster psychiatry is ethical and free of liability. No single chapter can provide a comprehensive list of all possible issues. Instead, this chapter lists issues that have been noted by the author to arise more frequently due to the often impromptu nature of disaster response. Although these issues require attention, this chapter should not discourage individuals from engaging in clinical work and research in the wake of disasters. Indeed, some may perceive an ethical responsibility to help those in need and to advance our collective understanding so that we may better help others in the future. Fortunately, when we are thoughtful about how to balance our urge to help with consideration of these liabilities and ethical imperatives, it is often possible to navigate a path that protects all parties and addresses profound needs.

▮ Teaching Points

- Disaster psychiatrists should be clear about whether they are serving an individual or an organization and should be vigilant about role conflicts, such as those created when one conducts impromptu fitness-for-duty evaluations.
- Despite the fluid nature of disaster work, it remains necessary to maintain confidentiality.
- Although the degree of charting should vary depending on the level of service provided, disaster psychiatrists still need to maintain a medical record of services that they provided and to whom.
- Disaster psychiatry is not always covered by Good Samaritan laws.
- Some states may allow doctors from other states to provide disaster medical services during a declared state of emergency, but neither the validity of licensure across state lines nor malpractice coverage should be assumed unless an individual is deployed under an established system such as the Emergency Management Assistance Compact.
- Psychiatrists working under the auspices of the government or established health care providers are more likely to have coverage than individuals who self-deploy.
- The American Psychiatric Association (APA) can help psychiatrists identify opportunities to volunteer, but APA is not a formal health care provider, and volunteers should not assume that APA is providing malpractice coverage for their disaster work.
- The American Red Cross provides liability for psychiatrists for generic mental health services but does not cover the liability from physician-specific mental health care services, such as making diagnoses, prescribing medications, or hospitalizing a patient.

Review Questions

20.1 Which of the following statements about conducting ethical disaster psychiatry research is *true*?

A. Based on existing research, survivors of disasters should not be considered a vulnerable population requiring special protections for ethical research.

B. Conducting research immediately after a disaster better protects subjects than getting contact information that can be used for research later.

C. About an equal percentage of subjects report positive and negative experiences after engaging in disaster psychiatry research.

D. None of the above.

E. All of the above.

20.2 In which of the following scenarios should the psychiatrist be most concerned about liability coverage?

A. A psychiatrist employed by a state hospital who prescribes an antidepressant after being deployed by the hospital to a declared disaster in another state where he does not have a license.

B. A psychiatrist deployed by the American Red Cross who provides generic mental health services in a state where he does not have a license.

C. A psychiatrist who decides on her own to help out at a disaster site at the far end of her own state.

D. A psychiatrist sent by his state office of emergency management to respond to a disaster within his own state.

E. None of the above; all of these psychiatrists are covered by well-established mechanisms as long as they are not acting maliciously.

20.3 Which of the following circumstances would increase the risk of ethical or legal problems for a disaster psychiatrist?

A. Lack of clarity about roles.

B. Countertransference in the psychiatrist.

C. Helping a patient who will need to sue to get paid for pain and suffering by emphasizing problems since the disaster and not mentioning problems that predate the disaster.

D. Avoiding any documentation of one's psychiatric services to ensure that there is no risk of loss of confidentiality.

E. All of the above.

20.4 Which of the following statements about fitness-for-duty evaluations is *true*?

A. A psychiatrist who conducts such evaluations at a disaster site should act as an advocate to make sure that a patient is not removed from his or her job.

B. A psychiatrist should conduct such evaluations when it is in the best interest of the disaster response to remove an impaired responder.

C. Even if one has not conducted such evaluations before, it is more important to show sufficient flexibility to conduct these when they are requested by a commanding police officer.

D. A psychiatrist who is treating an essential first responder who has a serious addiction has an obligation to inform the authorities that they are available to conduct a fitness-for-duty evaluation.

E. None of the above.

20.5 Which of the following is recommended to protect against legal liability?

A. Responding to a disaster through a request from any district branch of the American Psychiatric Association.

B. Maintaining a log of the names for anyone whom the psychiatrist treats.

C. Waiting to deploy under the auspices of an authorized agency only if this does not delay one's ability to respond to a disaster within 48 hours of the event.

D. All of the above.

E. None of the above.

References

American Psychiatric Association: Guidelines for Psychiatric "Fitness for Duty" Evaluations of Physicians: Resource Document. Washington, DC, American Psychiatric Association, 2004

Collogan L, Tuma F, Dolan-Sewell R, et al: Ethical issues pertaining to research in the aftermath of a disaster. J Trauma Stress 17:363–372, 2004

Disaster Psychiatry Outreach: The Essentials of Disaster Psychiatry: A Training Course for Mental Health Professionals (Course Syllabus). New York, Disaster Psychiatry Outreach, 2008. Available as DPOCourseSyllabus_052108.pdf at: https://sites.google.com/a/disasterpsych.org/blog/File-Cabinet. Accessed December 28, 2009.

Dwyer J, Shih A: The ethics of tailoring the patient's chart. Psychiatr Serv 49:1309–1312, 1998

Emergency Management Assistance Compact: Homepage. Available at: http://www.emacweb.org. Accessed March 14, 2009.

Health Insurance Portability and Accountability Act of 1996, Pub. L. No. 104-191, 110 Stat. 1936 (1996)

Kantor EM: Liability issues, in Hidden Impact: What You Need to Know for the Next Disaster. A Practical Mental Health Guide for Clinicians. Edited by Stoddard FJ, Katz CL, Merlino JP. Sudbury, MA, Jones & Bartlett, 2010, pp 195–206

Kilpatrick DG: The ethics of disaster research: a special section. J Trauma Stress 17:361–362, 2004

Merlino JP: Ethics, in Hidden Impact: What You Need to Know for the Next Disaster. A Practical Mental Health Guide for Clinicians. Edited by Stoddard FJ, Katz CL, Merlino JP. Sudbury, MA, Jones & Bartlett, 2010, pp 207–217

Newman E, Kaloupek DG: The risks and benefits of participating in trauma-focused research studies. J Trauma Stress 17:383–394, 2004

Norris DM, Gutheil TG, Strasburger LH: This couldn't happen to me: boundary problems and sexual misconduct in the psychotherapy relationship. Psychiatr Serv 54:517–522, 2003

North CS: Approaching disaster mental health research after the 9/11 World Trade Center terrorist attacks. Psychiatr Clin North Am 27:589–602, 2004

North CS, Weaver JD, Dingman RL, et al: The American Red Cross Disaster Mental Health Services: development of a cooperative, single function, multidisciplinary service model. J Behav Health Serv Res 27:314–320, 2000

North CS, Pfefferbaum B, Tucker P: Ethical and methodological issues in academic mental health research in populations affected by disasters: the Oklahoma City experience relevant to September 11, 2001. CNS Spectr 7:580–584, 2002

Pandya A: Reconsidering the role of a disaster psychiatrist. Psychiatr Serv 61:449–450, 2010

Resnick PJ: Guidelines for the evaluation of malingering in posttraumatic stress disorder, in Posttraumatic Stress Disorder in Litigation. Edited by Simon RI. Washington, DC, American Psychiatric Press, 1995, pp 121–134

Rosenstein DL: Decision-making capacity and disaster research. J Trauma Stress 17:373–381, 2004

Volunteer Protection Act of 1997, Pub. L. 105-19, 42 USC sec. 14501 (1997)

21

Telepsychiatry in Disasters and Public Health Emergencies

Anthony T. Ng, M.D.

One of the challenging health management issues in the aftermath of disasters and public health emergencies is the shortage of resources, including facilities, such as hospitals and clinics, and health professionals of all disciplines. Psychiatric clinicians are especially in short supply. The psychiatrist, however, has an important role in a team approach to disaster psychiatric care, by being a leader in a multidisciplinary team approach. The psychiatrist also has important consultative roles with other health professionals, such as primary care providers or emergency medicine physicians (Ng 2010; Ruzek et al. 2004). As noted in Chapter 19, "Psychiatrists as Ambassadors," the psychiatrist can make significant contributions through consultation with disaster response and management entities as well as through public health leadership.

Despite the importance of psychiatry being included as an integral part of disaster response, access to psychiatric resources remains a challenge. Although increasing numbers of psychiatrists are receiving training in disaster psychiatry, not enough psychiatrists are available who can respond to disasters. Telepsychiatry may have a role in addressing this need. Telepsychiatry has been increasingly used as an effective tool in providing access to psychiatric care, especially in rural settings (Hilty et al. 2002; Norman 2006). The effectiveness of interventions delivered via telepsychiatry for patients with posttraumatic stress disorder (PTSD) has also been demonstrated (Frueh et al. 2007a, 2007b). Many of the roles that a psychiatrist may fulfill in the field may be performed via telepsychiatry when infrastructure for it is in place and not enough psychiatric clinicians are in the field.

Although the increased role of telepsychiatry has been described, limited data are available on the applicability of telepsychiatry in disaster settings (Merrell et al. 2008; Reissman et al. 2006). Much can be extrapolated, however, from existing literature on telepsychiatry in emergency psychiatry (Shore et al. 2007b; Sorvaniemi et al. 2005). Although clinicians may readily think of Internet video links as telepsychiatry, telephone and electronic mail may also be used as tools to supplement traditional telepsychiatry (Hilty et al. 2006).

The use of telepsychiatry has significant benefits in disaster psychiatry. The primary one is clinician accessibility. Due to often massive postdisaster disruptions to infrastructure, such as transportation and utilities, clinicians may not be able to access the affected area to help. Telepsychiatry can minimize the need for clinicians to travel to distant, inaccessible, or remote disaster locations. Telepsychiatry can also potentially lessen psychiatric volunteer surge burden and resultant chaos at the affected area. Telepsychiatry makes it possible for clinicians to access psychiatric expertise in specialty areas such as trauma, disaster psychiatry, substance abuse, specific topics in psychopharmacology, cross-cultural psychiatry, or working with special populations (Ng 2010). Telepsychiatry can be a safer alternative for clinicians and individuals. The use of telepsychiatry can be an excellent tool to provide psychiatric evaluations and interventions in public health emergencies such as disease outbreaks, where either the community or the clinician or both may be quarantined or have their movement restricted.

Although telepsychiatry can be an effective tool in delivering psychiatric services to affected individuals who may not otherwise be able to obtain psychiatric services, the use of telepsychiatry in disaster settings presents several challenges. A primary problem is that in the immediate aftermath of disasters, infrastructure such as electricity and Internet/telephone systems may be disrupted. Also, clinicians and patients might be apprehensive about the use of telepsychiatry due to unfamiliarity with its use, especially in disaster settings. The issue of confidentiality may be challenged due to the often chaotic settings in the postdisaster environment in which telepsychiatric assessment may be conducted.

Disaster Telepsychiatry Application

Disaster planning and response can be categorized into three phases: the predisaster phase, in which much of disaster planning occurs; the acute phase; and the postacute phase, which focuses on disaster recovery. As discussed in the following subsections and summarized in Table 21–1, telepsychiatry is applicable in all three phases.

Predisaster Phase

Before disasters occur, the focus is on disaster planning and education. Planners need to identify how and when telepsychiatry might be used. Infrastructure needs to be in place, which includes appropriate and secure high-speed Internet connections and equipment such as videos, with careful planning for backups in case of disruptions of electricity and Internet. The use of portable videoconferencing, perhaps with the use of satellite phones, should be considered. Clinicians can develop a familiarity with the licensing and credentialing guidelines that may be necessary or encourage their professional organizations to help identify these guidelines. Individual psychiatrists will need to develop a competency base and a level of comfort with the use of telepsychiatry, both the techniques and the equipment.

Acute Phase

During the acute phase of a disaster, telepsychiatry can be used in multiple ways. It can be in the form of consultation by a clinician—psychiatric or nonpsychiatric—in the disaster area, with a psychiatric clinician located elsewhere. The initial emphasis is on the delivery of medical care to the affected population; therefore, the greater immediate need is for medical providers. These clinicians need support, however, to meet the challenges of some of the mental health demands from affected individuals. Psychiatric clinicians can provide consultation to the medical providers via telepsychiatry on how to assess for mental health issues, can assist them in triaging those who may need more direct psychiatric interventions, and can even assist in delivering those interventions.

Those who practice disaster telepsychiatry need to stay aware that there may be some ambivalence and even apprehension on the part of the medical provider in the field and disaster victims, who may feel they are unable to identify with and relate to the distant psychiatric clinician who is providing the consultation. The personal face-to-face contact, which is often an important piece of psychiatric care in the field after disaster, may not be possible. Affected individuals may feel that the use of telepsychiatry prevents them from connecting with the clinician. With face-to-face contact, individuals may feel a sense that care providers share a common disaster experience. This is hard when the clinician is removed from the disaster site. For some cases, especially with individuals from certain cultural groups or special populations, an advocate or someone who can act as a broker in the

TABLE 21-1.   Application of disaster telepsychiatry

Phase of disaster response	Roles of telepsychiatry
Predisaster	Training in postdisaster mental health issues Developing competence in the use of culturally aware telepsychiatry Learning to manage safety issues Developing supportive infrastructure Creating licensing and regulatory guidelines Creating emergency protocols for the use of telepsychiatry with clear delineation of roles and responsibilities
Acute	Consultation with medical providers Consultation with other mental health professionals Consultation with disaster human services providers or organizations Training Monitoring of wellness in disaster responders Direct triage, evaluation, and intervention
Postacute	Ongoing consultation with medical providers, including primary care physicians and emergency physicians Ongoing training and education of stakeholders Ongoing triage, evaluation, and intervention

field may help to maximize the benefit of disaster telepsychiatry by being present during the evaluation process. In instances where non-video-based telepsychiatry may be conducted, the consultant may need to make an increased effort to ascertain clinical data without the benefit of visual data.

Telepsychiatry can also be used for consultations between psychiatric clinicians and disaster human services agencies and senior disaster response leadership. Disaster telepsychiatry can assist medical providers and other disaster responders in providing services to maintain the psychiatric wellness of the medical providers themselves, who will be experiencing tremendous levels of stress due to the intense workload and to secondary traumatization from exposure to the disaster victims.

Postacute Phase

In the postacute phase, telepsychiatry can continue to have a significant role in providing psychiatric care. As noted in Chapter 5, "Psychiatric Evaluation," during the postacute phase, psychiatric needs evolve and many individuals may seek help for the first time. Despite the initial surge of psychiatric resources following disasters, these resources may diminish over time and no longer be as readily available. Telepsychiatry can be used for continued access to psychiatric expertise. For example, cognitive-behavioral interventions for PTSD have used videoconferencing (Frueh et al. 2007b).

Disaster telepsychiatry is also effective for ongoing education on the psychiatric consequences of disasters.

Issues With Telepsychiatry in Disaster

Psychiatric clinicians should consider several challenging issues related to the application of disaster telepsychiatry. Medicolegal issues are important concerns. In disaster telepsychiatry, a consulting clinician might be in one state and the individual being evaluated in another state. In such a case, the provider should confirm whether his or her services will be considered the practice of medicine in the location of the patient and the location of the long-distance psychiatrist. (See Chapter 20, "Legal and Ethical Issues," for more details about the licensing requirements during disasters.) It is important that agencies undertake efforts to identify the credentialing of potential disaster telepsychiatric clinicians as a means of maintaining a minimal standard of care. Clinicians need to maintain medical records when working with patients via telepsychiatry. Psychiatric clinicians also should ensure that their malpractice insurance will cover their clinical telepsychiatric work in disasters.

Access to the use of telepsychiatry may be influenced by cultural, language, ethnic, and socioeconomic issues, although some studies have demonstrated minimal differences in the effectiveness of telepsychiatry across cultural groups (Shore et al. 2006, 2007a). People from some cultures may not be as receptive to the use of telepsychiatry, because they cannot directly see a "real" person in a face-to-face interaction. In some cases, translators may need to be available at either end of the consultation. In international disasters, the need for translators is paramount. In such instances, a more consultative role with on-scene medical providers and disaster responders may be more effective than direct evaluation and assessment of distressed individuals.

Conclusion

The scarcity and inaccessibility of psychiatric resources will continue to be challenges in disasters and public health emergencies, despite the best planning efforts. Alternate effective means to meet this challenge must be identified. The use of telepsychiatry is one possible effective intervention. As more and more psychiatric clinicians are trained and the pool of those with disaster expertise increases, disaster telepsychiatry can help to bring these tremendous resources to affected communities. Advance planning will facilitate the accessing of these resources in a potentially organized and effective manner. Lastly, disaster telepsychiatry can greatly help to promote greater collaborative and integrated public health care, which is critical in the postdisaster environment.

■ Teaching Points

- Telepsychiatry is an effective means of supporting disaster mental health.
- The use of telepsychiatry can increase access to psychiatric care in disasters, with a lower burden on medical surge capacity.
- Disaster telepsychiatry can be employed to support clinical work, including triage, assessment, and interventions.
- Postacute collaboration between various disaster medical and human services providers can be enhanced by disaster telepsychiatry.
- Consideration should be given to issues such as liability, working with special populations, and training, when planning and implementing disaster telepsychiatry.

Review Questions

21.1 Disaster telepsychiatry is applicable in which stage of disaster response?

  A. Predisaster phase.
  B. Acute phase.
  C. Postacute phase.
  D. B and C only.
  E. A, B, and C.

21.2 The benefits of the use of telepsychiatry in disaster response include all of the following *except*

  A. Reducing the surge of mental health resources.
  B. Reducing the need for licensing and credentialing processes.
  C. Reducing disaster risks to mental health professionals.
  D. Increasing access to postdisaster psychiatric care.
  E. Minimizing the need for clinicians to travel to distant, inaccessible, or remote disaster locations.

21.3 Disaster telepsychiatry may be used in which of the following ways?

  A. Triage of patients.
  B. Consultation with emergency response workers.
  C. Direct clinical care.

    D. Provision of disaster psychiatric expertise from outside of the disaster area.

    E. All of the above.

21.4 Potential medicolegal concerns in regard to disaster telepsychiatry include all of the following *except*

    A. State licensure requirements.

    B. Malpractice.

    C. Whether the event is declared a federal emergency.

    D. Adequate documentation.

    E. Protection of patient confidentiality.

21.5 Which of the following is a potential challenge to the use of disaster psychiatry?

    A. Cultural concerns.

    B. Availability of infrastructure to support telepsychiatry.

    C. Stigma toward mental health.

    D. Lack of standards of practice in disaster psychiatry.

    E. All of the above.

References

Frueh BC, Monnier J, Yim E, et al: A randomized trial of telepsychiatry for posttraumatic stress disorder. J Telemed Telecare 13:142–147, 2007a

Frueh BC, Monnier J, Grubaugh AL, et al: Therapist adherence and competence with manualized cognitive-behavioral therapy for PTSD delivered via teleconferencing technology. Behav Modif 31:856–866, 2007b

Hilty DM, Luo JS, Morache C, et al: Telepsychiatry: an overview for psychiatrists. CNS Drugs 16:527–548, 2002

Hilty DM, Yellowless PM, Cobb HC, et al: Use of secure email and telephone psychiatric consultations to accelerate rural health care delivery. Telemed J E Health 12:490–495, 2006

Merrell RC, Cone SW, Rafiq A: Telemedicine in extreme conditions: disasters, war, remote sites. Stud Health Technol Inform 131:99–116, 2008

Ng AT: Use of telepsychiatry: implications in disaster, in Hidden Impact: What You Need to Know for the Next Disaster. A Practical Mental Health Guide for Clinicians. Edited by Stoddard FJ, Katz CL, Merlino JP. Sudbury, MA, Jones & Bartlett, 2010, pp 187–194

Norman S: The use of telemedicine in psychiatry. J Psychiatr Ment Health Nurs 13:771–777, 2006

Reissman DB, Schreiber M, Klomp RW, et al: The virtual network supporting the front lines: addressing emerging behavioral health problems following the tsunamis of 2004. Mil Med 171(suppl):40–43, 2006

Ruzek JI, Young BH, Cordova MJ, et al: Integration of disaster mental health services with emergency medicine. Prehosp Disast Med 19:46–53, 2004

Shore JH, Savin DM, Novins D, et al: Cultural aspects of telepsychiatry. J Telemed Telecare 12:116–121, 2006

Shore JH, Savin D, Orton H, et al: Diagnostic reliability of telepsychiatry in American Indian veterans. Am J Psychiatry 164:115–118, 2007a

Shore JH, Hilty DM, Yellowless P: Emergency management guidelines for telepsychiatry. Gen Hosp Psychiatry 29:199–206, 2007b

Sorvaniemi M, Ojanen E, Santamaki O: Telepsychiatry in emergency consultations: a follow-up study of sixty patients. Telemed J E Health 11:439–441, 2005

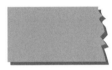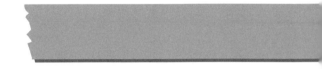

Appendixes

Appendix A

Key Readings and Resources

Print Publications

Bisson J, Andrew M: Psychological treatment of post-traumatic stress disorder (PTSD). Cochrane Database of Systematic Reviews 2007, Issue 3. Art. No.: CD003388. DOI: 10.1002/14651858.CD003388.pub3.

Blumenfield M, Ursano RJ (eds): Intervention and Resilience After Mass Trauma. New York, Cambridge University Press, 2008

Brenner G, Bush D, Moses J (eds): Creating Spiritual and Psychological Resilience: Integrating Care in Disaster Relief Work. New York, Routledge, 2009

Charney DS: Psychobiological mechanisms of resilience and vulnerability: implications for successful adaptation to extreme stress. Am J Psychiatry 161:195–216, 2004

Figley C, Nash W (eds): Combat Stress Injury. New York, Routledge, 2007

Foa EB, Keane TM, Friedman MJ, et al (eds): Effective Treatments for PTSD, 2nd Edition: Practice Guidelines From the International Society for Traumatic Stress Studies. New York, Guilford, 2009

Hobfoll SE, Watson P, Bell CC, et al: Five essential elements of immediate and mid-term mass trauma intervention: empirical evidence. Focus 7:221–242, 2009

Katz CL, Pandya A (guest eds): Disaster Psychiatry: A Closer Look. Psychiatr Clin North Am 27(3 [special issue]), 2004

Katz CL, Pellegrino L, Pandya A, et al: Research on psychiatric outcomes and interventions subsequent to disasters: a review of the literature. Psychiatry Res 110:201–217, 2002

Lindemann E: Symptomatology and management of acute grief. Am J Psychiatry 101:141–148, 1944

National Institutes of Mental Health: Mental Health and Mass Violence: Evidence-Based Early Intervention for Victims/Survivors of Mass Violence. A Workshop to Reach Consensus on Best Practices (NIH Publ No 02-5138). Washington, DC, U.S. Government Printing Office, 2002

Neria Y, Gross R, Marshall R, et al. (eds): 9/11: Mental Health in the Wake of Terrorist Attacks. Cambridge, UK, Cambridge University Press, 2006

Neria Y, Galea S, Norris FH (eds): Mental Health and Disasters. New York, Cambridge University Press, 2009

Norris FH, Friedman MJ, Watson PJ, et al: 60,000 Disaster victims speak, part I: an empirical review of the empirical literature, 1981–2001. Psychiatry 65:207–239, 2002

Norris FH, Friedman MJ, Watson PJ, et al: 60,000 Disaster victims speak, part II: summary and implications of the disaster mental health research. Psychiatry 65:240–260, 2002

Norris FH, Galea S, Friedman MJ, et al. (eds): Methods for Disaster Mental Health Research. New York, Guilford, 2006

Pandya AA, Katz CL (eds): Disaster Psychiatry: Intervening When Nightmares Come True. Hillsdale, NJ, Analytic Press, 2004

Ritchie EC, Watson PJ, Friedman MJ (eds): Interventions Following Mass Violence and Disasters: Strategies for Mental Health Practice. New York, Guilford, 2006

Rose SC, Bisson J, Churchill R, et al: Psychological debriefing for preventing post traumatic stress disorder (PTSD). Cochrane Database of Systematic Reviews 2002, Issue 2. Art. No.: CD000560. DOI: 10.1002/14651858.CD000560.

Stein DJ, Ipser JC, Seedat S: Pharmacotherapy for post traumatic stress disorder (PTSD). Cochrane Database of Systematic Reviews 2006, Issue 1. Art. No.: CD002795. DOI: 10.1002/14651858.CD002795.pub2.

Stoddard FJ, Saxe G: Ten-year research review of physical injuries. J Am Acad Child Adolesc Psychiatry 40:1128–1145, 2001

Stoddard FJ, Katz CL, Merlino JP (eds): Hidden Impact: What You Need to Know for the Next Disaster. A Practical Mental Health Guide for Clinicians. Sudbury, MA, Jones & Bartlett, 2010

Ursano RJ, Fullerton CS, Norwood AE (eds): Terrorism and Disaster: Individual and Community Mental Health Interventions. Cambridge, UK, Cambridge University Press, 2003

Ursano R, Fullerton CS, Weisaeth K, et al (eds): Textbook of Disaster Psychiatry. New York, Cambridge University Press, 2007

Wolfenstein M: Disaster: A Psychological Essay. Glencoe, IL, Free Press, 1957

Online Resources

General Disaster Mental Health

Center for the Study of Traumatic Stress (CSTS) of the Uniformed Services University of the Health Sciences (www.centerforthestudyoftraumaticstress.org)

Centers for Disease Control and Prevention—disaster mental health information for the general public and health care providers (www.bt.cdc.gov/mentalhealth)

National Center for Posttraumatic Stress Disorder (PTSD) of the U.S. Department of Veterans Affairs
(www.ptsd.va.gov)

Substance Abuse and Mental Health Services Administration—disaster mental health Web site; includes a link to SAMHSA's Disaster Technical Advisory Center (DTAC)
(http://mentalhealth.samhsa.gov/cmhs/emergencyservices)

Organizations Active in Disasters

American Psychiatric Association
(www.psych.org/Resources/DisasterPsychiatry.aspx)

American Red Cross
(www.redcross.org)

Disaster Psychiatry Outreach
(www.disasterpsych.org)

Federal Emergency Management Agency—provides information about disasters in the United States
(www.fema.gov)

Inter-Agency Standing Committee—provides information to coordinate United Nations (UN) and non-UN humanitarian activities internationally
(www.humanitarianinfo.org/iasc)

National Voluntary Organizations Active in Disasters—helps to coordinate nongovernmental organizations responding to disasters in the United States
(www.nvoad.org)

Risk Communication

General Guidance on Trauma and Disasters for Families

American Academy of Child and Adolescent Psychiatry
(www.aacap.org/cs/root/facts_for_families/posttraumatic_stress_disorder_ptsd)
(www.aacap.org/cs/root/facts_for_families/children_and_the_news)

Guidance on Talking to Children About Terrorism and War

American Academy of Child and Adolescent Psychiatry
(www.aacap.org/cs/root/facts_for_families/
talking_to_children_about_terrorism_and_war)

American Psychiatric Association
(www.psych.org/Resources/DisasterPsychiatry/APADisasterPsychiatryResources/
talkingtochildrenrewarterror.aspx)

Guidance for Journalists Covering Trauma

Dart Center for Journalism and Trauma
(www.dartcenter.org)
(dartcenter.org/files/covering_children_and_trauma_0.pdf)

Guidance for Public Officials

Substance Abuse and Mental Health Services Administration
(www.riskcommunication.samhsa.gov)

Courses and Guides on Psychological First Aid

Psychological First Aid Field Operations Guide—developed by the National Child
Traumatic Stress Network and the National Center for PTSD; non-English
versions and many adaptations for specific populations are available
(http://www.nctsn.org/content/psychological-first-aid)

Psychological First Aid: Helping People Cope During Disasters and Public Health
Emergencies—a self-study program from the Center for Disaster Medicine and
Emergency Preparedness at the University of Rochester, New York
(www.centerfordisastermedicine.org/disaster_mental_health.html)

Psychological First Aid Online—a 6-hour interactive course from the National
Child Traumatic Stress Network in which participant plays the role of a provider
in a postdisaster scene
(http://learn.nctsn.org)

Listen, Protect, and Connect—Model and Teach: Psychological First Aid for
Students and Teachers—guidance for teachers on helping themselves and their
students through their reactions to a disaster; produced in part by the U.S.
Department of Homeland Security
(www.ready.gov/kids/_downloads/PFA_SchoolCrisis.pdf)

Nebraska Psychological First Aid Curriculum—an adaptation of "Community-
Based Psychological Support" developed by the International Federation of
Red Cross and Red Crescent Societies
(www.disastermh.nebraska.edu/psychfirstaid.html)

Other Topics

TB-CBTWeb (Trauma-Focused Cognitive-Behavioral Therapy)—free 10-hour
Web-based training course from the National Crime Victims Research and
Treatment Center at the Medical University of South Carolina, Charleston
(http://tfcbt.musc.edu)

U.S. Department of Veterans Affairs/Department of Defense Clinical Practice
Guideline for Management of Concussion/Mild Traumatic Brain Injury (mTBI)
(http://www.healthquality.va.gov/management_of_concussion_mtbi.asp)

World Health Organization Model List of Essential Medications—may be helpful
for planning postdisaster pharmacological interventions
(www.who.int/medicines/publications/essentialmedicines/en/index.html)

Appendix B

Answers to Review Questions

Part I: Readiness

Chapter 1 (Preparation and Systems Issues: Integrating Into a Disaster Response)

1.1   Correct answer: **E**

1.2   Correct answer: **False**

1.3   Correct answer: **False**

1.4   Correct answer: **C**

1.5   Correct answer: **B**

Chapter 2 (Communicating Risk Before, During, and After a Disaster)

2.1   Correct answer: **E**

2.2   Correct answer: **C**

2.3   Correct answer: **E**

2.4   Correct answer: **E**

2.5   Correct answer: **E**

Chapter 3 (Rescuing Ourselves: Self-Care in the Disaster Response Community)

3.1   Correct answer: **B**

3.2   Correct answer: **A**

3.3   Correct answer: **C**

3.4   Correct answer: **A**

3.5   Correct answer: **B**

3.6   Correct answer: **A**

3.7   Correct answer: **A**

Chapter 4 (Needs Assessment)

4.1   Correct answer: **C**

4.2   Correct answer: **E**

4.3   Correct answer: **E**

4.4   Correct answer: **False**

4.5   Correct answer: **B**

Part II: Evaluation

Chapter 5 (Psychiatric Evaluation)

5.1   Correct answer: **E**

5.2   Correct answer: **C**

5.3   Correct answer: **A**

5.4   Correct answer: **False**

5.5   Correct answer: **D**

Chapter 6 (Special Populations)

6.1   Correct answer: **C**

6.2   Correct answer: **D**

6.3   Correct answer: **D**

6.4   Correct answer: **E**

6.5   Correct answer: **E**

Chapter 7 (Serious Mental Illness)

7.1   Correct answer: **E**

7.2   Correct answer: **B**

7.3   Correct answer: **A**

7.4   Correct answer: **B**

7.5   Correct answer: **C**

Chapter 8 (Substance Abuse)

8.1   Correct answer: **B**

8.2   Correct answer: **B**

8.3   Correct answer: **B**

8.4   Correct answer: **D**

8.5   Correct answer: **C**

Chapter 9 (Personality Issues)

9.1   Correct answer: **C**

9.2   Correct answer: **A**

9.3   Correct answer: **D**

9.4   Correct answer: **B**

9.5   Correct answer: **E**

Chapter 10 (Injuries and Triage of Medical Complaints)

10.1   Correct answer: **E**

10.2   Correct answer: **E**

10.3   Correct answer: **B**

10.4   Correct answer: **D**

10.5   Correct answer: **C**

Chapter 11 (Grief and Resilience)

11.1 Correct answer: **D**

11.2 Correct answer: **D**

11.3 Correct answer: **A**

11.4 Correct answer: **D**

11.5 Correct answer: **E**

Part III: Intervention

Chapter 12 (Psychological First Aid)

12.1 Correct answer: **D**

12.2 Correct answer: **B**

12.3 Correct answer: **E**

12.4 Correct answer: **True**

12.5 Correct answer: **C**

Chapter 13 (Group and Family Interventions)

13.1 Correct answer: **D**

13.2 Correct answer: **C**

13.3 Correct answer: **D**

13.4 Correct answer: **D**

13.5 Correct answer: **E**

Chapter 14 (Psychotherapies)

14.1 Correct answer: **C**

14.2 Correct answer: **A**

14.3 Correct answer: **E**

14.4 Correct answer: **D**

14.5 Correct answer: **A**

Chapter 15 (Psychopharmacology: Acute Phase)

15.1 Correct answer: **E**

15.2 Correct answer: **E**

15.3 Correct answer: **D**

15.4 Correct answer: **C**

15.5 Correct answer: **D**

Chapter 16 (Psychopharmacology: Postacute Phase)

16.1 Correct answer: **E**

16.2 Correct answer: **B**

16.3 Correct answer: **D**

16.4 Correct answer: **A**

16.5 Correct answer: **C**

Chapter 17 (Child and Adolescent Psychiatry Interventions)

17.1 Correct answer: **D**

17.2 Correct answer: **E**

17.3 Correct answer: **A**

17.4 Correct answer: **E**

17.5 Correct answer: **B**

Chapter 18 (Geriatric Psychiatry Interventions)

18.1 Correct answer: **B**

18.2 Correct answer: **C**

18.3 Correct answer: **A**

18.4 Correct answer: **B**

18.5 Correct answer: **B**

Part IV: Emerging and Other Topics

Chapter 19 (Psychiatrists as Ambassadors)

19.1 Correct answer: **E**

19.2 Correct answer: **B**

19.3 Correct answer: **D**

19.4 Correct answer: **C**

19.5 Correct answer: **D**

Chapter 20 (Legal and Ethical Issues)

20.1 Correct answer: **A**

20.2 Correct answer: **C**

20.3 Correct answer: **E**

20.4 Correct answer: **E**

20.5 Correct answer: **B**

Chapter 21 (Telepsychiatry in Disasters and Public Health Emergencies)

21.1 Correct answer: **E**

21.2 Correct answer: **B**

21.3 Correct answer: **E**

21.4 Correct answer: **C**

21.5 Correct answer: **D**

Index

*Page numbers printed in **boldface** type refer to tables or figures.*